Fundamental Skills in Patient Care

Lu Verne Wolff Lewis
r.n., m.a.

Formerly Consultant, College
of Nursing, Arizona State University,
Tempe, Arizona; Research Associate,
Institute of Research and Service in
Nursing Education, Teachers College,
Columbia University, New York

J. B. Lippincott Company
philadelphia
new york   san jose   toronto

Distributed in Great Britain by
Blackwell Scientific Publications
London · Oxford · Edinburgh

ISBN 0-397-54174-0
Library of Congress Catalog Card Number 75-26993

Printed in the United States of America

4 6 8 9 7 5

Library of Congress Cataloging in Publication Data

Lewis, LuVerne Wolff.
    Fundamental skills in patient care.

    Includes bibliographies.
    1. Nursing.   I. Title.   [DNLM: 1. Nursing
care. WY100 L674f]
RT41.L67   610.73   75-26993
ISBN 0-397-54174-0

preface

Educators frequently speak of a career ladder or of career mobility in educational programs for nursing. Many hold that each level of education is built on a previous level of learning so that students in nursing may go on to advanced study without repeating previous work. This philosophy also supports the belief that nursing has certain core content that all nurses must master before they can give competent patient care.

The purpose of this book is to present basic nursing skills which every nurse needs to know, regardless of the type of educational program in which she is enrolled—practical, associate degree, diploma, or baccalaureate. Once the nurse has mastered these skills, she can move on to more advanced study. This book also could serve as a reference for the practicing nurse as well as for nurses enrolled in refresher courses.

People have different views concerning how learning in one area of study is transferred to others. Many believe that transfer of learning occurs more readily when the student is helped to see how information acquired in one area is used in other areas. For example, knowledge from courses in anatomy and physiology is necessary in order to carry out nursing skills safely and competently. This book often touches upon material that students learn in courses other than that offered in fundamental nursing skills. These brief reviews are intended to trigger the nurse's memory so that she can see how she applies content learned in other areas to the performance of nursing skills. Hopefully, the reviews are sufficient for their intended purpose without being boring or overly detailed.

The following are additional concepts that reflect the philosophy on which this text is built:

- This text supports what many persons refer to as a holistic approach which states that man cannot be separated into psychological and physiological parts. Man is constantly under environmental influences, and, therefore, a patient is best considered in the context of the environment whence he comes.
- Today's nurse has an important role in helping people to stay well and to live a full life to the best of their abilities. Preventive and restorative nursing care are important aspects of this text.
- This text emphasizes that it is important for the nurse to know why she takes whatever action she does when giving nursing care. Memorizing a procedure prepares the nurse poorly for working anywhere except in one situation. Therefore, it is believed that knowing the reason for her action better prepares the nurse for any situation in which she gives care.
- The uniqueness of man is pointed out often. The best care is individualized care designed to meet a particular patient's needs. The reader is re-

minded that the exact details of care can rarely be stated precisely since each patient is different from all others.

- Most patients have families. This text points out ways in which the nurse can include relatives while giving nursing care and how she can help families of patients for whom she is caring.
- The nurse is a health teacher. Her opportunities for teaching are almost limitless, and information she can share with her patients and their families is called to the reader's attention frequently.
- Chapter 2 includes a brief overview of the law as applied to nursing. Nurses, including students, are accountable for their practice, and, therefore, this text stresses factors that help to promote safety and to prevent accidents and errors when giving care.

There are several features of this text that were designed to assist the reader to master content with greater ease.

- Each chapter begins with statements of behavioral objectives which describe abilities the student will have when she has mastered content. Learning is often described as having occurred when there is a change in behavior. Therefore, the objectives are stated in behavioral terms so that learning can be determined on the basis of a change in behavior.
- A glossary with definitions is included at the opening of each chapter.
- The text presents numerous charts that were prepared to assist the student to learn how to carry out basic nursing skills. These suggest appropriate actions together with reasons for so doing.
- The text contains a considerable amount of illustrative material. Many photographs are given in sequence to show how a particular skill is executed.

- Each chapter includes references, most of which refer the reader to periodicals commonly found in agency libraries. It is hoped the references will help the interested reader to enrich content presented in this book.
- There are numerous ways in which content could have been arranged. A final decision often must be made knowing that every arrangement presents advantages and disadvantages. The order of presentation is not intended as a course outline. Rather, it is hoped that the arrangement lends itself to easy adaptation to meet the reader's needs. There may be times when studying chapters out of order may be desired. For example, the reader may wish to consider Chapter 8, dealing with vital signs, before earlier chapters. Or, Chapters 4 and 15, dealing with practices of medical and surgical asepsis respectively, may be studied simultaneously.
- The table of contents lists the major sections of each chapter. These sections are also presented at the opening of each chapter. Hopefully, this will be useful when only part of a chapter's content is to be considered for study. For example, recording the patient's intake and output and offering the bedpan and urinal are main chapter sections that can be studied without necessarily considering other material in the chapters in which they are discussed.

Finally, it should be noted that the pronoun "she" is used to refer to the nurse, and that most patients are referred to as "he." This is done for convenience, in the absence of a bisexual third person singular, with no slight intended to the increasing ranks of male graduates in nursing.

It is my sincere hope that this text will serve its ultimate goal of helping to improve nursing care for the patient.

acknowledgments

The author wishes to express gratitude to these agencies and persons who made important contributions during the preparation of this book:

Dolores La Mothe, Instructor in Fundamentals of Nursing and Rehabilitation Nursing, Department of Practical Nursing, Area Vocational Center, Phoenix, Arizona, who reviewed the manuscript and assisted with photography for some of the figures in the book.

Barbara John, Instructor, Department of Nursing, Scottsdale Community College, Scottsdale, Arizona, who assisted with photography for some of the figures.

Cary L. Hilger, Nursing Coordinator, Good Samaritan Hospital, Phoenix, Arizona, for her help and advice with photography illustrating range of joint motion.

Students enrolled in the refresher course for registered nurses at Mesa Community College, Mesa, Arizona, and their instructor, Cheri Bradshaw, who assisted with figures describing the intravenous infusion.

Carolyn Hartman, Industrial Nurse, Western Electric Company, Phoenix, Arizona, and her photographer, Hal B. Becker, for their assistance with Figure 1-2.

Students enrolled in the Department of Practical Nursing, Area Vocational Center, Phoenix, Arizona, those enrolled in the Department of Nursing, Scottsdale Community College, Scottsdale, Arizona, graduate nurses, patients, and models who offered to be photographed for figures in this book.

Area Vocational Center, Phoenix, Arizona, Good Samaritan Hospital, Phoenix, Arizona, Scottsdale Memorial Hospital, Scottsdale, Arizona, Desert Samaritan Hospital, Mesa, Arizona, and Western Electric Company, Phoenix, Arizona, which offered facilities for photography.

David T. Miller, Managing Editor, Nursing Department, J. B. Lippincott Company, Philadelphia, Pennsylvania, for editorial assistance and guidance.

My friends and my family who offered endless support and patience during the book's preparation.

contents

4 practices of medical asepsis 40

5 principles of body mechanics 58

charts

1 the nurse and her patient

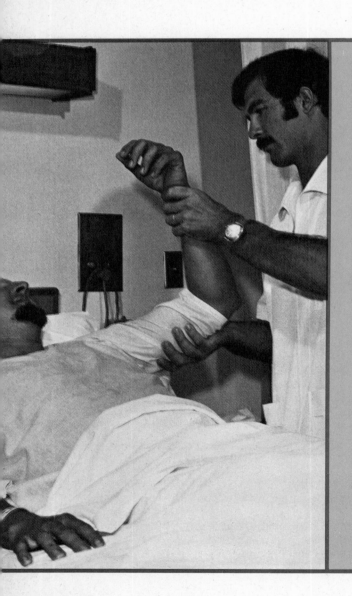

chapter outline

behavioral objectives

When mastery of content in this chapter is reached, the student will be able to

Define terms appearing in the glossary.

Describe three or four differences in nursing of years past and nursing today.

List several examples of curative nursing care, of preventive nursing care, of restorative nursing care, and of supportive nursing care.

Describe three guides to nursing action and list an example of each.

Discuss briefly two or three reasons why health and nursing teams are important for providing patients with total health care.

Describe the major responsibilities of the nursing team.

List the major responsibilities of the nursing team leader.

List two or three independent functions of the nurse.

List two or three dependent functions of the nurse.

Describe the four areas that make up comprehensive health care services.

Describe how the health practitioner provides for continuity of care for patients.

List two reasons why the amount of money spent on health care in this country is on the increase.

glossary

Activities of Daily Living Common acts which people carry out each day in the normal course of living.

Acute Illness One that lasts a relatively short period of time.

Chronic Illness One that lasts a relatively long period of time.

Comprehensive Health Care Services Services that include promoting health, preventing disease, discovering and treating disease, and rehabilitation.

Continuing Education Education, formal or informal, offered to nurses who have completed basic programs in nursing.

Continuity of Care A continuum of health care, offered whether the patient is in a state of health or illness.

Continuum A continuous whole.

Curative Nursing Care Care intended primarily to help people regain health.

Dependent Functions of the Nurse Actions of the nurse which cannot be carried out without a physician's order.

Health Optimum physical, mental, and social efficiency and well-being.

Health Agency An institution or organization that offers health services.

Health-Illness Continuum States of health and illness that fluctuate within a whole.

Health Practitioner One engaged in the practice of giving health care services.

Health Team An organization of health practitioners representing various professions that work cooperatively in planning and giving total health care services.

High-Level Wellness A state of health in which the body is functioning at its best level in relation to the individual's abilities.

Independent Functions of the Nurse Actions of the nurse which can be carried out without a physician's order.

Nursing Team A group of nursing personnel under the leadership of a qualified nurse, having the responsibility of giving total nursing care service.

Patient Any person receiving services from a health practitioner.

Policy A directive or regulation.

Preventive Nursing Care Care intended primarily to help people stay well.

Principle A truth developed after careful study of a particular event or process.

Procedure A method or way of doing something.

Rehabilitation The art and skill of helping handicapped persons regain function and/or of helping them to use remaining abilities in the best way possible.

Restorative Nursing Care Care intended primarily to help the handicapped person make the best possible use of remaining abilities.

Supportive Nursing Care Care intended primarily to offer psychological comfort to the patient.

Theory Explanation of a process or an event which is based on careful observations, but which lacks absolute or direct proof.

Well-Being Experiencing health and happiness.

introduction

Nurses care for patients. A **patient** is anyone receiving care by a physician, nurse, or other health professionals. This chapter will present a brief overview of nursing and of common needs of patients.

Nursing described

Caring for the sick and helpless can be traced back in history for thousands of years. Until approximately the middle of the 19th century, nursing was usually practiced by people without formal education, mostly by those dedicated to giving aid and comfort to the less fortunate.

The nurse and her patient

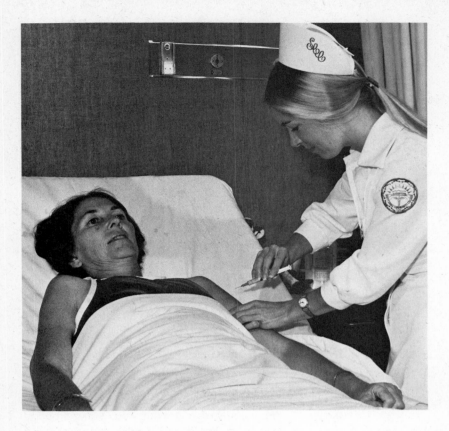

Fig. 1-1 The nurse's services include care intended to help people regain health. The medication the patient is receiving was prescribed to promote the healing process.

Florence Nightingale is usually given credit for guiding nursing from a poorly defined craft to the status of an occupation. She described the duties of the nurse and then set up a school to prepare young women for a nursing career.

A typical dictionary definition states that nurses take care of the sick by giving aid, comfort, nourishment, protection, and support. This kind of nursing emphasizes helping sick people regain their health. It is often referred to as **curative nursing care.** Figure 1-1 illustrates an example. However, nursing is a good deal more.

Nurses today play an important part in helping people stay well. This is often called **preventive nursing care,** since its primary purpose is to help prevent illness. A nurse is giving preventive care, for example, when she assists in a program to protect children against diphtheria, tetanus (lockjaw), and whooping cough. An example of this type of care is given in Figure 1-2.

Assisting people to overcome handicaps by helping to return function to a part of the body or by making the best possible use of remaining abilities is often referred to as **rehabilitation.** Until recently, rehabilitation was usually thought of as a specialized field of work done by people who helped severely handicapped patients. However, today, nursing includes many responsibilities that are intended to help patients overcome handicaps. Some refer to this kind of nursing as **restorative nursing care.** For example, a nurse is giving restorative care when she exercises a partially paralyzed arm to help bring back its normal functioning, as Figure 1-3 illustrates.

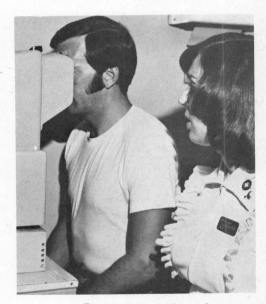

Fig. 1-2 The industrial nurse is conducting an eye examination as part of the employee's routine physical examination. The results of such examinations often help to prevent illnesses and problems long before they become debilitating.

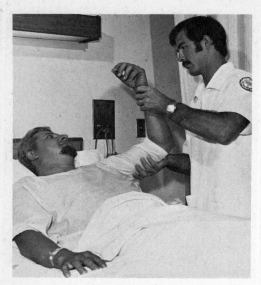

Fig. 1-3 The patient is helped to regain full use of his arm as the nurse assists him in moving it through its range of motion.

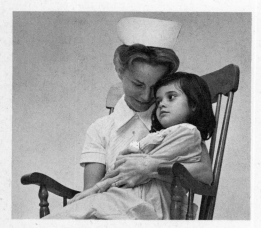

Fig. 1-4 This child cried as her parents left for the day. The nurse offers emotional support and demonstrates that she cares by holding the patient securely, and by rocking and speaking to her. As a result, having to be hospitalized and away from her family becomes a little easier.

There will be times when nursing care will help to support the patient psychologically. Possibly, this can be expressed by the words nursing is *caring.* Caring is more than giving curative, preventive, or restorative care. It takes one further step that shows the nurse has sincere interest and concern for the patient as a person. Nursing is really not nursing unless it is caring. There may be times when the nurse does no more than offer the patient comfort with a firm handclasp or a smile, but even by such simple gestures she is giving what may be called **supportive nursing care.** Figure 1-4 illustrates an example.

In the past nursing care was concerned mostly with the physical care of the sick in hospitals. Nurses spent their time doing "things" *to* or *for* patients and carrying out tasks to help keep the patients' rooms clean and tidy. It soon could be seen that emphasizing tasks as the center of nursing was too narrow. Today, the center of interest is the *patient,* and nurses have learned the importance of doing things *with* the patient. This kind of care emphasizes the person being served rather than tasks and how to do procedures. Nursing care that centers on the patient requires that the nurse not only be able to carry out nursing skills well; it also requires her to know about people and to know the reasons for the care she gives.

The phrase **activities of daily living** is often used to describe acts which people do in the normal course of living. Such activities include eating, sleeping, working, moving about, playing, socializing, and so on. In all of her care, the nurse helps patients to perform activities of daily living, and later chapters in this book will describe how she does so.

Nurses are teachers. While giving care, the nurse finds many opportunities to teach patients how to encourage the healing process, how to stay well and prevent illness, and how to carry out activities of daily living in the best possible way. The nurse teaches not only by telling and explaining things to her patient, but also through the examples she sets by her own behavior. For example, she may wish to teach a mother how to help in preventing the spread of colds. She may explain how colds spread from person to person and that it is best to keep children with colds home from school. However, her teaching will be less than successful if she is on duty when she has a bad cold. Patients notice what nurses do. Many are heard to say that they do something in a particular manner because they saw a nurse do it that way.

Nurses recognize differences in people and, therefore, treat each patient as a unique individual. Although in some ways, we are all alike—for example, we all need food, water, and oxygen to live, and we need to be able to get rid of wastes from our bodies—each of us is different from every other person. We react differently to events in our lives; we have different levels of intelligence; we play and work in different ways; we believe different things; we have different values; and so on. The nurse offers her services to everyone regardless of his color, creed, sex, age, or social or economic status. She is interested in seeing that her patient's health needs are well met and in a way that shows concern for him as an individual. Understanding people and respecting their beliefs and rights come with experience. Knowledge of the social sciences, such as psychology and sociology, heightens understanding. This will be discussed further in Chapter 3.

Nurses offer their services to people in many different situations.

Hospitals employ the largest number, but nurses work in clinics, nursing homes, community health agencies, private homes, physicians' offices, schools, stores, factories, in the armed forces, on board ship—in other words, wherever care is needed. The various institutions and organizations that offer health services are often called **health agencies.**

Nursing welcomes men and women of every color and creed. It offers not only a wide range of work opportunities, but daily satisfaction to those entering it who have a genuine desire to help others.

Guides to nursing action

Earlier in this chapter, it was pointed out that it is important for nurses to know *why* they take whatever action they do when giving care. For example, the nurse learns to cover her nose and mouth when sneezing or coughing and teaches others to do so because microorganisms expelled from the nose and mouth during sneezing and coughing can be spread to others. The reason for the action—the *why*—is often referred to as a principle. Although definitions vary, this book defines a **principle** as a truth developed after careful study of a particular event or process.

Consider the preceding example. Study has shown that the moist particles, called droplets, expelled during sneezing and coughing can carry live organisms from the person's nose and throat. These droplets are often carried considerable distances, and if someone else breathes them in, he may become infected with microorganisms. But by trapping the droplets with a tissue, these microorganisms do not reach others. The suggested action, then, is to cover the nose and mouth when sneezing and coughing. The reason for the action, that is, the principle guiding action, is that microorganisms expelled in the droplets can be spread to others. It can be seen that the principle does not tell the nurse *what* to do; rather, it tells her *why* she takes a particular action.

Consider another example. From the science of microbiology, it is learned that cold hinders the growth of bacteria. Knowing this, any number of actions can be based on it, depending on the desired results. The bacteriologist will keep some specimens in a warm place to help the growth of bacteria he wishes to study. On the other hand, the homemaker will keep foods refrigerated to prevent spoilage by bacterial growth.

Sometimes, a theory is used to guide action. A **theory** lacks absolute or direct proof, but it may be used as a guide to action until research finds that it is wrong. Certain theories about the moon, for example, were changed after the astronauts made findings that no longer supported them.

An example of a theory used as a guide to action in the field of health concerns cigarette smoking. There is evidence that heavy smoking is often present in the history of patients who develop lung cancer. Yet, some heavy smokers do not develop lung cancer, and some nonsmokers do. There is no direct or absolute proof yet that smoking causes cancer, but because of what is known, it seems best to go on the theory that reducing irritation to the lungs caused by smoking is helpful in preventing lung cancer.

Procedures and policies sometimes are used to guide nursing action.

A **procedure** is a method or way of doing things. Most places where nurses work have a procedure book which tells how something is carried out, and states what equipment and supplies the nurse will use. For instance, a hospital procedure book will describe how a cleansing enema is given, what equipment is to be used, where to obtain the equipment, and how to care for it after use.

A **policy** usually refers to a directive or regulation which a health agency follows. A hospital usually has a policy concerning visiting hours, and a school has a policy concerning what the school nurse does when she needs the help of a physician. Procedures and policies are intended to help run a health agency smoothly and efficiently, and employees (students as well) are expected to follow them.

The following example shows how a nurse is guided by principles, procedures, and policies. A nurse is caring for a 71-year-old patient who is limited in what he is allowed to do because of a heart disease. He needs a bath, and the nurse plans to give him a complete bed bath. The reason for giving the bath in bed (i.e., the principle that guides the nurse in her action) is that this will help to prevent the patient from placing unnecessary strain on his diseased heart muscles. The nurse will use equipment and linen as the hospital's procedure indicates. This hospital has a policy which states that patients over 65 years of age are to have bed siderails up at all times. When the nurse has completed caring for the patient, she places siderails on the bed according to hospital policy.

This book will not describe procedures and policies as health agencies do. However, it will describe suggested action a nurse will take in order to carry out nursing care and give the reason for the action. In many cases, the suggested action and the reason will be described in a chart with two columns, one column describing the action, and the other the reason. An example can be found on pages 47 through 50.

In nursing today, it would be difficult for the nurse to function without knowing the reasons for her actions. Memorizing a particular procedure would prepare her poorly for working anywhere except in one health agency. Equipment and supplies differ from place to place, and in home situations, the nurse may need to improvise in order to use equipment on hand. Therefore, knowing the reason for her action makes it possible to work in any situation.

In addition, this chapter has emphasized that no two people are exactly alike and good nursing care makes adjustments to meet each individual's needs. Knowing the *why* of one's action and being able to predict with a degree of safety what will result when a particular action is taken help to adjust care to fit each patient. Good nursing care requires sound judgment. This becomes possible only when the nurse knows why she is doing something and what results she can expect from her actions.

The health and the nursing teams

There are many people who offer services of various sorts to help patients overcome illnesses and stay well: physicians, registered nurses, licensed practical/vocational nurses, dietitians, pharmacists, social workers, occupational therapists, physical therapists, clinical psychologists, students in these various occupations, and so on. These people are often called **health practitioners,** since, in general, they practice their professions by offering services to meet the various health needs of society. Depending on their backgrounds, health practitioners offer patients many different kinds of services. However if each group worked independently, there would be utter chaos in giving service, and the patient would probably rarely have complete and total care. To offer services in an orderly and coordinated fashion, the **health team** has developed. The result is a cooperative venture offering total health care. A community health team usually is concerned with broad overall aspects of programs that mean better health for all citizens. A hospital health team usually is concerned primarily with patients' problems during hospitalization and immediately before and after discharge.

Each group of practitioners brings its particular arts and skills to the health team: the physician is responsible for diagnosing and prescribing therapy; the dietitian plans a diet appropriate to the patient's needs; the nurse is responsible for planning and carrying out nursing care; and so on.

As was true of the health team, if all persons who offer nursing care worked independently of other nursing personnel, patients would rarely receive complete or total nursing care. Therefore, the **nursing team** has developed. It is responsible for seeing that patients' total nursing needs are met. It is headed by a qualified nurse, usually called the team leader, who plans, supervises, and assists with care and evaluates the team's work. The team leader has as her assistants registered nurses, licensed practical nurses, students from various nursing programs, nursing assistants, nursing aides, home health aides, volunteers, clerical assistants, and possibly others.

Figure 1-5 illustrates the health and the nursing teams. As can be seen, the center of attention is the patient and *his* needs.

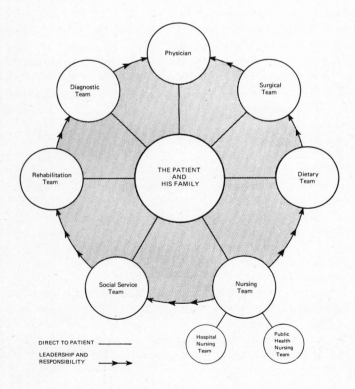

Fig. 1-5 An illustration of the health team whose members represent a variety of professions working collaboratively to aid in meeting the needs of the patient. Also illustrated is the nursing team whose members are responsible for planning and administering nursing care required by the patient.

The functions of the nurse are sometimes classed as dependent and independent. **Dependent functions** are those which are carried out only with a physician's order. For example, a nurse does not give drugs without a physician's order; therefore, giving a patient a drug is a dependent function of the nurse. **Independent functions** are those which can be carried out without a physician's order. Tending to the patient's hygienic needs, such as giving a bath, does not require a physician's order and, therefore, is an independent function. The independent functions of the nurse have tended to increase in the past few decades. This is true for both registered and licensed practical nurses. As this trend continues, nurses find that they must continue to study as they work in order to keep up with changes in their practice. No one course of study is enough to see a nurse through a lifetime of work. Therefore, continuing education has become an important part of the nurse's career. **Continuing education** is education offered nurses who have completed basic educational programs in nursing.

The health-illness continuum

Well-being means that an individual is experiencing health and happiness. Today, well-being is generally accepted as the right of everyone. Health care is no longer reserved for a privileged few; rather, health practitioners pledge themselves to the care of all people.

Health may be defined in many ways. In the preamble of its constitution, the World Health Organization defined health as ". . . a state of complete physical, mental and social well-being and not merely the absence of disease or infirmity." In addition, the World Health Organization stated that health is ". . . one of the fundamental rights of every human being."

While most people think of themselves as being well when they are not sick, health and illness usually fluctuate within a rather wide range. In other words, well-being may not necessarily be constant in nature. At times people who are considered healthy may not feel as well as they do at other times. For example, you may have a headache and not do as well as usual in school. While you may not feel "tops," you probably would not think of yourself as being sick unless your headache continues or returns frequently. Sometimes, people who are sick may find that they feel better at times and can do more for themselves than they can at other times. But they still may be considered sick and unable to go to work or school.

A **continuum** is defined as a continuous whole. Changes in health and illness can be described on a health-illness continuum, as illustrated in Figure 1-6. As can be seen, there is no exact point at which health ends and illness begins. Health and illness are different for each individual and there may be considerable range in which any one individual may be considered ill or well.

Death | ILLNESS AREA | WELL AREA | Optimum Well-being

Fig. 1-6 The health-illness continuum.

The nurse and her patient

Health practitioners have found the continuum helpful in viewing a patient's state of health and illness. Thus when a person functions well, he may be considered in the health area of the continuum even though he may have diabetes. When the body functions poorly, illness is present. When the body fails and damage to important organs occurs, death eventually results.

High-level wellness

High-level wellness means that the body is working at its best and the person is enjoying being well.

Assume that you are caring for a man in the hospital who is well on the road to recovery after having a stroke. He has partial paralysis in his left arm and leg but has learned to walk with the help of a cane. He eats well and, in general, feels good. The physician has ordered certain drugs which are intended to help prevent another stroke and has told the patient that he can return to work in another week or so. This man who was ill now appears to be enjoying well-being. He also may be said to be enjoying high-level wellness even though he walks with a cane and has had a stroke. His body is functioning at its best level.

Helping patients reach and stay at high-level wellness is the goal of every health practitioner. Patients also look for high-level wellness, even though they may not call it that, when they go to health practitioners for care. It is no longer enough to think a job is well done when the "sick are made well" and discharged from a hospital. Hospital care is planned primarily for the care of the sick. But the hospital is only one place where health practitioners work to help patients reach and maintain high-level wellness.

Comprehensive health care services

Helping patients reach the goal of high-level wellness requires many services and many different kinds of people. **Comprehensive health care services** generally are considered to include promoting health, preventing disease, discovering and treating disease, and rehabilitation. These various services overlap, and it is often difficult to determine where one ends and another starts. Nor do health practitioners generally deal with only one of these services. Many practitioners, including nurses, help in all four areas.

Promoting Health. Great progress has been made in describing what good health is. It is generally agreed that it includes both mental and physical health. For example, psychologists and psychiatrists have studied how stress and strain are handled by the human body. Based on these studies, programs that help us deal with stress are making it possible for more people to enjoy better mental health. The numerous counseling programs are examples of services that help to promote mental health.

An example of promoting physical health may be given from the field of nutrition. The body's food requirements are well known and the results of poor eating have been demonstrated. Through teaching programs, nurses as well as other health practitioners are promoting health by helping people learn how to select and prepare nutritious diets.

Preventing Disease. Even with care that promotes health, disease attacks man. Fortunately, many illnesses, such as smallpox, which can be prevented with vaccination, have practically disappeared. What work is being done to fight diseases that continue to strike man? A few examples will illustrate.

Two of the most common causes of death in man are heart disease and cancer. Both are being studied in many different places by many different people. Nurses often assist in these research programs. The purposes of such programs are to find how these diseases are caused, how they can be prevented, and how they can best be treated when present.

A **chronic illness** is defined as one that lasts a long time, for example arthritis. Researchers are constantly at work trying to find causes of chronic diseases. The number of elderly people in our population is increasing, and it is these people especially who tend to suffer with chronic diseases. The aging process itself is under study. The more that is learned about chronic illnesses, the more we can do to prevent them. Also, when they do appear, every effort is being made to start early treatment so that the effects on the body can be decreased. Thus, with early discovery and treatment, many of the crippling effects of arthritis can be prevented.

An **acute illness** is one that lasts a short time. Since discovery of antibiotic drugs, many acute illnesses, such as streptococcal sore throats (strep throats), are handled with relative ease. Nevertheless, many acute illnesses, such as infectious hepatitis, an acute illness that affects the liver, and the common cold, still remain difficult to treat, and science continues to look for their cure.

Within recent years, health practitioners have become interested in our environment and its effects on health. Pollution and its effects on health are front-page news almost daily. Also, health practitioners are concerned with safe working conditions as they strive to prevent illnesses.

Discovering and Treating Disease. While caring for her patients, the nurse plays an important part in helping to treat disease. For example, she usually gives prescribed medications, applies heat or cold to various parts of the body, and carries out other therapeutic measures.

Through her observations while caring for patients, the nurse often notices signs that help in discovering a particular problem a patient has. For instance, while bathing the patient, the nurse may see that his skin is reddened over the lower part of his back. This sign may mean that the patient is likely to develop a bedsore, and the nurse takes action to help prevent it.

Rehabilitation. Rehabilitation and restorative nursing were described earlier in this chapter. Helping a disabled person to overcome a handicap so that he may function to the best of his ability is not limited to that time when the nurse may, for example, help a patient learn how to use crutches. It begins with the first contact a nurse has with her patient, and it continues throughout the period of illness and thereafter until the person reaches a high level of wellness.

It was once believed that nurses should give complete personal care to patients. Health practitioners now agree that the best care is that which helps the patient to become independent, and that he should be taught how he can best help himself. Most patients appear to be happiest as they make progress toward helping themselves to the fullest extent possible and many have overcome tremendous handicaps with great pride. The nurse who stands in the way of this kind of progress by giving the patient too much "tender loving care" may delay his move toward wellness.

Continuity of care

Continuity of care is a continuum of health care, and it is important whether the patient is in a state of health or illness.

Continuity of care requires the smooth transfer and follow-up of care among health practitioners and health agencies. It means that any type of care will be available to everyone as needed. In far too many cases, persons may be dropped from care when an immediate problem has been solved. In such instances, there is lack of follow-up and of obtaining help from health practitioners who may well have services to offer that would result in better health for the patient.

In later chapters, there will be discussion of how nurses communicate among themselves in order that the patient's nursing care is both continuous and complete. There will also be discussion of how nurses assist in referring patients from one health agency to another, or from one unit in an agency to another, so that continuity of care is possible.

Delivering and financing health care

A topic of great concern today is how to provide and pay for health services for all people. Almost daily, there is news about health care delivery which should be of special interest to nurses.

With more people wanting and needing health care, efforts are being made to increase the number of health practitioners and to improve their education. Your teachers, for example, are constantly trying to find ways to help you become a good nurse. In addition, in various ways, we are trying to bring health services to everyone—those living in the city, in country areas, on the farm, in rundown neighborhoods.

However, it helps little to make health care available if the patient cannot afford it. Health care is big business in the United States. In 1950, it was estimated that approximately 15 to 20 billion dollars were spent on health care. It is predicted by some experts that as much as 200 billion dollars will be spent by 1980. Not only are people buying more health care, but the cost of the care has risen sharply. There are many ways health care is paid for in this country. As you follow the news, you will learn of additional ways being suggested to further help people pay for the care they need.

Many nursing journals carry articles regularly on how nurses can help provide services for people at a cost they can afford. State and federal governments are working on the problems. As a student, you can do your part by keeping informed on ways to help all people receive the health care they need at a cost they can afford.

Conclusion

Nurses are the largest single group of health practitioners in the United States today. They are found at work wherever care is needed. Nurses work collaboratively with other health practitioners to help meet the patient's total health care needs. As the population increases and people demand and expect more health services, additional health practitioners and health agencies will be needed.

This chapter has given you a brief overview of what nursing is, who the patient is, and what the patient needs and expects in terms of health care. Nurses play an important part in helping patients receive their ever-increasing needs and demands for health services. They are looked to for care that is high in quality, that takes into account a great variety of needs, and that shows respect for each patient as a unique individual.

References

"Accountability: How, for What, and to Whom," Editorial, *Nursing Outlook*, 20:315, May 1972.

"Bill of Rights for Patients," *Nursing Outlook*, 21:82, February 1973.

Carnegie, M. Elizabeth, "The Patient's Bill of Rights and the Nurse," *The Nursing Clinics of North America*, 9:557–562, September 1974.

Chaney, Patricia, Ed., "Ordeal," *Nursing 75*, 5:27–40, June 1975.

Dunn, Halbert L., "What High-Level Wellness Means," pp. 1–7, in *High-Level Wellness*, Beatty, Arlington, Virginia, 1971.

Echeveste, Dolores W. and Schlacter, John L., "Marketing: A Strategic Framework for Health Care," *Nursing Outlook*, 22:377–381, June 1974.

Extending the Scope of Nursing Practice: A Report of the Secretary's Committee to Study Extended Roles for Nurses, U. S. Government Printing Office, Washington, D.C., 1971, 17 p. (Reproduced, except for Preface and Appendix, in the *American Journal of Nursing*, 71:2346–2351, December 1971.

Keller, Nancy S., "Care Without Coordination: A True Story," *Nursing Forum*, 6:280–323, No. 3, 1967.

Kelly, Dorothy, "One Town's One-Nurse Service," *American Journal of Nursing*, 73:1536–1538, September 1973.

Kron, Thora, "Patient Care Management and Team Nursing," pp. 169–205, in *The Management of Patient Care: Putting Leadership Skills to Work*, W. B. Saunders Company, Philadelphia, 1971.

Lenarz, Dorothea M., "Caring is the Essence of Practice," *American Journal of Nursing*, 71:704–707, April 1971.

Lewis, Edith P., "The Care of the Sick," Editorial, *Nursing Outlook*, 22:625, October 1974.

———, "The Stuff of Which Nursing is Made," Editorial, *Nursing Outlook*, 23:89, February 1975.

McLaren, Phyllis M. and Tappan, Ruth M., "The Community Nurse Goes to Jail," *Nursing Outlook*, 22:35–39, January 1974.

Naugle, Ethel H., "The Difference Caring Makes," *American Journal of Nursing*, 73:1890–1891, November 1973.

Schorr, Thelma M., "Interdisciplinary Is As Autonomous Does," Editorial, *American Journal of Nursing*, 73:807, May 1973.

———, "Show and Tell," Editorial, *American Journal of Nursing*, 73:997, June 1973.

Somers, Anne R., *Health Care in Transition: Directions for the Future*, Hospital Research and Educational Trust, Chicago, Illinois, 1971, 176 p.

Steen, Joyce, "Liaison Nurse: Ombudsman for the Chronically Ill," *American Journal of Nursing,* 73:2102–2104, December 1973.

Storlie, Frances, *Nursing and the Social Conscience,* Appleton-Century-Crofts, New York, 1970, 222 p.

Todd, Malcolm C., "U.S. Health Care and You," *The Journal of Practical Nursing,* 24:14–15, 36, July 1974.

2 the nurse, the law, and ethics

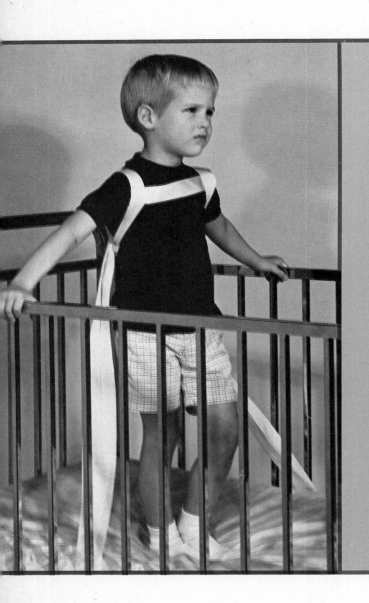

behavioral objectives

When mastery of content in this chapter is reached, the student will be able to

Define terms appearing in the glossary.

List four sources of laws and give an example of a law from each of these sources.

Describe an example of a wrong that, in the eyes of the law, could be considered a felony; a misdemeanor negligence; assault; battery; slander; libel; false imprisonment; and invasion of privacy.

Describe responsibilities of a person who witnesses the signing of a will.

Describe an example of a privileged act.

Discuss how privilege is present when Good Samaritan Laws are observed.

Describe an act that a Good Samaritan Law could not be expected to excuse.

Discuss why students in nursing can be expected to be held responsible for their acts while caring for patients.

List where student and graduate practical and registered nurses can obtain liability insurance.

Determine whether the laws are permissive or mandatory for practical nurses and for registered nurses after reading the nurse practice act in the state in which she is studying or working.

List three typical responsibilities of state boards of nursing.

Describe in a sentence or two how a code of ethics is best enforced. Describe the purpose of a code of ethics.

glossary

Administrative Law A law made by executive agencies of the government.

Assault A threat or an attempt to make bodily contact with another person without that person's consent.

Battery An assault that is carried out.

Common Law A law that results from court decisions that are then followed when other cases involving similar circumstances arise.

Constitutional Law A law in the federal and/or state constitution.

Crime A wrong committed against persons or property. The act is considered to be against the public also and is prosecuted by the government.

Defendant A person accused of breaking a law.

Ethics A system that defines actions with respect to their being right or wrong.

False Imprisonment Unjustifiable restraint or prevention of the movement of a person without proper consent.

Felony A crime considered to be of a serious nature. See also misdemeanor.

Good Samaritan Law A law that gives certain persons legal protection when giving aid to someone in an emergency situation.

Invasion of Privacy A wrongful act that violates the right of a person to be let alone.

Law A rule of conduct established and enforced by the government of a society.

Lawsuit A legal action in a court.

Liable Being accountable, responsible, or answerable for an act.

Libel An untruthful written statement about a person that subjects him to ridicule or contempt.

Malpractice An act of negligence. Commonly used when speaking of negli-

gent acts committed by persons working in certain professions, such as medicine and nursing.

Mandatory Nurse Practice Act A law requiring a nurse to be licensed in order to practice nursing.

Misdemeanor A wrong considered to be less serious than a felony.

Negligence Performing an act that a reasonable and comparable person under similar circumstances would not do, or, failing to perform an act that a reasonable and comparable person under similar circumstances would do.

Permissive Nurse Practice Act A law that allows a licensed nurse to refer to herself as a licensed practical nurse or a registered nurse but does not require that the nurse be licensed to practice nursing.

Plaintiff A person (or government) bringing a lawsuit against another person.

Privilege Special rights that grant freedom from a lawsuit for certain people in specific situations.

Slander An untruthful oral statement about a person that subjects him to ridicule or contempt.

Statutory Law A law enacted by a legislative body.

Tort A wrong committed by a person against another person or his property. A tort is less serious than a crime.

Will A statement of a person's wishes about what shall be done with his property after his death.

introduction

A full discussion of the legal and ethical aspects of nursing usually occurs when students are nearing graduation. However, since certain laws affect nurses from the time they begin their study, this brief chapter will give an overview of the law and ethics as they apply to nursing.

The word **liable** means being accountable, responsible, or answerable for an act. Nurses are liable for their acts when they give patients nursing care. For example, a patient falls out of bed and breaks his hip when a nurse forgot to replace the siderails after giving the patient a bath; the

The nurse, the law, and ethics

nurse can be held legally liable for her careless act. Other examples of actions that can lead to problems if done incorrectly include making entries on the patient's records, caring for the patient's personal clothing and valuables, and reporting accidents and errors in nursing care.

Sources of laws

A **law** is a rule of conduct established and enforced by the government of a society. Laws are intended primarily to protect the rights and privileges of people. For example, nurse practice acts are laws planned primarily to protect the public from persons considered unfit to practice.

There are four main sources of laws in the United States. They are the constitutions, the legislatures, the judiciary system, and administrative agencies.

Constitutions. In any society there must be authority if chaos is to be prevented. Countries have governments which are given authority to maintain order and to protect the people.

In the United States, the federal and state constitutions describe how government is created and given authority. These constitutions contain laws which are called **constitutional laws.** For example, the federal Constitution forbids religious tests for those holding office in this country, and it defines the word treason, which guides the courts to decide whether a person accused of having committed treason is guilty.

Legislatures. Under the Constitution our government has created legislatures that are responsible for making laws. Legislative bodies are called the Congress at the federal level and legislatures at the state level. Certain legislative bodies at the local level (county, municipal, and so on) may be established also. A law made by a legislative body is referred to as **statutory law.** These laws must be in keeping with the federal Constitution and, within each state, with that state's constitution as well. The nurse practice acts are statutory laws.

The Judiciary System. Our government provides for a judiciary system which is responsible for settling controversies and conflicts in the courts. Over the years a body of law, known as **common law,** has grown out of legal decisions reached in the courts. Once a decision has been made in a court of law, it becomes the rule to follow when other cases involving similar circumstances arise. Court decisions can be changed, but only when there is good reason for doing so. Common law prevents one set of rules being used to judge one person and another set being used to judge another person when the circumstances are similar.

Common law concerned with nursing exists. Under common law, for example, students in hospital-controlled schools of nursing have been considered employees of the hospital.

Administrative Agencies. A responsibility of the executive branch of the federal and state governments is to execute the law of the land. Executive power is placed in the hands of the President of the United States, the governors of states, and the mayors, or their equivalents, at lower levels of government. These chief executives have power to create various agencies to assist them that, among other things, can make and enforce certain rules and regulations. These rules and regulations are called **administrative laws.**

The boards of nursing are examples of administrative agencies at the state level. An example of a municipal agency is a city's board of health. Rules and regulations by boards of nursing and boards of health are examples of administrative laws.

Torts and crimes

A **tort** is a wrong committed by a person against another person or his property. A **crime** is also a wrong against a person or his property, but the act is considered to be against the public as well. In criminal cases, the government (called "The People") takes the accused offender to court for trial. When a crime is committed, intention to commit the wrong is present. Persons found guilty of wrongs are punished by fines or imprisonment or both.

A wrong of a serious nature is often referred to as a **felony;** imprisonment is for more than one year. A wrong of less seriousness is called a **misdemeanor;** imprisonment is for less than one year. A person who is practicing nursing unlawfully and whose patient dies as a result can be tried for a felony. Disturbing the peace and breaking traffic laws are examples of misdemeanors.

Negligence and malpractice

Negligence occurs when a person performs an act that a reasonable and comparable person under similar circumstances would not do; or conversely, fails to do what reasonably should be done. Comparable persons are those with much the same education and experience. For example, a nurse can be held liable for negligence when a patient is burned with a hot-water bottle.

Malpractice is also negligence. The prefix *mal* comes from a Latin word meaning bad. Malpractice is the term generally used to describe negligence when persons working in professions are involved. It is commonly used when speaking of negligent acts of physicians and nurses.

Assault and battery

Assault is a threat to, or an attempt to, make bodily contact with another person without that person's consent. A **battery** is an assault that is carried out. Every person is granted freedom from bodily contact by another unless consent has been granted. In the field of health, a person operated on without his consent can sue the physician and/or the health agency involved. Health practitioners cannot force patients to do things against their will, unless consent has been granted, without fear of a legal suit. The use of certain consent forms, discussed later in this book, is important to avoid problems related to assault and battery.

The nurse, the law, and ethics

Slander and libel

Slander is an untruthful oral statement about a person that subjects him to ridicule or contempt. **Libel** is the same, except that the statement is in writing, signs, pictures, or the like. Untrue statements that indicate someone is not fit for the practice of his profession can be held as slander or libel. Falsely accusing someone of committing a crime can constitute slander or libel. Nurses who gossip or make false statements about their patients or coworkers run the risk of being sued for slander or libel.

False imprisonment

Preventing the movement of a person without proper consent can constitute **false imprisonment.** Such a wrong would be committed if any person were forcibly held in a health agency because he did not pay for the services he received. Protective restraints are discussed in Chapter 6. Using them with poor judgment can constitute false imprisonment. If an adult patient is sound of mind, he can leave a health agency even if health practitioners believe that he should remain for additional care. In such instances, health agencies use a form for the patient to sign indicating that he is leaving of his own will and against medical advice. This form is further discussed in Chapter 7. Some mentally ill patients and patients with certain communicable diseases can legally be kept in a health agency against their will, if it can be shown that they present a danger to society.

Invasion of privacy

Everyone has the right to withhold himself from public exposure. If a person is exposed to the public, either personally or through pictures, the person responsible for such exposure could be sued for **invasion of privacy.** However, this would not hold true if the person granted permission for the exposure.

Exposure necessary while caring for a patient does not constitute invasion of privacy. However, nurses should recognize that unnecessary exposure of patients while moving them through corridors or while giving them care in a room where other patients or visitors are present can constitute invasion of privacy.

Health practitioners who gossip about patients can be charged with invasion of privacy. Information on patients' records is considered confidential and should not be discussed with unauthorized persons. Students who prepare class assignments (oral or written) are advised not to reveal the identity of patients in order to prevent what could be considered invasion of privacy. Gossiping about patients with classmates and coworkers can be a dangerous practice.

Defenses for the accused

A **lawsuit** is a legal action in a court of law. The one being accused of breaking the law is called the **defendant.** The person (or government) bringing the suit against a defendant is called the **plaintiff.**

A defendant has every opportunity to defend himself in court and is presumed innocent until proven guilty. Hence, being accused of wrongdoing does not necessarily mean that the person is guilty.

The law also provides for what is called **privilege** in certain instances. Privilege grants certain persons special rights for their acts, in which case grounds for a lawsuit may not be present. For example, if a patient of sound mind has signed a proper consent for an operation, he is in no position to sue the physician for having done it.

A law which states that persons have certain privileges in emergency situations is often called a **Good Samaritan Law.** It is named after a traveler (described in the Bible as the good Samaritan) who helped another traveler who had been beaten and robbed. These laws vary from state to state. Nurses are covered in some states, while in others they are not.

Good Samaritan Laws tend to encourage persons to give assistance at the scene of an emergency. However, they do not make it legally necessary to do so. When health practitioners do assist and when consent to give care is not forthcoming from the victim, they can be expected to use good judgment in deciding whether an emergency does indeed exist. Also, they can be expected to give care that a reasonable and comparable person in similar circumstances would give. If they give emergency care that can be shown to be grossly careless in nature, a Good Samaritan Law will not necessarily excuse them.

Wills

A **will** is a statement of a person's wishes about what shall be done with his property after his death. State laws give requirements for a legal will.

Nurses are sometimes asked to witness a will. By so doing, the nurse indicates that the will was signed by the person who made it. Also, the witness indicates that to the best of his knowledge, the person signing the will is of sound mind and that he acted without force when he signed it.

The nursing student's legal status

In hospital-controlled programs, the nursing student has been considered an employee of the hospital. A student is still liable for her acts, but the hospital as the employer may also be held liable. The status of students caring for patients while enrolled in high school, college, and university programs for nursing is not clear since there appears to be no common law on this subject.

It may seem severe to hold a student responsible for her nursing care. Yet, in fairness to the patient, he should be able to expect safe care no matter who gives it to him. If a student feels that her assignment is beyond her ability, it is recommended that she go to her supervising nurse to discuss the assignment before attempting to carry it out.

Health agencies generally carry liability insurance to protect themselves in case of a lawsuit. However, students and graduate nurses may also wish to carry their own insurance. Many health agencies and schools recommend that they do so. Liability insurance is available from many commercial insurance companies, some of which advertise in nursing magazines. It is also available through the National Nursing Students' Association, the American Nurses' Association, and the National Federation of Licensed Practical Nurses.

Nurse practice acts

The first law dealing with the practice of nursing in this country was enacted in North Carolina in 1903. At present, there are nurse practice acts in all of the 50 states, the District of Columbia, Guam, Samoa, Puerto Rico, and the Virgin Islands. In general, the laws are intended to protect the public from people who are unfit to practice nursing.

The laws vary considerably from state to state. Some laws define nursing while others describe what a nurse may or may not do in the practice of nursing. In some states, the law requires that a nurse be licensed in order to practice. Such a law is called a **mandatory nurse practice act.** In other states, the law allows a licensed nurse to refer to herself as a licensed practical nurse (licensed vocational nurse) or a registered nurse; however, it does not require that the nurse be licensed to practice. Such a law is called a **permissive nurse practice act.**

The agency in each state that has power to make regulations concerning nurse practice acts is the state board of nursing. The regulations made by these boards are like laws, as described earlier in this chapter. Some typical responsibilities of the state boards of nursing include setting standards for educational programs for nursing, setting requirements for obtaining a license, and deciding when a nurse's license may be suspended or revoked.

Codes of ethics

The word ethics comes from the Greek word *ethos,* meaning customs or modes of conduct. **Ethics** may be defined as a system that defines actions with respect to their being right or wrong.

The ethics of various professional groups are described in codes. For example, nurses have set up standards of conduct in their codes of ethics. The purpose of a code is to encourage high standards of conduct among the group's members. When a nurse agrees to uphold a code of ethics, she accepts the trust and responsibility the patient has placed in her.

It is difficult for codes of ethics to be enforced by committees and panels. Rather, each nurse is expected to uphold and abide by the code. Enforcement depends more on one's conscience and heart than on law enforcement officials.

The following are three codes of ethics adopted by nurses:

Code for nurses

Adopted by the American Nurses' Association in 1950 and revised in 1960 and 1968.

- The nurse provides services with respect for the dignity of man, unrestricted by considerations of nationality, race, creed, color, or status.
- The nurse safeguards the individual's right to privacy by judiciously protecting information of a confidential nature, sharing only that information relevant to his care.
- The nurse maintains individual competence in nursing practice, recognizing and accepting responsibility for individual actions and judgments.
- The nurse acts to safeguard the patient when his care and safety are affected by incompetent, unethical, or illegal conduct of any person.
- The nurse uses individual competence as a criterion in accepting delegated responsibilities and assigning nursing activities to others.
- The nurse participates in research activities when assured that the rights of individual subjects are protected.
- The nurse participates in the efforts of the profession to define and upgrade standards of nursing practice and education.
- The nurse, acting through the professional organization, participates in establishing and maintaining conditions of employment conducive to high-quality nursing care.
- The nurse works with members of health professions and other citizens in promoting efforts to meet health needs of the public.
- The nurse refuses to give or imply endorsement to advertising, promotion, or sales for commercial products, services, or enterprises.

Code of ethics for the licensed practical nurse

Adopted by The National Federation of Licensed Practical Nurses. The licensed practical nurse shall:

- Practice her profession with integrity.
- Be loyal to the physician, to the patient, and to her employer.
- Strive to know her limitations and to stay within the bounds of these limitations.
- Be sincere in the performance of her duties and generous in rendering service.
- Consider no duty too menial if it contributes to the welfare and comfort of her patient.
- Accept only that monetary compensation which is provided for in the contract under which she is employed, and she does not solicit gifts.
- Hold in confidence all information entrusted to her.
- Be a good citizen.
- Participate in and share responsibility of meeting health needs.
- Faithfully carry out the orders of the physician or registered nurse under whom she serves.
- Abstain from administering self-medications, and in event of personal illness, take only those medications prescribed by a licensed physician.
- Respect the dignity of the uniform by never wearing it in public.
- Respect the religious beliefs of all patients.
- Abide by the Golden Rule in her daily relationship with people in all walks of life.

- Be a member of The National Federation of Licensed Practical Nurses, Inc. and the state and local membership associations.
- Not identify herself with advertising, sales, or promotion of commercial products or service.

ICN Code for nurses

Adopted by the International Council of Nurses in 1973.

The fundamental responsibility of the nurse is fourfold: to promote health, to prevent illness, to restore health, and to alleviate suffering.

The need for nursing is universal. Inherent in nursing is respect for life, dignity, and rights of man. It is unrestricted by considerations of nationality, race, creed, colour, age, sex, politics, or social status.

Nurses render health services to the individual, the family and the community and coordinate their services with those of related groups.

- **Nurses and People**
  The nurse's primary responsibility is to those people who require nursing care.
  The nurse, in providing care, respects the beliefs, values, and customs of the individual.
  The nurse holds in confidence personal information and uses judgment in sharing this information.

- **Nurses and Practice**
  The nurse carries personal responsibility for nursing practice and for maintaining competence by continual learning.
  The nurse maintains the highest standards of nursing care possible within the reality of a specific situation.
  The nurse uses judgment in relation to individual competence when accepting and delegating responsibilities.
  The nurse when acting in a professional capacity should at all times maintain standards of personal conduct that would reflect credit upon the profession.

- **Nurses and Society**
  The nurse shares with other citizens the responsibility for initiating and supporting action to meet the health and social needs of the public.

- **Nurses and Coworkers**
  The nurse sustains a cooperative relationship with coworkers in nursing and other fields.
  The nurse takes appropriate action to safeguard the individual when his care is endangered by a coworker or any other person.

- **Nurses and the Profession**
  The nurse plays the major role in determining and implementing desirable standards of nursing practice and nursing education.
  The nurse is active in developing a core of professional knowledge.
  The nurse, acting through the professional organization, participates in establishing and maintaining equitable social and economic working conditions in nursing.

Conclusion

Students and graduate nurses are legally and ethically responsible for their acts while giving nursing care, as well as in their daily living as responsible citizens. While the discussion here has been brief, the student is urged to continue her study in this area throughout her career and to keep herself up-to-date on legal and ethical matters as they relate to nursing. Many nursing publications and the news media offer good sources of information for continuing education in this area.

References

Agree, Betty C., "The Threat of Institutional Licensure," *American Journal of Nursing,* 73:1758–1763, October 1973.

"Code for Nurses," *American Journal of Nursing,* 68:2581–2585, December 1968.

Creighton, Helen, "Legal Aspects of Expanding LP/VN Roles," *The Journal of Practical Nursing,* 23:16–19, August 1973.

———, "Ten Commandments in Nursing," *Nursing '73,* 3:7–8, January 1973.

———, "The Malpractice Problem," *The Nursing Clinics of North America,* 9:425–433, September 1974.

———, "Your Legal Risks in Emergency Nursing Care," *Nursing '73,* 3:23–25, April 1973.

Feld, Lipman G., "The Nurse's Liability for Faulty Injections," *Nursing Care,* 7:25, April 1974.

Hershey, Nathan, "When Is A Communication Privileged?" *American Journal of Nursing,* 70:112–113, January 1970.

Kelly, Lucie Young, "Institutional Licensure," *Nursing Outlook,* 21:566–572, September 1973.

———, "Nursing Practice Acts," *American Journal of Nursing,* 74:1310–1319, July 1974.

Kerr, Avice H., "Nurses' Notes: 'That's Where the Goodies Are!'", *Nursing '75,* 5:34–41, February 1975.

Lambertsen, Eleanor C., "The Changing Role of Nursing and Its Regulation," *The Nursing Clinics of North America,* 9:395–402, September 1974.

Lipman, Michel, "Can You Afford to be a Good Samaritan? Yes!" *RN,* 37:90–91, September 1974.

———, "Defamation: A Rash Comment Could Get You Sued," *RN,* 38:48–51, February 1975.

McGriff, Erline P., "A Case for Mandatory Continuing Education in Nursing," *Nursing Outlook,* 20:712–713, November 1972.

"Nursing Ethics: The Admirable Professional Standards of Nurses: A Survey Report," *Nursing '74,* 4:34–44, September 1974.

"Nursing Ethics: The Admirable Professional Conduct of Nurses: A Survey Report. Part 2. Honesty, Confidentiality, Termination of Life, and Other Decisions in Nursing," *Nursing '74.* 4:56–66, October 1974.

Peterson, Paul and Guy, Joan S., "Should Institutional Licensure Replace Individual Licensure?" *American Journal of Nursing,* 74:444–447, March 1974.

Pratt, Richard Putnam, "The Nurse and Her Money: Do You Need Malpractice Insurance?" *RN,* 36:65–67, June 1973.

Reinders, Agnes A., "Nursing and Some Large Moral Issues," *The Nursing Clinics of North America,* 9:547–556, September 1974.

Schorr, Thelma M., "Outrage in Massachusetts," Editorial, *American Journal of Nursing,* 73:1167, July 1973.

Silva, Mary Cipriano, "Science, Ethics, and Nursing," *American Journal of Nursing,* 74:2004–2007, November 1974.

Stahl, Adele G., "State Boards of Nursing: Legal Aspects," *The Nursing Clinics of North America,* 9:505–512, September 1974.

"The ICN Meets in Mexico City," *American Journal of Nursing,* 73:1344–1359, August 1973.

References   27

3 developing good nurse-patient relationships

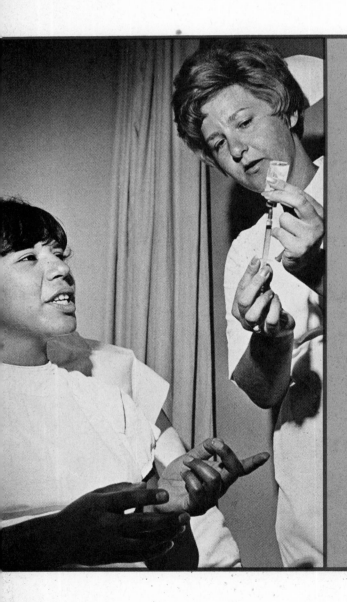

behavioral objectives

When mastery of content in this chapter is reached, the student will be able to

Define terms in the glossary.

List three signs that would suggest that a good nurse-patient relationship is developing.

Describe three or four acts typical of her own behavior and discuss briefly why she thinks she acts in that particular way.

List three basic physical needs of man; list six basic psychosocial needs of man.

List the three most commonly practiced religious faiths in this country.

List five common activities of every person that are learned from the culture into which he was born.

Describe a cultural factor that would help to promote healthful living; describe one that would stand in the way of healthful living.

List three examples of verbal communica-tion; list six examples of nonverbal communication.

List two purposes of observation.

Describe two ways in which a patient can determine when a nurse is not listening to him.

Describe what basic psychosocial need is often met when the nurse explains a procedure to a patient.

List three examples of times when a patient is unlikely to be ready for learning.

List five expectations patients often have of nurses who care for them.

List five activities which would demonstrate that a nurse is showing respect for the patient as an individual.

glossary

Communication An exchange of information.

glossary cont.

Culture Everything an individual learns from the groups of people of which he is a part.

Nonverbal Communication Exchange of information without using words.

Psychology The study of the mind and mental processes that helps explain why people act, think, and feel as they do.

Psychosocial Pertaining to both mental and social processes.

Relationship An association between people.

Sociology The study of social processes and of social relationships among people.

Nurse-Patient Relationship An association between a patient and a nurse.

Verbal Communication Exchange of information through the use of words.

introduction

The material in this chapter is usually dealt with in fuller detail in other nursing courses. However, it has been included here to serve as a brief overview and as a "bringing together" of some of the factors that influence the kind of relationships nurses have with patients. It is information that you will wish to be familiar with before starting the care of patients since the relationships you develop with patients begin at the moment you have your first contact with them.

Description of a good nurse-patient relationship

The word **relationship** refers to an association between people. This chapter will discuss associations between patients and nurses. A relationship that is unsatisfactory can stand in the way of a patient's progress toward wellness. A good relationship is one that helps the patient *feel* better as a result of his associations with the nurse.

It is not always easy to see when the patient feels better as a result of his relationship with the nurse. It cannot be measured as can his body temperature or blood pressure. Often the patient's behavior—the tone of his voice, the stride of his walk, a smile, or the twinkle in his eyes—will tell the nurse how he feels. Figure 3-1 illustrates methods one nurse used to develop a good relationship with her young patient.

In other courses, you have no doubt learned that **psychology** is often described as the science that studies the mind and mental processes. It examines why people act, think, and feel as they do. **Sociology** deals with social processes, in other words, with relationships among people. The word **psychosocial** refers to both mental and social processes.

You have also studied how the body functions as a living organism. This is often referred to as the physical portion of the human being.

Often the body is thought of as having two parts: a psychosocial part and a physical part. However, no person can be separated into these parts because what affects one will affect the other. The two are completely intertwined and the body functions as a whole. For example, a physical handicap, such as a leg amputation, affects the person in a psychosocial as well as in a physical manner. Likewise, a person living

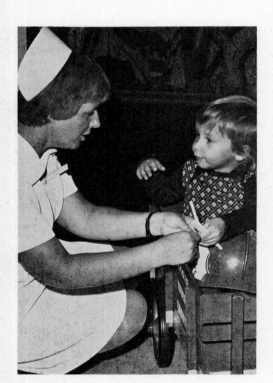

Fig. 3-1 Ingenuity and patience are often required to build a good nurse-patient relationship. This nurse found that a few simple toys and positioning herself near the child helped to put him at ease as she prepared to admit him for hospital care.

under much strain and having many worries due to psychosocial problems may eventually develop physical signs, such as nausea, headaches, or chest pains. For the sake of discussion, psychosocial aspects will be discussed here while the student is cautioned to remember that these aspects of a person cannot function separately from his physical being.

The remainder of this chapter deals with factors that help to promote good nurse-patient relationships.

Knowing oneself

Getting along with others and respecting differences among people begin with knowing oneself. It is a good idea to look at yourself and see what attitudes and prejudices you have and why you act as you do. This is not necessarily an easy experience for it means looking closely at our shortcomings as well as our strengths. But until we are ready to look at ourselves honestly, we cannot take steps to change for the better. Nor are we in a position to understand our patients well.

As the nurse learns to know herself, she will learn to respect each patient for himself and accept him as he is. While doing so, she will usually see an atmosphere of trust and respect develop. Also, her patients will be more likely to feel that she is indeed a real and dependable person.

It is easy to dismiss a patient as being uncooperative, difficult, or irritable. At the same time, the patient may be thinking the same things of the nurse. There is always a reason for behavior—for the nurse's as well as the patient's.

For the patient, illness is nearly always a difficult experience. The independent person suddenly needs to be cared for; the patient is separated from his family; he probably feels sick; he worries about recovery; he wonders what will happen to him and those he cares for at home; he wants something to eat and the nurse brings water; he wants to be left alone, but the nurse wants to take his temperature; he would like a shower when the nurse insists on giving him a bed bath. It is little wonder that patients feel irritable. The nurse is of limited help if she does not understand. This understanding will come as she begins to understand herself and how she would feel if she were in the patient's position.

Knowing needs of the patient

Man has certain basic physical needs. For example, oxygen, food, and water are basic to life itself.

Man also has certain basic psychosocial needs. While there are differences in the way these needs are sometimes described, in general, they are as follows, in order of priority:

- The need for security and survival.
- The need for affection and love and a feeling of belonging.
- The need for self-respect and self-esteem.
- The need for self-fulfillment.

- The need to know and understand.
- The need for enjoying beauty.

When these needs are not being well met, human beings usually feel lonely, friendless, and rejected. They often become fearful and feel inferior to others. They may worry and become depressed.

Nurses also have these same basic needs. When you are trying to learn to know yourself, you will wish to see how you satisfy these basic needs in your life. The nurse will wish to be careful not to use her patients to meet her needs. For example, if she is trying to make the patient respect her by forcing him to do as he is told, she may be trying to meet *her* needs rather than his.

When the relationship between nurse and patient is warm and comfortable, when it demonstrates accepting the patient as he is, when it illustrates feelings of understanding for his basic needs, and when the nurse's needs are not taking over, a good nurse-patient relationship can grow and develop.

Knowing the patient's religious beliefs

Religion helps man to understand his relationship with the universe about him. There are countless religious beliefs in the world. In this country, the most commonly practiced religions are Christianity (Protestantism and Roman Catholicism) and Judaism. However, the nurse can expect to care for persons holding other beliefs as well. Examples include Jehovah's Witnesses, Moslems, Buddists, and Shintoists.

Some people do not accept any particular religious faith. They too deserve respect for what they choose to believe.

It is common for patients who practice a religion to seek support from their faith when ill. Prayer, devotional readings, and other practices often do for the patient spiritually what medicine may do for him physically. Patients have been known to face serious illness and illness-related problems because of strong faith. Spiritual support is often the key to hope and determination when illness is present.

The presence of religious items at the patient's bedside tells the nurse that he is practicing a religious faith. He may wish to spend part of his day in prayer or other religious practices. Since some patients prefer privacy, it is a thoughtful gesture for the nurse to provide such privacy when desired.

Many hospitals have chapels in which patients may worship, such as the one illustrated in Figure 3-2. When regular services are not held, patients usually are permitted to go to the chapel when they wish if their condition permits. Frequently, it is the nurse who can tell the patient of such facilities.

Although a person's religious faith often appears to help recovery, there are times when beliefs conflict with care the patient needs. For example, the doctrine of Jehovah's Witnesses does not permit blood transfusions. If a particular religious practice presents a problem in relation to the patient's care, the nursing team may wish to turn to a clergyman. He may very well be the person who can best help the patient to accept necessary care. In many hospitals, clergymen of various faiths are available at all times.

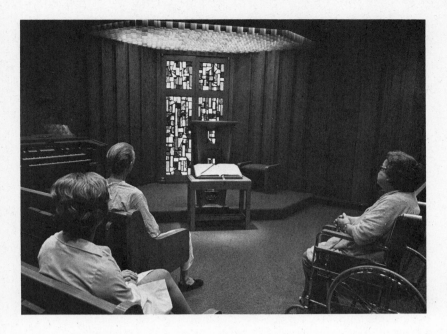

Fig. 3-2 The chapel is often a place where patients as well as staff may wish to meditate quietly.

The clergyman's visit is usually an important part of the patient's day. The thoughtful nurse will assist the clergyman to locate the patient and see whether he is able to receive the visit. Having the clergyman visit at an unsuitable or inconvenient time is embarrassing to both the patient and the clergyman. The nurse also will provide privacy if desired.

Knowing the patient's cultural background

Culture is everything that an individual learns from the groups of people of which he is a part. It includes understandings and values. It is made up of certain ways of acting, thinking, and feeling. For example, we are born into a culture, that, over a period of time, teaches us what to eat, how and when to eat, what to wear, how to get along with others, and how to care for ourselves. It includes such activities as using a language, running a government, getting married, rearing children, and making a living. Even though our bodies function in much the same way, we act and think differently, mostly because of what we learn from our culture.

It is important for the nurse to learn something about her patients' cultural backgrounds. Recognizing differences in backgrounds helps to decrease prejudices and helps the nurse to accept people as they are.

Attitudes and values are generally deep and firmly fixed. For instance, a vegetarian does not eat meat, fish, or poultry. If the patient refuses meat, even though the nurse thinks he needs it for his health, he is not being stubborn. He has reasons for his belief. Rather than trying to convince him to eat meat, a better course of action is to serve him a meat substitute, such as cheese or eggs.

Cultural factors often influence health and illness. In the United States, health in general is highly valued and illness is considered unpleasant and undesirable. In some cultures, illness is regarded with much less concern, almost as an acceptable way of life.

The following are some of the cultural differences seen in this country: wanting to eat the main meal of the day in the evening rather than at noon, liking highly spiced food, refusing to undress before a stranger, being upset because it is necessary to sleep in a room with a strange person, avoiding the use of a bedpan because someone else has to take care of the contents, refusing to have a bath during the menstrual period, and refusing a vaginal examination done by a male.

Trying to understand the patient's cultural background helps the nurse to understand his behavior. The nurse who feels her own cultural background is the best will tend to judge others harshly as she closes her mind to understanding her patient's behavior. Efforts to develop a good nurse-patient relationship in such instances are almost certain to fail.

Using communication skills

Communication is an exchange of information by means of hearing, seeing, tasting, smelling, and touching. Everything an individual does communicates something—his work, the food he eats, the clothes he wears, a handshake, a wink of the eye, a smile, a glance, or a gesture. Communication is essential in the development of a nurse-patient relationship, and it is a continuous process, occurring with every contact the nurse has with her patients.

Communication can be either verbal or nonverbal. **Verbal communication** uses words, and includes speaking, reading, and writing.

Nonverbal communication is the exchange of information without using words. It is what is *not* said. People communicate nonverbally through facial expressions, body movement, tone of voice, gestures, and so on. Crying and moaning are considered nonverbal communication since they do not use a language or words.

A person has less control over nonverbal than verbal communication. We can use words with care, but a facial expression is harder to control. As a result, feelings are often communicated more accurately through nonverbal communications. For example, a patient may say that he does not feel lonely but the expression on his face, the way he moves, and the tone of his voice all show signs of loneliness.

Messages of verbal communication may not be what we think they are. A patient may say that he is not eating because he has no appetite. Yet, when the nurse begins to feed him, he starts to eat. Does he want the attention of being fed?

A word of caution is offered. It would be unwise to assume that everything the patient says must be viewed with suspicion and as a reason for probing and prying to try to find true meanings. Rather, the nurse will wish to be alert to the possibility that the patient may not always be able or willing to say what he really feels. Therefore, the nurse will want to observe nonverbal communication carefully while still listening closely to what is said.

Touch is common in nursing because of the many times when nurses and patients are in close physical contact. Thus, how the nurse gives an injection tells the patient that she is either very skilled or unskilled.

The nurse who holds a crying child in her arms gives the child a feeling of security and affection through the sense of touch. A patient once said that her nurse gave a backrub that showed "a lot of love."

Silence is often part of nonverbal communication. Periods of silence can have any number of meanings. A patient may use silence as an escape; he may be afraid of an examination and remain silent in order to avoid talking about his fears. A husband and wife can often sit quietly without talking and yet, tell each other much about their love for one another. A comfortable and happy person may prefer silence to talking as an expression of his contentment. Silence may be a time when someone is exploring his feelings; to interrupt with conversation when someone is deep in thought disturbs his thinking process.

Certain patients present special communication problems. The nurse may need to use special means, such as gestures, touch, and written notes, when communicating with patients who are deaf, blind, or mute. When caring for patients who speak a language with which the nurse is unfamiliar, nonverbal communication is helpful, but an interpreter may also be necessary.

As this brief discussion shows, communication is an important ingredient in the nurse-patient relationship. In fact, without communication, a relationship could not even be developed. Observing and listening are important when communicating with others and will be discussed in the following section.

Observing and listening to the patient

To observe is to take notice of something. Observation includes being aware of a situation and then interpreting it. In its broadest sense, it includes seeing, touching, listening, and smelling. For example, the nurse sees a rash on the patient's skin. She observes, through her sense of smell, that the drainage on a dressing has a foul odor. While giving a backrub, she feels, through her sense of touch, that the patient has a lump on his back. She hears that a patient's breathing is noisy.

Some observations must be made by using instruments. For example, the nurse obtains body temperature by using a thermometer and observes that the patient's temperature is above normal. Similarly she uses a scale to determine the patient's weight.

The purpose of observing is twofold. First, it helps guide care for which the nursing team is responsible. The nurse observes a particular patient need and reports it to the team, whose members then adjust nursing care to meet that need. For instance, a patient who has been allowed out of bed to take his own shower bath appears unsteady when he walks and tells the nurse that he feels dizzy. She reports this symptom and nursing care is changed; the patient is given a bed bath.

A second purpose of observation is to assist coworkers on the health team so its members may adjust their care also to better meet the patient's needs. For instance, when the nurse observes that a patient who is taking a drug because he has a heart disease has a very slow pulse rate, she reports this symptom promptly so that the physician may adjust the drug dosage as necessary.

It is important for the nurse to know which signs and symptoms are not normal. Without such knowledge, she cannot observe intelligently and report accurately. This book will often describe the normal as well as the abnormal. Other nursing courses will also help the student learn abnormal and normal signs. If she is in doubt, she will report to her supervising nurse promptly for assistance in making a judgment.

Observation goes on whenever a nurse-patient relationship occurs. It includes knowing what to observe, how and when to observe, and what to report as important.

Listening involves the act of hearing and interpreting what is heard. A good listener pays close attention to what is said. She forgets about herself and concentrates on the speaker.

It is difficult to overstress the importance of listening to patients. During the course of a busy day, it is easy to think about what must be done and forget to listen to the patient. Many important signs of the patient's condition and how he feels are missed because the nurse failed to listen when the patient spoke.

Most people quickly learn when someone is pretending to listen. They usually can tell also when the listener is bored or impatient to get on with something else. For example, the nurse may look out the window, interrupt the patient, or have a faraway look while the patient speaks. It is easy to see that if the nurse becomes careless and does not listen, a good nurse-patient relationship cannot be expected to develop.

●

Teaching the patient

It was pointed out previously that a basic psychosocial need of humans is to know and to understand. The nurse helps meet this need when she teaches her patients.

Teaching can be formal in nature. For example, students often attend a specific class with a planned lesson. A classroom is set up for a lecture or demonstration. Nurses sometimes plan specific classes for groups of patients, such as for a group of pregnant women. But teaching can also be informal, occurring spontaneously at the patient's bedside with only a patient and a nurse present. As a health teacher, the nurse often teaches in an informal manner. She takes advantage of helping the patient learn what he needs and wants to know whenever the opportunity arises.

Informal teaching does not mean that there is little or no planning. On the contrary, a nursing team will want to include teaching in its nursing care plan. But teaching may often occur on the spur-of-the-moment and in a manner that meets the patient's needs at the time.

Teaching includes explaining things to patients. Whenever the nurse carries out nursing care, she explains what she is going to do. Place yourself in a strange situation, having various people doing things to you, none of which you understand. Think of how quickly you might become frightened—and, how quickly you could be put at ease if someone just stopped to explain. Would you agree that explaining to the patient is an important part of a good nurse-patient relationship? What nurses may take for granted, even such a simple procedure as obtaining the patient's temperature, may not be simple for the patient unless the nurse explains what she is about to do.

The nurse will adjust her teaching so that the patient understands. It is of little value to use terminology which is not familiar to the patient, or to teach in such depth that he becomes confused. The patient who is learning how to take his own insulin, for instance, wants to know how to inject himself safely and with minimum discomfort. He is rarely interested in a detailed explanation of the anatomy of the skin and underlying body tissues.

A good teacher avoids teaching when the patient is not ready for learning or appears uninterested at that moment. A very ill patient is rarely ready to be taught how he can make adjustments in his daily living at home until he is on the road to recovery. Similarly, most patients are not interested in being instructed when visitors are present.

High-quality nursing always includes teaching. As a nurse, you will wish to take advantage of situations when you can teach. Also, as you do so, your skills will grow and you will be helping to develop a good nurse-patient relationship.

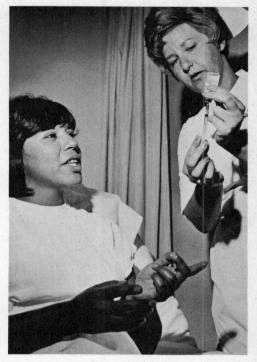

Fig. 3-3 Instruction is often necessary for the patient who will be managing at home. This nurse is teaching the patient how to prepare and give herself an injection.

What patients expect of nurses

There have been investigations on what patients expect of nurses. Also, much has been learned on the subject from what patients have written and said about nurses who cared for them. The following is a brief summary of the findings.

- Patients expect the nurse to be skilled in her work.
- Patients expect the nurse to be serious about her work. They appreciate a nurse who is cheerful and can enjoy humor, but only when used appropriately and while still being serious about what she is doing.
- Patients expect the nurse to be thoughtful, understanding, and accepting of them.
- When patients are unable to care for themselves, they expect the nurse to assist them.
- Patients expect the nurse to insure their privacy.
- Patients expect the nurse to listen to them and to believe what they say.
- Patients expect the nurse to explain the nursing care she gives them.
- Patients expect the nurse to consider their own suggestions concerning the care they are to receive.
- Although patients anticipate hospital routines, they expect that reasonable and fair exceptions should be made when necessary in order that their needs can be met satisfactorily.

While none of these findings may come as a surprise, the nurse who remembers the patient's expectations will help good relationships to grow.

Conclusion

Hopefully, this chapter has helped you understand what is meant by respecting each patient as an individual. Most of the remaining chapters discuss specific care that nurses carry out with patients. You will not be told each time a procedure is described to respect the patient, to be familiar with his background, to explain what will be done, to provide privacy, and so on. Rather, after studying this chapter, it will be assumed that you will remember to do so without additional reminders. It may be helpful to review this chapter from time to time so that its content becomes a part of all of your nursing care.

References

Aiken, Linda and Aiken, James L., "A Systematic Approach to the Evaluation of Interpersonal Relationships," *American Journal of Nursing*, 73:863–867, May 1973.

Amacher, Nancy Jean, "Touch Is a Way of Caring," *American Journal of Nursing*, 73:852–854, May 1973.

Beaumont, Estelle and Wiley, Loy; Eds., "Trusting Patients to Teach Themselves," *Nursing '74*, 4:15–16, March 1974.

Burkett, Alice D., "A Way to Communicate," *American Journal of Nursing*, 74:2185–2187, December 1974.

Carrington, Lawrence W., "The Therapeutic Community: All Relationships Relevant," *The Journal of Practical Nursing*, 25:16–17, 33, April 1975.

Durm, Mary, "Empathy," *American Journal of Nursing*, 73:683, April 1973.

Fuchs, Lucy, "Talking to the Elderly," *Nursing Care*, 8:16–17, March 1975.

Glittenberg, Joann, "Adapting Health Care to a Cultural Setting," *American Journal of Nursing*, 74:2218–2221, December 1974.

Gruendemann, Barbara J., "Hospital Chaplain: The "Now" Member of the Health Team," *RN*, 36:38–40, 42, 46, 48, 52, October 1973.

"Is Patient Care Too Impersonal? You Can Bring Back the Human Quality By Touching," *Nursing Care*, 8:32–33, February 1975.

Kalisch, Beatrice J., "What Is Empathy?" *American Journal of Nursing*, 73:1548–1552, September 1973.

Lore, Ann, "Adolescents: People, Not Problems," *American Journal of Nursing*, 73:1232–1234, July 1973.

Luckmann, Joan and Sorensen, Karon Creason, "What Patients' Actions Tell You About Their Feelings, Fears & Needs," *Nursing '75*, 5:54–61, February 1975.

Mangen, Sister Kathryn, "'It's a Family Affair,'" *The Journal of Practical Nursing*, 24:18–20, August 1974.

Marram, Gwen D., "Patients' Evaluation of Their Care: Importance to the Nurse," *Nursing Outlook*, 21:322–324, May 1973.

Nehring, Virginia and Geach, Barbara, "Patients' Evaluation of Their Care: Why They Don't Complain," *Nursing Outlook*, 21:317–321, May 1973.

Rickles, Nathan S. and Finkle, Betty C., "Anxiety: Yours . . . And Your Patient's," *Nursing '73*, 3:23–26, March 1973.

Robinson, Vera M., "The Tactful Use of Humor in Nursing," *RN*, 37:38–39, October 1974.

Sharp, Alice E., "Four Steps to Better Patient-Teaching," *RN*, 37:62–63, May 1974.

Veninga, Robert, "Communications: A Patient's Eye View," *American Journal of Nursing*, 73:320–322, February 1973.

White, Earnestine Huffmann, "Health and the Black Person: An Annotated Bibliography," *American Journal of Nursing*, 74:1839–1841, October 1974.

Wood, M. Marion, "Part 1. (A-L). 300 Valuable Booklets to Give to Patients & Their Families: A Source Guide," *Nursing '74*, 4:43–50, April 1974.

————, "Part 2. (M-Z). 300 Valuable Booklets to Give to Patients & Their Families: A Source Guide," *Nursing '74*, 4:59–66, May 1974.

4 practices of medical asepsis

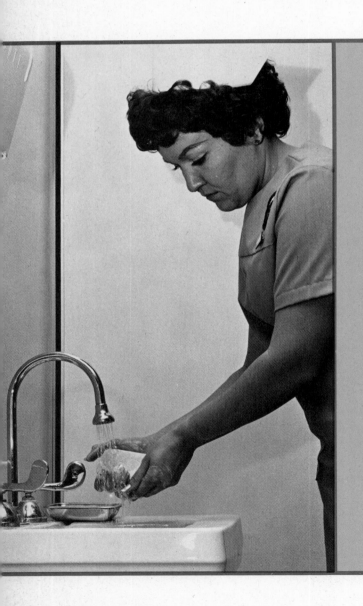

behavioral objectives

When mastery of content in this chapter is reached, the student will be able to

Define terms appearing in the glossary.

List at least eight examples of good practices of medical asepsis from everyday living; list at least eight additional practices when caring for patients in a health agency.

Explain why a sterilized item is also a disinfected item but a disinfected item is not necessarily a sterilized item.

Describe why spores are difficult to destroy.

List the four basic needs that most microorganisms require in order to live and reproduce.

Describe the cycle that explains how microorganisms move from place to place and give examples to illustrate.

Discuss briefly why frequent and good handwashing is essential to help prevent the spread of microorganisms.

Demonstrate how to wash forearms, wrists, and hands and explain the reason for her actions.

List at least ten guides to follow when cleaning equipment and supplies with soap or detergent and water and give the reason for each.

List four guides that help to select a proper sterilization or disinfection method.

List two methods of chemical disinfection/sterilization.

List four methods of physical disinfection/sterilization.

Demonstrate how to clean, disinfect, and sterilize several contaminated items, following guides given in this chapter and policy where the nurse studies or works.

List three methods of disinfection/sterilization that can be used conveniently in most homes.

Demonstrate how to clean a patient's supplies and equipment after he is discharged and explain the reason for her actions.

glossary

Aerobe A microorganism requiring free oxygen to live.

Anaerobe A microorganism that does not require free oxygen to live.

Antibiotic A drug that destroys or inhibits growth of microorganisms.

Antiseptic A substance used to destroy pathogens. In general, safe for use on persons.

Asepsis The absence of organisms causing disease.

Bacteriocide A substance capable of destroying microorganisms but not spores.

Bacteriostatic A substance that prevents growth of microorganisms.

Coagulate A process that thickens or congeals a substance.

Communicable Disease Technique Practices to prevent transfer of microorganisms. Synonym for isolation technique.

Contaminate To render something unclean or unsterile.

Disinfectant A substance used to destroy pathogens. In general, not intended for use on persons.

Disinfection A process by which pathogens but not necessarily spores are destroyed.

Germicide A substance that helps prevent growth of microorganisms.

Host An animal or a person on which or in which microorganisms live.

Isolation Technique Practices to prevent transfer of microorganisms. Synonym for communicable disease technique.

Medical Asepsis Practices that help reduce the number and spread of microorganisms.

Microorganism (Organism) A tiny living animal or plant that can cause disease. Most are visible only with a microscope.

Nonpathogen A microorganism that does not ordinarily cause disease.

Pathogen A microorganism that causes disease.

Reservoir A place on which or in which microorganisms grow and reproduce.

Spore A cell produced by a microorganism which develops into active microorganisms under proper conditions.

Sterile An item on which all microorganisms have been destroyed.

Sterilization A process by which all microorganisms, including spores, are destroyed.

Surgical Asepsis Practices that render and keep objects and areas free of all microorganisms.

introduction

Medical asepsis is discussed early in this text because an important part of nursing is to give care in a way that will help prevent the spread of disease.

The word "germ" is a popular term for microorganism. A **microorganism** is a tiny living animal or plant. Most are harmless but some can cause disease. Most can be seen only with a microscope. Microorganism is often shortened to the word organism. There are microorganisms everywhere about us. Often, a sick person is more likely to develop an illness from microorganisms his body could fight off with ease if he were well. For example, a person may not catch a cold from another person when he is in good health, but he may become very ill if he catches a cold when he is already sick. Therefore, it is especially important for health practitioners to use every possible way to prevent the spread of microorganisms. In addition, the nurse will wish to teach her patients and their visitors how they, too, can help.

Description of asepsis

Asepsis is defined as the absence of organisms causing disease. Such organisms are called **pathogens.** For example, a virus is the pathogen causing German measles, and the *Neisseria gonorrhoeae* is the pathogen that causes gonorrhea. A **nonpathogen** is a microorganism that does not ordinarily cause disease. For example, the organism *Escherichia coli* is normally found in the intestinal tract where it does not cause disease. However, if the organism is spread to another part of the body, such as the urinary bladder, it may cause infection there. A **host** is a person or an animal upon which or in which microorganisms live.

Asepsis is divided into two forms: surgical asepsis and medical asepsis. **Surgical asepsis** refers to practices that eliminate *all* microorganisms, nonpathogenic as well as pathogenic. An item, such as a needle used for injecting a drug, is called **sterile** after all microorganisms on it have been destroyed. Practices of surgical asepsis are discussed in Chapter 15.

Medical asepsis refers to practices that help reduce the number and the spread of microorganisms. The following are some good medical aseptic practices that we observe in our everyday living: covering the nose and mouth when coughing or sneezing; washing hands before handling food; using individual personal care items, such as towels, toothbrushes, combs, brushes, shaving gear, and the like; washing hands after using the bathroom; using water fountains instead of public drinking cups; using pasteurized milk; licensing food handlers and inspecting public eating places; controlling pests that may spread disease, such as rats and mosquitoes; and having regulations for immigrants who otherwise may enter our country with infectious diseases.

Certain practices are followed when persons are ill with infections. For example, a patient who has an active case of tuberculosis is often isolated from others, and a procedure known as **isolation** or **communicable disease technique** is used when caring for him. Isolation techniques use practices of medical asepsis plus certain other practices that will be discussed in Chapter 22.

The following are additional terms commonly used when discussing medical and surgical asepsis:

To **contaminate** means to make something unclean or unsterile. In medical asepsis, areas and equipment are considered to be contaminated if it is believed they contain microorganisms that cause disease. For example, the inside of a sink, the floor, and all items used by or for patients are considered contaminated. The hands are considered contaminated after giving nursing care. In surgical asepsis, areas are considered contaminated if they have been touched by anything that is unsterile.

Disinfection refers to the process by which pathogenic organisms, but not spores, are destroyed. Spores are discussed in the following section. A **disinfectant** is a substance used to destroy pathogens. Disinfectants are not intended for use on persons. An **antiseptic** is a disinfectant also but usually can be used on the living person.

Sterilization refers to the process by which all microorganisms, including spores, are destroyed.

Study the definitions of sterilization and disinfection. These conclusions can be made: anything that is sterilized is also automatically disinfected, but if an item is disinfected, it cannot safely be considered sterile also.

A **bacteriocidal** agent is a substance that is capable of destroying microorganisms. A **bacteriostatic** agent is a substance that prevents the growth and reproduction of microorganisms.

An important part of medical and surgical asepsis depends on the individual. If the nurse takes shortcuts in medical and surgical aseptic practices, possibly no one will be the wiser. However, she risks her own health as well as that of her patients. Thus, conscientiousness, honesty, and faithfulness are important ingredients of all aseptic practices.

Preventing the spread of microorganisms

Before discussing some of the ways to prevent their spread, it may be helpful to recall a few characteristics of microorganisms.

Just as man does, a microorganism has certain basic needs in order to live. It needs warmth, food, and water or moisture. Microorganisms that are **aerobes** require oxygen to live. **Anaerobes** grow best where there is no free oxygen. Some anaerobes are very dangerous because they can grow rapidly in deep wounds, such as nail punctures. The microorganism causing tetanus (lockjaw) is of this kind.

Certain microorganisms produce cells called **spores.** Spores have thick walls and can live through extremes of heat, cold, dryness, or lack of food. They are especially difficult to destroy. Spores develop into active microorganisms when conditions are right for their growth. Unbroken skin can usually handle spores well, but when the skin is broken, especially if a wound is deep, an infection with spores can be very dangerous. The organism causing tetanus produces spores. Plant seeds are examples of spores also.

Most microorganisms grow best in darkness and will die when exposed to light and dryness. For this reason, sunning articles and airing them well are good ways to destroy many organisms. One can see that they have a poor chance to live in a room that is dry, clean, bright, and airy.

One method to control disease-causing microorganisms is to take away their basic needs so that they cannot grow, reproduce, and spread. Many practices of medical and surgical asepsis are intended to destroy microorganisms in this manner.

Microorganisms move from place to place in a cycle, as shown in Figure 4-1. If that cycle is broken anywhere, the organism cannot grow, spread, and cause disease. For example, a person has a cold and coughs and sneezes. Microorganisms are carried in the expelled droplets. They enter another person's body when that person inhales the droplets and he then develops a cold. This sequence is illustrated in Figure 4-1 between points 3 and 5. If the droplets are trapped in tissues which are

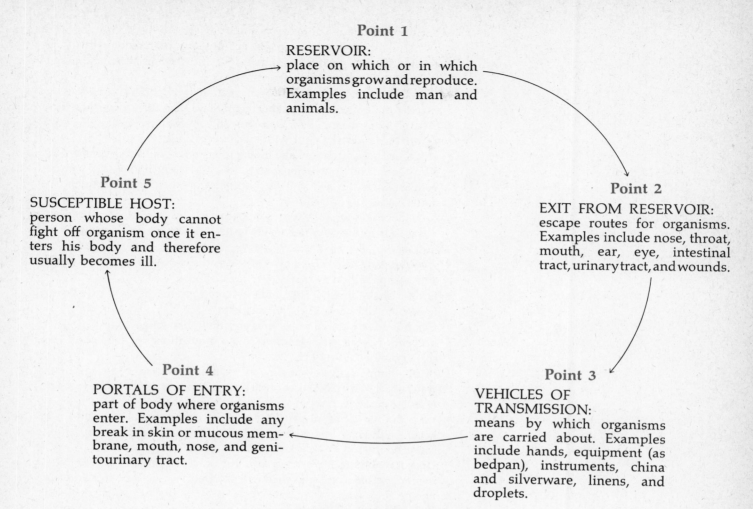

Point 1
RESERVOIR:
place on which or in which organisms grow and reproduce. Examples include man and animals.

Point 5
SUSCEPTIBLE HOST:
person whose body cannot fight off organism once it enters his body and therefore usually becomes ill.

Point 2
EXIT FROM RESERVOIR:
escape routes for organisms. Examples include nose, throat, mouth, ear, eye, intestinal tract, urinary tract, and wounds.

Point 4
PORTALS OF ENTRY:
part of body where organisms enter. Examples include any break in skin or mucous membrane, mouth, nose, and genitourinary tract.

Point 3
VEHICLES OF TRANSMISSION:
means by which organisms are carried about. Examples include hands, equipment (as bedpan), instruments, china and silverware, linens, and droplets.

Fig. 4-1 Infection process cycle.

then properly destroyed, the organisms have no way of getting to another person. The cycle has been broken and the organisms cannot spread. Many practices are directed toward interrupting the cycle, thus preventing the spread of microorganisms.

Some examples of medical aseptic practices that break this cycle have already been given. Below are additional common practices that should be observed.

- Wash hands before and after giving nursing care or after handling equipment and supplies used for care. A detailed discussion of handwashing will be found in the next section.
- Handle discharges as though they always contain disease-producing organisms. Discard them promptly and according to agency policy. Bandages, dressings, tissues, and cotton balls are commonly used to absorb body discharges. They can very easily spread organisms if not discarded properly.
- Discard disposable equipment according to agency policy. All equipment used for patient care is considered contaminated after use.

- Flush away contents of bedpans and urinals promptly, unless they are being saved for a specimen. Except possibly in remote areas, it is considered safe to flush contents into the sewage system. Sewage treatment destroys microorganisms.
- Use equipment and supplies for one patient only. If they are reused by another patient, clean them thoroughly and then disinfect or sterilize them in the manner described later in this chapter.
- Cover breaks in the skin with sterile dressings.
- Use every precaution to keep food and water supplies clean and fresh.
- Keep soiled equipment and supplies, especially linens, away from your uniform so that you do not carry organisms from patient to patient and to yourself.
- Consider the floor as heavily contaminated. Discard any item or clean it if it falls to the floor before using it. Also, disinfect or sterilize it as necessary.
- Avoid raising dust which can carry organisms. Use a vacuum cleaner and dampened or treated cloths for cleaning.
- Do not shake linens. This tends to create drafts that will carry contaminated dust and lint from place to place.
- Clean the least soiled areas first and the most soiled areas last. This prevents having cleaner areas soiled even more by material from dirtier areas.
- Wrap damp or wet items, such as dressings and bandages, in a waterproof bag before discarding so that handlers of trash and garbage will not come in contact with body discharges.
- Pour liquids to be discarded, such as bath water and mouthwash rinsings, directly into a drain or toilet. Avoid spilling and splashing these liquids on yourself, the floor, and other equipment.
- Do not wear rings other than a plain band. Microorganisms can lodge in stone settings and in etched and grooved areas and be carried from person to person.
- Keep the patient's room as clean, bright, dry, and airy as possible.
- If you are in doubt about whether an item is clean (or sterile if necessary), do not use it until you have cared for it properly.

Return to point 5 in Figure 4-1. When efforts have failed to prevent organisms from spreading to a susceptible person, that person may become ill as the organisms grow and reproduce. He then becomes the reservoir for organisms, as Figure 4-1 illustrates. Keeping oneself in the best possible health helps the body fight off microorganisms. Eating nutritious meals and getting enough rest, for example, are important ways to prevent an infection from developing or becoming severe, even though the organisms have entered the body. These protective measures are important for patients and health workers alike.

Antibiotics are drugs that destroy microorganisms or prevent their growth. They are often used to fight infections, and their use has been a life-saving measure for many patients. However, not all organisms can be handled with antibiotics. They are not effective against most viruses, such as the ones that cause the common cold. Also, they often are not particularly helpful when the infection is caused by staphylococci, or "staph" as they are frequently called. Staphylococci are commonly found in health agencies and are usually spread by the hands. They are the organisms that often cause boils, styes, and food poisoning.

Chart 4-1 Washing the hands, wrists, and forearms

The purpose is to clean the hands, wrists, and forearms of contamination

Suggested Action	Reason for Action	Figure to Illustrate
Approach sink. Do not allow uniform to touch sink during washing procedure.	Sink is considered contaminated. Uniform may carry organisms from place to place.	
Turn on water with foot or knee control. If hand-operated faucet is used, open faucets with paper towel and discard towel properly.	Organisms can accumulate on faucets and spread to others.	
Regulate temperature of water so that it is comfortably warm.	Warm water makes better soap suds than cold water. Hot water tends to dry and chap skin. Organisms can lodge in roughened and broken areas of chapped skin.	
Regulate flow of water so that it does not splash from sink.	Water splashed from sink will contaminate uniform.	
During entire procedure, keep hands and forearms lower than elbows as illustrated in Figures 4-2 through 4-6.	Gravity will allow water and rinsings to drain from an area of less contamination (forearms) to an area of more contamination (hands) into sink.	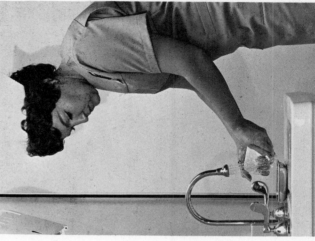
Wet hands and soap them well. Apply a teaspoon or so if liquid soap is used. When bar soap is used, hold bar in hands during entire washing period. If bar is dropped accidently into soap dish, sink, or floor, start washing procedure from beginning.	Soap dish, sink, and floor are considered contaminated. Contaminated soap will contaminate hands.	

Fig. 4-2 Nurse wetting and soaping hands well. Note precautions she observes: she stands a safe distance from sink to prevent contaminating her uniform; she holds hands below level of her elbows and makes certain she does not touch sink; and she regulates the water so that it does not splash from sink.

Chart 4-1 continued

Suggested Action	Reason for Action	Figure to Illustrate
With firm rubbing and circular motions, wash hands (palm and back), each finger, area between fingers, and knuckles.	Friction caused by firm rubbing and circular motions helps to loosen dirt and organisms. Dirt and organisms lodge between fingers and in skin crevices of knuckles, as well as on palm and back of hands.	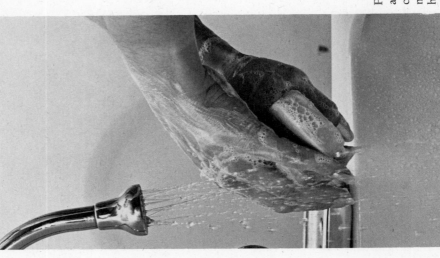
Rinse hands and fingers well under running water.	Running water rinses dirt and organisms loosened with soap, water, and friction into sink.	Fig. 4-3 The hands, knuckles, and areas between the fingers are cleaned with firm, rubbing motions. Note nurse continues to hold the soap during the procedure.

Wash forearms and wrists. Wash forearms at least as high as contamination is likely. Use firm rubbing and circular motions.

Organisms can be present on wrists and forearms as well as on hands. Friction helps to loosen dirt and organisms. Cleaning least contaminated areas (forearms and wrists) after hands are clean prevents spreading organisms from hands to forearms and wrists.

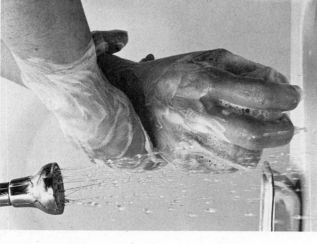

Fig. 4-4 The wrists and forearms are cleaned with firm circular motions.

After washing, rinse soap well under running water and drop bar into soap dish without touching dish.

Rinse forearms, wrists, and hands well under running water.

Dirt and organisms can accumulate on bar of soap and be spread to next user. Soap dish is considered contaminated.

Running water rinses dirt and organisms loosened with soap, water, and friction into sink.

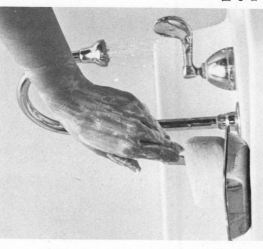

Fig. 4-5 To prevent contaminating her hands, the nurse drops the soap into the soap dish.

Chart 4-1 continued

Suggested Action	Reason for Action	Figure to Illustrate
Clean under nails with orange stick or flat toothpick carefully when hands are heavily contaminated and at least once a day before beginning work. Rinse fingers well under running water.	Organisms can lodge and remain under nails where they can grow and be spread to others. If cleaning instrument is used carelessly, organisms and dirt may lodge in injured areas and cause infection. Running water rinses organisms and dirt loosened with cleaning instrument into sink.	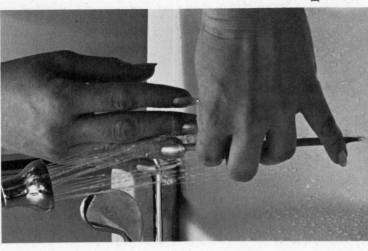 Fig. 4-6 The area under the fingernails is cleaned with an orange stick, and the running water continuously flushes dirt and organisms into sink.
Repeat washing procedure as indicated and especially if hands are contaminated with blood, pus, or drainage from wounds or body openings.	When hands are heavily contaminated, a second and even a third washing are necessary to assure that all dirt and organisms have been removed.	
A sterile brush may be used to scrub hands if they are heavily contaminated. Use brush carefully.	Brush causes friction which helps to loosen dirt and organisms. If brush is used carelessly, organisms and dirt may lodge in injured areas and cause infection.	
If hand-operated faucets are used, protect hands well with paper towel and turn off faucets.	Hands will remain clean if protected with towel when faucets have become contaminated.	
Dry forearms, wrists, and hands well with paper towel.	Drying skin well prevents chapping. Dirt and organisms can lodge in roughened and broken skin areas.	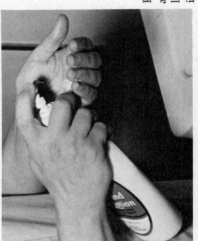 Fig. 4-7 To keep the skin soft and prevent chapping, hand lotion is applied after the washing procedure.
Apply lotion to forearms, wrists, and hands.	Lotion helps to keep skin soft and easier to clean. It helps prevent chapping. Chapped skin is difficult to keep clean since dirt and organisms can lodge in roughened areas.	

Any person who is careless about observing good medical aseptic practices has given poor care. And anyone who cuts corners while thinking that antibiotics are handy if an infection spreads and develops is guilty of the poorest kind of care!

Handwashing

The handwashing procedure described here is used when medical asepsis is being practiced. The procedure used in operating and delivery rooms, frequently called the surgical scrub, will be described in other nursing courses.

Of all procedures to prevent the spread of microorganisms, possibly none is more important than handwashing. Many authorities believe the hands are responsible for most instances of spreading infections. We are constantly being warned about the importance of washing hands frequently and well. Yet, carelessness continues. The hands of persons working around patients are in constant use. A few examples will illustrate: a nurse giving a patient a bath; a physician examining a patient; a maid folding linen; a nurse's aide making a bed; an engineer repairing a patient's television set; a volunteer taking a patient from his room to the x-ray department; a laboratory technician taking a sample of blood; and an x-ray technician taking an x-ray picture.

Keeping the hands clean is largely up to the individual. The amount of respect the nurse has for her own health as well as for that of others determines to a large extent how well she cleans her hands. Conscientiousness cannot be overstressed.

Chart 4-1 describes handwashing and Figures 4-2 through 4-7 illustrate the procedure. It should take one to two minutes to wash the forearms, wrists, and hands well. If they are heavily contaminated, the procedure should take at least two, three, or even four minutes. A timer placed near the sink is convenient, and will help time the washing period accurately.

Cleaning supplies and equipment

The nurse's duties in relation to cleaning supplies and equipment will vary from agency to agency. This section is included to assist the nurse in those situations when the responsibility is hers. Supplies and equipment should be cleaned before they are disinfected or sterilized. This will be discussed later in this chapter.

Soap or detergent and water remain among the best cleaning agents available. Both break up dirt into tiny particles which can be rinsed off more easily with water. Detergents have several advantages over soap. For example, they can be used in hard water or in cold water with better results than can soap. Studies have shown that soaps are about equal in ability to clean. Those containing perfume may be pleasant to use but appear to be no better than plain green or odorless soap.

Some soaps and detergents contain a **germicide,** that is, a substance that helps prevent the growth of microorganisms. However, studies have found that germicides can be harmful. Therefore, many of them are available only with a physician's prescription or within a hospital operating or delivery room.

The following guides will help make the procedure effective and safe when using soap or detergent and water to clean supplies and equipment:

- Wear waterproof gloves if items are heavily contaminated or if you have any breaks in your skin.
- Rinse items first under cool, running water. Hot water causes many substances to **coagulate,** that is, to thicken or congeal, making them difficult to remove.
- Use hot water and soap or detergent for cleaning purposes. Hot water and soap or detergent break up dirt into tiny particles which can be more easily rinsed off with water.
- A sponge or cloth may be used for many surfaces. They create friction which helps to loosen dirt and organisms.
- Use a brush with stiff bristles as necessary to remove dirt. A brush is necessary to get into small grooves and joints in instruments. Brushes designed especially to clean barrels of reusable syringes are particularly helpful.
- Abrasive cleaners are helpful for removing stubborn stains, as on a wash basin or emesis basin.
- Force sudsy water through reusable needles. Alcohol or ether may be used also and will help to break up oily substances.
- Disassemble and rinse reusable needles and syringes immediately after use, especially when time does not permit a thorough cleaning immediately. This prevents parts from becoming locked together.
- Rinse catheters and rectal tubes immediately after use, and leave them to soak if a thorough cleaning is not possible immediately. Force sudsy water through them frequently for thorough cleaning.
- Rinse items well under running water after cleaning with soap or detergent and water. This will rinse away loosened dirt and organisms into the sink.
- Dry equipment well to prevent rusting.
- Handle gloves, brushes, sponges, cleaning cloths, and water as contaminated and clean or discard accordingly.
- Avoid splashing or spilling water on yourself or on the floor or other equipment during entire procedure.
- Consider your hands heavily contaminated after cleaning equipment and wash them as described above.
- For most purposes, thorough laundering of linen is sufficiently safe for cleaning. For heavily contaminated linen, special precautions, which will be discussed in Chapter 22, are necessary.

Certain items cannot be washed without ruining them. These include instruments used for taking the blood pressure, and for examining the eyes and the ears, and the cuff which is part of the apparatus to obtain blood pressure. Follow agency policy concerning the handling of such pieces of equipment. Wipe them with a small cloth or a cotton ball dampened with a disinfectant. Some items, such as a blood pressure cuff, are best cleaned by sunning and airing them.

When supplies and equipment are thoroughly clean, they are ready for disinfection or sterilization.

Practices of medical asepsis

Methods of disinfection and sterilization

The nurse's duties concerning sterilization and disinfection will vary, depending on agency policy. Most hospitals have central supply units where equipment and supplies are cleaned, kept in good working order, and disinfected and sterilized. In addition, most health agencies are using many more items for patient care that are disposable, that is, used only once or only for one patient and then discarded. The use of central supply units and disposable equipment has helped cut down on both the spread of organisms in health agencies and work for nurses and others.

This section is included since nurses are responsible for cleaning, sterilizing, and disinfecting equipment in some agencies. Also, the nurse has these responsibilities in most cases when she cares for patients in their homes.

There are several basic guides to help select a proper sterilization or disinfection method. As has been mentioned, some organisms are easier to destroy than others. Spores and the organism causing tuberculosis are especially difficult to destroy, while the organism causing the common cold is relatively easy to destroy. However, we are rarely sure exactly which microorganisms are present. Therefore, it is poor practice for the nurse to eliminate disinfecting or sterilizing items and cleaning them only because she thinks she knows what organisms are present. Shortening the time required for adequate disinfection or sterilization is also unwise for the same reason. The conclusion is that when selecting disinfection and sterilization methods, it is better for the nurse to overdo than underdo the procedure, because she can never be absolutely sure of the organisms that are present.

The more organisms that are present, the longer it takes to destroy them. This makes cleaning items before disinfecting or sterilizing them particularly important. When organisms are protected under layers of grease or oil or are in blood and pus, disinfecting and sterilizing items becomes more difficult and therefore less safe.

The type of equipment used makes a difference. For example, equipment with small grooves, as a lifting forceps, or items with small lumens, such as hypodermic needles or catheters, require special care. Such items must be cleaned thoroughly first and then completely covered with solutions or exposed to steam or gas when disinfected or sterilized.

Items used for certain procedures must be sterile. If they are not, the patient is apt to develop an infection. All equipment used during operations must be sterile, for example. So also must the catheter that will be introduced into the urinary bladder. Other equipment, such as bedpans, urinals, bath basins, rectal tubes, and the like, need not necessarily be sterile. But we are not always sure what organisms may be present on these items. Except in home situations, cleaning such items may not be safe. Therefore, health agencies sterilize articles used for patients in order to make certain that they are entirely safe.

Chemical Means for Disinfection and Sterilization. Chemical sterilization uses chemical solutions or gases. Items to be sterilized are placed in a solution or exposed to fumes (gas) in a chamber for a specified period of time. However, many studies have shown that chemical sterilization is difficult to accomplish. In fact, some authorities believe that chemical solutions and gases are not safe for sterilization purposes. Therefore, their use is generally limited to items that are likely to be damaged by other methods. Or they are used in situations where a better method is not available. Nevertheless they are commonly used as disinfectants.

There is a variety of chemical solutions on the market for disinfection and sterilization. Some claim to be bacteriocidal; some are advertised as antiseptics, some as disinfectants, and so on. Agencies differ in their choices. It is recommended that you examine those used in the agency where you study and work and carefully follow the agency's policies concerning how they are to be used.

Physical Means for Disinfection and Sterilization. Physical sterilization and disinfection use heat. The most common methods are steam under pressure, dry heat, free-flowing steam, and boiling water. Sterilization and disinfection occur when there is enough heat to kill organisms. In short, the higher the temperature, the quicker the organisms will die.

As was true with chemical sterilization and disinfection, any of these methods require a certain amount of *time.* Organisms do not die instantly. The time varies depending on the method used, the type of equipment, and so on. Therefore, be sure to follow agency policies carefully, whichever method you use.

Steam sterilizers use moist heat and pressure. This is the most dependable method for destroying all forms of microorganisms. The autoclave is a pressure steam sterilizer which most hospitals and many other health agencies use. The amount of pressure used has nothing to do with destroying the organisms. Rather, the pressure makes it possible to develop a higher temperature which is responsible for killing the organisms.

The pressure cooker used in many homes operates just as an autoclave does. Foods cooked in them are prepared more quickly than if prepared in an open kettle because of the higher temperature developed in the cooker. Pressure cookers can be used for sterilizing equipment in the home. Articles are placed on a rack above the level of water in the cooker.

Dry heat, or hot-air sterilization, uses equipment similar to an ordinary baking oven. It is a good way to sterilize sharp instruments and syringes because moist heat damages cutting edges and the ground surfaces of glass. It is also a good way to sterilize linens, especially when this becomes necessary in a home.

Free-flowing steam has the same temperature as boiling water. It is not a particularly practical way to sterilize since it is difficult to expose all surfaces of equipment well in a free-flowing steam sterilizer. Some hospitals use steam sterilizers as part of the procedure for cleaning bedpans. However, they have not been found entirely safe for sterilizing bedpans.

Placing equipment in boiling water for a period of time is a common method for disinfection and sterilization. Boiling water does not kill spores and other organisms that are particularly difficult to destroy unless items are boiled for a very long time. It is a convenient way to disinfect and sterilize items in the home.

Care of the patient's supplies and equipment after discharge

Policy will differ from agency to agency concerning who is responsible for cleaning the patient's supplies and equipment after he is discharged. Chart 4-2 is offered to assist the nurse when it is her duty.

Chart 4-2. Care of supplies and equipment after patient is discharged

The purpose is to render equipment and supplies free from pathogenic organisms after the patient is discharged

Suggested Action	Reason for Action
Remove one piece of linen at a time to be sure possessions of patient or agency are not accidently sent to laundry.	This precaution can save costs for agency as well as unpleasantness if patient's personal belongings were accidently left among bed linens.
Roll each piece of linen carefully so that surface that was not in direct contact with patient is on outside.	Friction and motion can create lint which may transport organisms. Confining more contaminated areas reduces amount of contamination that could escape into air.
Roll or fold soiled linens away from uniform.	Organisms can be carried by air currents in dust and lint to uniform and then carried to self or others.
Hold soiled linens away from uniform.	Organisms picked up on uniform from contaminated linens can be carried to self and others.
Avoid raising dust and lint by using cleaning methods to help prevent this, such as a dampened or treated cloth.	Organisms can be carried about on dust particles.
Wash surfaces of furniture, using soap or detergent and water; rinse with clear water and dry.	Cleaning with soap or detergent and water loosens dirt and organisms which can then be removed with rinsing. Drying items helps prevent damage to finish.
Wash cleaner areas before more contaminated areas, as the bed first, then overbed table and bedside stand.	Cleaning areas where there are fewer organisms before cleaning ones with more organisms helps reduce spread of organisms.
Wash with soap or detergent and water and rinse personal care items, such as basins, bedpan, urinal, and so on, before sterilizing them.	The fewer the organsims on an article, the easier it is to sterilize it.
Clean mattress and pillows according to agency procedure. Those with waterproof outer coverings may be cleaned with soap or detergent and water. Airing and sunning them outdoors is also a good way to clean them before reuse.	

After the patient's equipment and supplies are cleaned and sterilized, the bed is made and the room is prepared to receive another patient, as will be described in Chapter 6.

Conclusion

Observing good practices of medical asepsis is basic to good nursing care. It requires constant work, conscientiousness, and attention. Spreading infection is a great hazard in every health agency when health practitioners are careless.

You will find it an interesting and educational experience to study items on the market advertised for use as disinfectants in the home. A supermarket is a good place for this since there are many different products readily available for study. See what the products contain and read what they are advertised to do. Does the label tell what to do if someones swallows any of the product? Compare the active ingredients in the products. Would you conclude that some may help to clean one's conscience but little else? Possibly you may come to the conclusion that some of them are no better than using soap or detergent and water with old-fashioned elbow grease!

Table 4-1 illustrates the importance of cleaning equipment and supplies before sterilizing or disinfecting them. It also illustrates the importance of the time factor when disinfecting and sterilizing articles.

Table 4-1 Theoretical example of the order of death of a bacterial population

Minute	Bacteria living at beginning of new minute	Bacteria killed in 1 minute	Bacteria surviving at end of 1 minute
First	1,000,000	90% = 900,000	100,000
Second	100,000	= 90,000	10,000
Third	10,000	= 9,000	1,000
Fourth	1,000	= 900	100
Fifth	100	= 90	10
Sixth	10	= 9	1
Seventh	1	= 0.9	0.1
Eighth	0.1	= 0.09	0.01
Ninth	0.01	= 0.009	0.001
Tenth	0.001	= 0.0009	0.0001
Eleventh	0.0001	= 0.00009	0.00001
Twelfth	0.00001	= 0.000009	0.000001

From Perkins, J. J.: Principles and Methods of Sterilization. p. 35. Springfield, Ill., Thomas, 1956.

References

Flannagan, Jill, "A Student Writes: A View From Within," *The Journal of Practical Nursing,* 24:32–33, 35, April 1974.

Fox, Marion K., et al, "How Good Are Hand Washing Practices?" *American Journal of Nursing,* 74:1676–1678, September 1974.

Ginsberg, Frances and Clarke, Barbara, "When to Use Disinfectants and Which Ones Not To Use," *Modern Hospital*, 119:110, August 1972.

Marples, Mary J., "Life On The Human Skin," *Scientific American*, 220:108–115, January 1969.

Rendell-Baker, Leslie and Roberts, Robert B., "Gas Versus Steam Sterilization: When to Use Which," *Hospital Topics*, 48:81–83, 86, 87, 88, November 1970.

5 principles of body mechanics

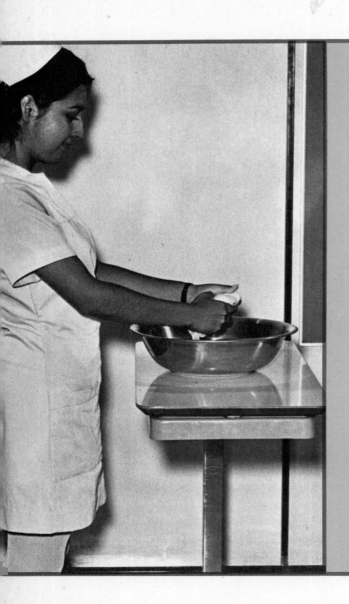

behavioral objectives

When mastery of content in this chapter is reached, the student will be able to

Define terms appearing in the glossary.

List three reasons for using good body mechanics.

Describe the base of support, the line of gravity, and the center of gravity when the body is in good sitting and standing position.

Demonstrate good posture in the standing and sitting positions.

Demonstrate each of the suggested actions listed in Chart 5-1 while using good body mechanics; and explain briefly how each action helps avoid strain and injury to the body.

glossary

Alignment Having parts in proper relationship to each other.

Balance Bringing an object into or keeping it in a steady position.

Base of Support The area on which an object rests.

Body Mechanics Efficient use of the body as a machine.

Center of Gravity The point at which the mass of a body is centered.

Gravity The force that pulls toward the center of the earth.

Line of Gravity An imaginary, vertical line which passes through the center of gravity.

Musculoskeletal System Pertaining to the body's bones, joints, and muscles.

Posture The position of the body, or the way in which it is held.

introduction

In activities of daily living, we reach, lift, stoop, pull, push, walk, sit, stand, and so on. These movements are also used when giving nursing care. We will need less energy, prevent strain and injury to ourselves, and appear more attractive as we work when we use our body well.

Body mechanics is defined as the efficient use of the body as a machine. Using good body mechanics is important for the nurse as well as for the patient. This chapter will discuss basic principles of body mechanics and illustrate how they are used by the nurse in her work.

Basic terminology and concepts of body mechanics

Gravity is a force that pulls objects toward the center of the earth. Gravity is at work, for example, when objects fall to the ground and when water drains to the lowest level it can find. Whenever movement is made, energy is required to overcome gravity.

Balance means to bring an object into or to keep it in a steady position. It is present when an object is firm and stable. When an object is off balance, it will topple as gravity pulls it down and out of position.

The **center of gravity** is defined as the point at which the mass of a body is centered. For the standing person, the center of gravity is the center of the pelvis and about half way between the umbilicus and the pubic bone.

The **line of gravity** is an imaginary, vertical line which passes through the center of gravity.

The **base of support** is that area on which an object rests. The feet are the base of support in the standing position.

Alignment means to bring parts into a proper relationship. The body,

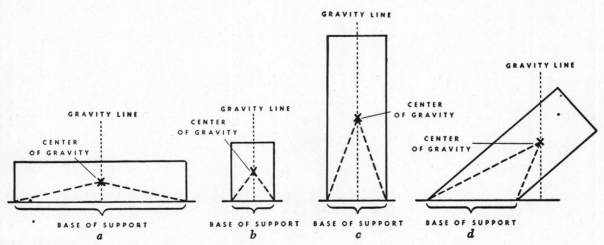

Fig. 5-1 The effect of the base of support and gravity on balance. (Winters, M. C.: Protective Body Mechanics in Daily Life and in Nursing, Philadelphia, Saunders, p. 20)

Principles of body mechanics

for example, is said to be in good alignment when its parts are in proper relationship to each other.

Figure 5-1 illustrates the terms just described.

The skeletal system of the body consists of bones and joints. It forms the body's framework. The muscles of the body produce movement. The term **musculoskeletal system** is often used to refer to the body's bones, joints, and muscles. Good body mechanics uses the musculoskeletal system efficiently.

Using body mechanics starts with good posture. **Posture** refers to the position of the body, or the way in which it is held. Good posture means positioning the body so that there is good body alignment and balance. In this position, the musculoskeletal system can be used in the best way possible. In addition, good posture makes it possible for other systems of the body to work more effectively. For example, slouching when standing or sitting makes it more difficult for the lungs to work at their best. It is also more difficult for the blood to circulate well through all parts of the body when posture is poor.

The following is a description of good posture in the standing position:

- Keep the feet parallel, at right angles to the lower legs, and about 4 to 8 inches apart. Distribute weight equally on both feet. This position of the feet gives the body a good base of support.
- Bend the knees slightly. This position of the knees avoids the strain of "locked knees" and acts like a shock absorber for the entire body.
- Pull in the buttocks and hold the abdomen up and in. This position is often referred to as putting on an internal girdle. It will help keep the back straight by preventing swayback which, in turn, keeps the spine properly aligned. It supports the abdominal organs and causes less strain on both back and abdominal muscles.
- Hold the chest up and slightly forward and extend the waist. This position is often described as putting on a long midriff. It gives internal organs, such as the lungs, the most amount of space for effective work. It also helps maintain good alignment of the spine by preventing a humped back. The shoulders may be relaxed but held back slightly.
- Hold the head erect with the chin in slightly. In a sense, the head is balancing at the top of the spine in this position. The position also helps keep the spine in good alignment by preventing a curve in the neck area.

As you study and practice good posture in the standing position, you will soon discover that you have a good base of support, the line of gravity goes through your base of support, and the body is in proper alignment. You will be in good balance, and the position is restful as well as attractive in appearance.

A good sitting position is like that just described except the buttocks become the base of support on the chair and the knees are bent. Practice not crossing your legs at the knees. The position interferes with proper circulation of blood in the feet and legs.

Having the framework of the body in good position is important. But equally important is using muscles correctly and to their best advantage. The first guide is to use the longest and strongest muscles to provide the energy you need. For example, it is best to use the long and strong

Chart 5-1 Using body mechanics

The purpose is to use the musculoskeletal system of the body as effectively as possible

Suggested Action	Reason for Action	Figure to Illustrate
Maintain good posture.	Good posture reduces strain and helps prevent injury to musculoskeletal system. It helps maintain balance and keeps body in good alignment.	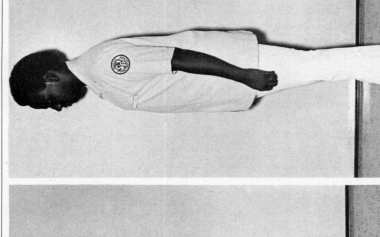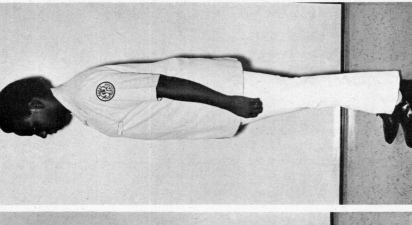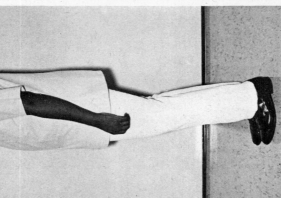

Fig. 5-2 (Left) The nurse in slouched position has relaxed abdominal muscles; his body is in poor alignment. (Right) A good standing position, as described on page 61.

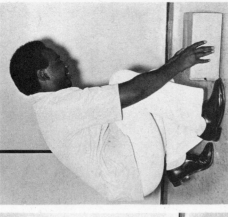

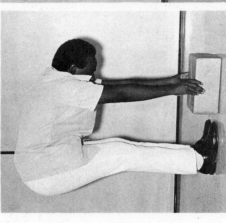

These movements make use of longest and strongest muscles of body and reduce strain on back. They provide good base of support, proper back alignment, and balance.

When stooping, place one foot in front of other; lower body while bending knees. Keep body weight on front foot and ball of back foot. Keep back straight. Return to standing position by lifting body with muscles of thighs and hips.

Fig. 5-3 (Left) The nurse reaches down to pick up the package. This results in poor body alignment and strain on back muscles. (Right) The nurse stoops down to pick up the package, using long and strong muscles to lift the package and himself into the standing position.

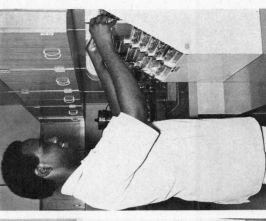

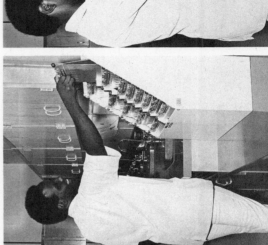

Keep work area close to body.

Stretching and reaching fatigue muscles quickly. When stretching, balance will be poor as line of gravity falls outside base of support.

Fig. 5-4 (Left) Stretching and twisting places the nurse's body in poor alignment and strains muscles. (Right) Keeping the work area close to the body minimizes stretching and twisting.

Chart 5-1 continued

Suggested Action	Reason for Action	Figure to Illustrate

Face working area.

A position that requires twisting strains and tires muscles.

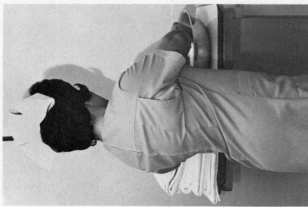 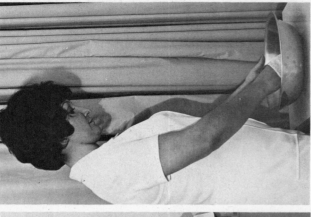

Fig. 5-5 (Left) The nurse twists her body and strains muscles when she does not face her work area. (Right) The nurse avoids twisting by facing her work area.

Pivot to turn body. When pivoting, with feet apart and body weight on ball of each foot (heels slightly raised), turn in desired direction. Keep body straight.

Twisting body causes strain on muscles. Turning is easier when weight is off heels and helps prevent twisting knees.

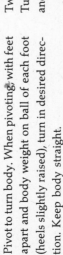 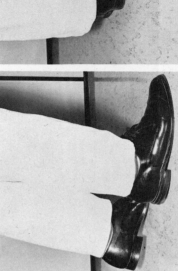 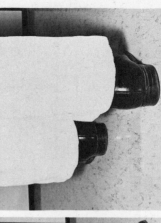

Fig. 5-6 (Left) Before pivoting, the nurse places his weight on the ball of each foot by raising his heels slightly. To pivot right, he places his right foot forward. (Right) The position of the feet after the pivot.

Carry objects close to body but without contaminating uniform.

Carrying objects close to body helps place line of gravity within base of support. Stretching arms outward while carrying object strains arm muscles.

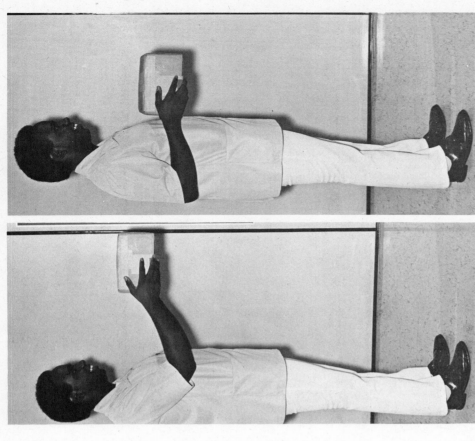

Fig. 5-7 (Left) The nurse strains his arms as he carries the package. He does not have the line of gravity well within his base of support which results in poor balance. (Right) By bringing the line of gravity closer to his base of support, he improves his balance and reduces strain on his arm muscles.

Chart 5-1 continued

Suggested Action

Keep work area at comfortable height.

Use longest and strongest muscles of body whenever possible.

Use sturdy stepping stool when obtaining articles out of easy reach.

Move muscles smoothly and evenly while working.

Reason for Action

Body alignment and balance are easier to maintain when work area is at comfortable height. When work area is too high, arm muscles are strained by stretching. When work area is too low, back muscles are strained when bending over work.

These muscles are less likely to become strained and injured than smaller muscles.

Stretching causes strain on muscles. As center of gravity is raised while in stretching position, body is placed in poor balance.

Jerky movements produce more strain on muscles and are uncomfortable for nurse and patient.

Figure to Illustrate

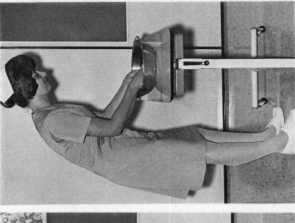
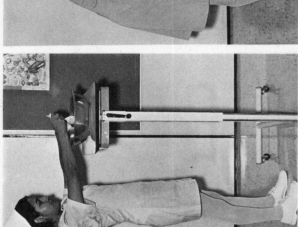
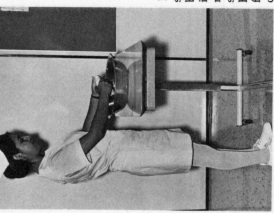

Fig. 5-8 (Upper left) The nurse stretches her arms and throws her back out of alignment by reaching to the work area. (Upper right) Bending over the work area strains back muscles. (Bottom) Having the work area at a comfortable height prevents the strain of bending or stretching.

Lean toward objects being pushed and away from objects being pulled. Use muscles of legs as much as possible.

Body weight adds force to muscle action. Using long and strong muscles of legs relieves strain on arms and back.

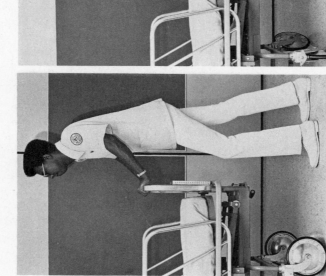

Fig. 5-9 The nurse leans toward the object he pushes (left) and away from the object he pulls (right). His body weight assists muscles to move the object.

muscles in the arms, legs, and hips whenever possible. Small and less strong muscles will strain and injure quickly if forced to work beyond their ability. One of the most common injuries affects the muscles in the lower part of the back. It is a painful injury and usually slow to heal. But it is preventable when proper body mechanics is used.

To protect the muscles of the abdomen and pelvis, use your internal girdle and make a long midriff. This use of muscles prevents strain and injury to the abdominal wall.

Whenever possible, push, pull, or roll objects rather than lift them. The muscles are working the most when you lift an object since you are working to overcome gravity. Use the weight of your body to assist when you push or pull an object. This too reduces the strain you place on muscles.

Muscles function best when they are rested between periods of exertion. For example, you are using your muscles to their best advantage by resting occasionally when working or exercising strenuously.

The body at work

From the discussion in this chapter, some general guides for good use of the musculoskeletal system of the body can be identified. These guides are summarized and illustrated in Chart 5-1 on pages 62 through 67. The guides given in Chart 5-1 are not limited for use by the nurse only when she gives nursing care. Rather, the nurse will find them helpful in all of her activities of daily living.

Conclusion

In every nursing care activity, the nurse uses her body. When she does so efficiently, she is less likely to injure herself, cause unnecessary strain and work for muscles, and become tired.

There will be reminders from time to time in this text concerning good body mechanics while giving nursing care. However, you are encouraged to become familiar with content in this chapter before starting to give care. You are further encouraged to practice good body mechanics while carrying out your daily activities of living. Keep Chart 5-1 handy until the proper use of the body becomes a natural part of all of your activities.

References

Carbary, Lorraine Judson, "Low Back Pain," *Nursing Care*, 7:12–15, August 1974.

Foss, Georgia, "Use Your Head & Your Back . . . Body Mechanics," *Nursing '73*, 3:25–32, May 1973.

"Medical Highlights: Head Over Heels . . . ," *American Journal of Nursing*, 75:1035, June 1975.

Merton, P. A., "How We Control the Contraction of Our Muscles," *Scientific American*, 226:30–37, May 1972.

Millen, Helen M., "Physically Fit for Nursing," *American Journal of Nursing,* 70:520–523, March 1970.

"Stop Think-Then Lift," *Nursing Mirror,* 134:9–11, June 23, 1972.

Winters, Margaret Campbell, *Protective Body Mechanics in Daily Living: A Manual for Nurses and Their Co-workers,* W. B. Saunders Company, Philadelphia, 1952, 150 p.

Works, Roberta F., "Hints on Lifting and Pulling," *American Journal of Nursing,* 72:260–261, February 1972.

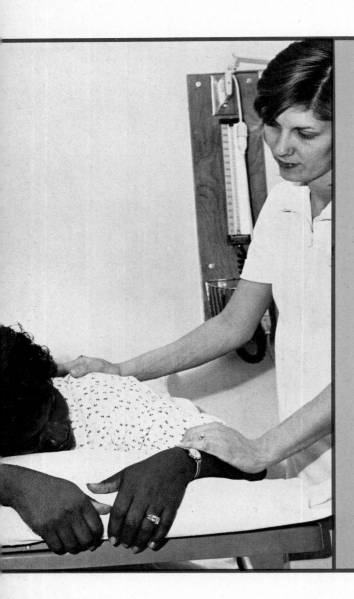

6 the patient's environment

behavioral objectives

When mastery of content in this chapter is reached, the student will be able to

Define terms appearing in the glossary.

Give an example from everyday living which illustrates how a person shows he prizes the space he has.

Describe a personal item the nurse would want to keep with her if hospitalized; describe how she might feel if it were lost or damaged.

Describe a comfortable, attractive, and practical room for a patient in terms of furniture, decor, temperature, humidity, ventilation, and privacy.

List common equipment in a patient's room, such as an adjustable bed, bed siderails, and a signal device, and describe how each operates.

List five or six ways in which noise can be controlled in the patient's environment; in which odors can be controlled.

Describe a safe patient unit, using the section on providing for safety in this chapter as a guide.

List ten examples of accidents that commonly occur in the patient's environment.

Describe times when bed siderails and/or protective restraints are necessary; describe advantages and disadvantages of protective restraints.

Explain the steps to take when an accident occurs.

List five ways in which the nurse can conserve time and energy while making an unoccupied bed.

glossary

Accident Report A written report that describes an accident or error in the patient's care. Synonym for incident report.

Asphyxiation Suffocation caused by lack of oxygen in the blood.

Environment All that surrounds us and influences life and development.

Humidity The amount of moisture in the air.

Incident Report A written report that describes an accident or error in the patient's care. Synonym for accident report.

Relative Humidity The ratio between the amount of moisture in the air and the greatest amount the air could contain at the same temperature.

Ventilation Movement of air.

introduction

The word **environment** means our surroundings and includes anything that influences our life and development. When our environment is safe, comfortable, and attractive, we can more readily enjoy well-being. Therefore, nurses are interested in helping to provide the best possible environment for their patients.

The patient's room is that area in which the nurse carries out most personal patient care. It may be in a hospital, in the home, in a clinic—wherever the patient receives care. The word unit is usually used to describe an area in a hospital where patients with similar illnesses are housed.

Many things in a patient's room or in a hospital unit cannot be changed by the nurse. She usually is not able to do much about the color of paint on the walls, the size of a room or window, or the design of draperies. However, she can sometimes do things that help to make a room more comfortable, safe, and pleasant for the patient without major alterations.

The need for space

All of us need space in our environment. This need varies among individuals, some requiring much more for their comfort than others. For instance, the city dweller may be lost in the open space of a farm, while, on the other hand, a country dweller may feel uncomfortable in a studio apartment.

It has been observed that people will fight for the space they have, and usually the less space they have, the more they will fight for it. We zealously claim and guard the space we have in a checkout line at the supermarket, for example.

The nurse should take the patient's need for space into account and demonstrate respect for the space he calls his own. For example, the patient will often express the feeling of owning his room and even call it his home. He will guard and prize personal items, such as a religious article, cards and letters, a family picture, a piece of handicraft, or in the case of a child, his favorite toy. The nurse shows respect for the patient's feelings by recognizing his need for space and by seeing to it that personal items are not lost or damaged. A beatup, tattered book which may seem of little value to the nurse may be the patient's prized possession.

The room

Walls and Floor. It is no longer necessary for health agencies to appear bare and sterile-looking. White walls and equipment are being replaced by more colorful furnishings and tastefully decorated floors and walls. However, there is still need for careful planning in the use of color and design. Most patients prefer decor that is modest and inconspicuous. Many patients have been disturbed by wall coverings with large and distinct designs because they have seen faces and other objects in them. Pictures, bedspreads, and draperies may have the same effect if not selected carefully. Some patients feel dizzy when they look at floor or wall coverings with small designs, parallel lines, or tiny squares. Bright and stimulating colors are often annoying. Nurses who help set up a patient's room in the home will wish to consider how best to assist the family in preparing the room for the patient's comfort while still keeping the decorating pleasant.

Lighting. Good lighting, natural and artificial, is important to patients and health workers alike. Light bulbs, shades, and lamps usually are easily adjusted so that good lighting is generally available. Many health agencies are now being built with large windows that can be shaded as needed. In addition to providing much more natural light, they make it pleasant for patients to enjoy looking out of doors. Also, most persons find bright rooms cheerful.

Looking into a light, glare from artificial lights, and reflected light from linens can be uncomfortable for patients and workers. In particular, older persons and those wearing glasses are bothered by glaring lights. Often, moving furniture a bit and adjusting shades on lights will help decrease glare.

While light that brightens the entire room may be best for health workers, it may still not be satisfactory for the patient when he wishes to read. A lamp at his bedside which is adjustable for brightness of light and for maintaining different angles is best. Most health agencies now provide such lamps in the patient's room.

Most persons prefer that a room be darkened when they rest and sleep. This can usually be accomplished with ease by adjusting shades and draperies and by turning off artificial lights.

At night, a dim light is valuable as a comfort and safety measure. It should be placed so that it does not shine in the patient's eyes but so that the floor around the bed is illuminated. Elderly patients in particular appreciate some light in the room at night so that they can orient themselves with greater ease should they waken and become confused.

Humidity, Temperature, and Ventilation. Humidity refers to the amount of moisture in the air. **Relative humidity** is the ratio between the amount of moisture in the air and the greatest amount the air could contain at the same temperature. Most people are comfortable in a temperature range of 68 to 74°F. and a relative humidity of 30 to 60 per cent. Illness may influence the patient's comfort, and he may feel too warm or too cold even when the temperature and humidity are within average normal ranges. Older persons generally prefer a warmer room and usually are more sensitive to drafts than younger people.

Most health agencies and many homes have air-conditioning units that regulate temperature and humidity. In climates or buildings where humidity is very low, humidifiers or steam from boiling water may be used. When humidity is unusually high, a dehumidifier is helpful.

Ventilation refers to the movement of air. A room with fresh air is comfortable, while a room with stale air is almost always uncomfortable. Air-conditioning units help to keep the air fresh and clean. Windows may be used for ventilation when weather permits. An electric fan is also helpful in ventilating a room. Attention to the patient's covering is important when ventilation creates drafts, and an extra blanket or a shawl may be necessary for comfort.

The furniture

Furniture used in health agencies is often as attractive as any used at home. It is generally designed according to the type of care the patient needs. For example, in units where patients are largely responsible for their own personal care, low beds, desks, comfortable chairs, and reading lamps are available. Also, dining areas and cafeterias are often provided for patients who can be up and about.

The Bed. For the convenience of health practitioners, health agencies generally use beds that are considerably higher than those used at home. Most health agencies now have adjustable beds on which the head and the foot can be raised and lowered as necessary. The height of the bed can be lowered (for those times when the patient is getting in and out of bed) and raised (for those times when care is being given). Adjustable beds may be operated electrically or mechanically. If the bed is not adjustable and is a high hospital bed, a stepstool should be provided so that the patient can get in and out of bed with greater ease and with less danger of falling. For patients at home who must remain in bed for long periods of time, the family may wish to consider renting a hospital bed. Or, one may be borrowed, for example, from the local Red Cross chapter. Also, the bed can be raised on solid blocks of wood for the convenience of those caring for the patient.

Beds designed for particular patient needs are discussed in Chapter 12.

Mattresses. A good mattress adjusts to the shape of the body to the degree that it permits the body to be in good position. A mattress that is too soft allows the body to sag and the patient may become tired and suffer backaches. Springs in mattresses should be of good structure and quality so that they keep their resiliency. Broken springs are uncomfortable. Figure 6-1 illustrates the effects of a good and poor mattress and springs on the patient's alignment.

The covering of the mattress should be of good quality so that it will not tear or separate easily. It is not general practice to sterilize mattresses between patient uses. Rather, they are generally vacuumed thoroughly. Since mattresses have some filling, such as horsehair, cotton, or kapok, which is difficult to clean, they are usually protected with coverings. These covers may be cotton-quilted pads that are washed after use. Or, because of laundry problems with washable covers, various kinds of plastic covers may be used. Plasticized covers have the disadvantage of being slippery which causes bed linens to slide about easily. They also impede air circulation and may cause patients to perspire excessively.

The patient's environment

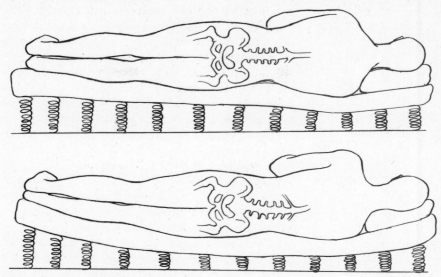

Fig. 6-1   Illustration of the effects of a good and a poor mattress and spring on body alignment.

Many health agencies now use mattresses with a special waterproof coating. These mattresses can be washed after each patient use. A rubber or plastic drawsheet is unnecessary although mattress pads are still used.

Pillows. Pillows, like mattresses, may be filled with any one of several materials and will vary in the comfort they give. Foam rubber pillows are often used by persons who are allergic to kapok, feathers, and other commonly used materials. They are not easily molded, and, therefore, are often difficult to arrange in the most comfortable position for the patient. Also, they tend to absorb and retain heat, causing the patient to perspire.

Most persons use pillows under the head for comfort. Nurses also find pillows helpful in aiding the patient to maintain a comfortable position in bed. This will be discussed further in Chapter 12.

As was true of mattresses, pillows are generally not sterilized between patient uses. Therefore, it is general practice to protect them in some way. Certain pillows are made from material that is resistant to dirt and moisture which is a great help in keeping them clean. Others require a separate cover to protect them. Plastic covers are commonly used. Their disadvantages include being slippery and hot.

Overbed Table. Overbed tables are convenient for patients for eating, reading, writing, or working. They can also be used to support the patient in a forward-leaning position while he rests the upper part of his body on the table, as illustrated in Figure 6-2. Health practitioners also find overbed tables convenient when carrying out certain care.

The type of table which is supported by a wide footpiece that fits under the bed and has only one post is convenient when bed siderails are in place or when cumbersome equipment is being used at the bedside. Most overbed tables are designed so that they can be lowered for the patient while he is in a chair. There is often a portion of the table that can

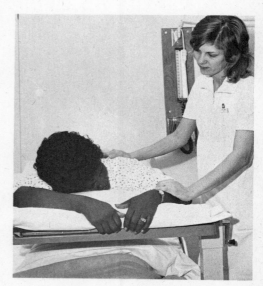

Fig. 6-2   This patient is made comfortable by being supported on her overbed table in a forward-leaning position. The position is often a welcomed one after long periods of being flat in bed.

The furniture

be tilted and will support a book or newspaper. Some have mirrors on the back of the tilt portion which are convenient for the patient to use when combing hair, shaving, or applying makeup.

A bedside stand is used for storing the patient's personal care items. While stands may vary among health agencies, certain features are handy for both patients and health personnel. The patient can handle the stand with greater ease when it is mounted on wheels. A drawer in the table usually is used for the patient's personal possessions. The inside of the stand is used for the storage of such items as a wash basin, oral hygiene equipment, soap dish, bedpan, urinal, bath blanket, and so on. Most stands have a rod on the outside for hanging the patient's towels and washcloth which allows them to dry between uses.

Some bedside stands have a paper bag frame and a "catch-all" which a patient may use for such items as occupational therapy work, handicraft projects, newspapers, and so on.

Chairs. A straight chair with good arm and back support is comfortable for most patients. For very short patients, a footstool, or other suitable object, can be placed under their feet. Having chairs available without arms is desirable. For instance, they are more suitable when patients must be lifted out of bed and into chairs since there are no arms to get in the way of those who are lifting.

Upholstered chairs are often very comfortable but are not practical for patients who find it difficult to raise themselves out of them. Elderly patients and those with limited movement, for example, usually find upholstered chairs difficult to use.

Personal care items

The following items are basic for personal care: water container and drinking glass, wash basin, soap dish, mouthwash cup, emesis basin, bedpan, and a urinal for the male patient.

Manufacturers provide a wide selection of equipment for personal care that is both attractive and safe to use. Plastic items are in common use. Glass items are dangerous because they may break. Monel is noisy when handled, and enamel chips readily and, therefore, is hard to keep clean. Disposable equipment is becoming more common and its use has greatly reduced the work of cleaning and sterilizing. Some health agencies send plastic items home with patients. When reusable items are used, they are cleaned and sterilized as described in Chapter 4.

Few agencies supply patients with personal items such as combs, brushes, shaving cream, razors, and toothpaste. Patients generally bring these items with them. In some agencies, kits containing these items are available from an agency drug store, a central supply unit, or a service shop.

Diversional items

Most health agencies have radios, television sets, and telephones for patient use. While these items offer patients much diversion and comfort, the nurse will wish to remember the hazards they can cause. Wiring

The patient's environment

on the floor, loose plugs, frayed cords, and television stands in doorways are some of the dangers they can present. Also, some patients are disturbed by the noise of radios and television. The nurse will wish to be alert to help prevent accidents and noise when the patient's room includes these common diversional items.

Privacy

Anyone who is being interviewed, examined, or cared for deserves and appreciates the comfort of privacy, even though many patients do not complain when privacy is not extended. It is very easy for nurses and other health practitioners to feel that anything routine for them is also accepted casually by patients. Therefore, the nurse will want to remain alert in preventing unnecessary exposure. For example, cubicle drapes should be used when the nurse is caring for patients who are not in private rooms; doors should be kept closed during care when patients are in private rooms; patients should be draped carefully when the nurse is giving care; whenever it is safe, the patient should be left when he is using the bedpan or urinal; and the nurse should knock when entering a closed door.

Patients also enjoy privacy when they have visitors. Every attempt should be made to avoid giving care in the presence of visitors. If care is necessary, the situation should be explained and visitors shown where they may wait comfortably until care is finished. It is a thoughtful gesture to notify visitors when care has been completed.

There was discussion in Chapter 2 concerning legal problems that can develop when patients are exposed unnecessarily. Review that section concerning the nurse's responsibilities when invasion of privacy could result from her actions.

The control of noise and odors

Many patients complain of noises that often seem to be a part of every health agency. Much money and effort have gone into the design of buildings and the use of carpeting, draperies, and accoustical ceilings to help reduce noise. The posting of signs has helped to remind visitors and health practitioners to refrain from making unnecessary noise.

These are some of the noises that patients complain about most frequently and that the nurse will wish to help keep at a minimum: careless handling of equipment and machinery in service areas; careless handling of dishes and trays; loud talking on the telephone; calling down corridors; laughing and talking in corridors and lounges; loud radios and television; dropping equipment; and noisy call systems. The nurse will wish to remember that sick persons generally are more sensitive to noise than well persons, especially to noises to which they are not accustomed.

Patients often hear much more than health practitioners think they do! Therefore, it is wise to keep conversation levels low and to avoid calling down corridors. Unfortunately, patients often misinterpret what they overhear and may become unnecessarily worried and concerned.

Illness tends to alter the sense of smell and hence, mild odors and odors that are usually pleasant may become disagreeable. For example, the smell of good cooking is pleasant for a well person but may nauseate an ill person. There are various air deodorants on the market, but in general, they seem to do little more than substitute one odor for another. However, they are frequently the only help when odors are hard to control and ventilation is insufficient.

Nurses can take the following measures to help cut down on odors in the patient's room: discard waste and refuse promptly; remove old flowers and stagnant water; empty bedpans, urinals, and emesis basins promptly and clean them carefully; change soiled linen promptly; and remove leftover food from rooms.

Most patients do not find it comfortable to have nurses giving care who are in need of a deodorant, whose perfume is strong, or who have been smoking recently.

Helping to make the environment safe

While nurses work to make the patient's environment as comfortable and attractive as possible, they also do whatever they can to see to it that the environment is **safe.** The following discussion includes practices that the nurse will wish to observe in order that the patient can enjoy a safe environment.

Making It Possible for the Patient to Call for Assistance. Health agencies use a signal system so that patients can call for assistance. A device, usually with a push button, is placed on the bed near the patient. It may be attached to the bed linen with a clasp. When the patient pushes the button, a light or bell signals for the nurse. Some devices have an attachment that when activated, sounds a loud buzzer, indicating that an emergency exists and help is needed immediately. Some health agencies use intercom systems that are used to communicate with the nurse. Signal devices are usually also placed in bathrooms, lounge areas, and other places where patients gather.

It is very important to make certain that a signal device is convenient for the patient's use and that it is in working order. Health practitioners are guilty of negligence when accidents occur because a patient could not reach his signal device or did not know how to use it.

In the home, a bell placed at the patient's bedside can be used. Patients who must be left alone for any reason should have a telephone within easy reach so that they can call for help if necessary.

Being Able to Identify Patients Accurately. One type of identification bracelet is illustrated in Chapter 7. It is important to check the patient's identification bracelet before giving nursing care so that treatments and drugs are not given to the wrong patient. Having the patient identify himself is not considered sufficient for safety purposes. It is important to be extremely cautious when caring for patients in clinics and also in the home where identification bracelets are not usually used. Legal problems can be very serious when health practitioners confuse one patient for another.

Helping to Prevent Falls. Falls are among the most frequent causes of injuries for people of all ages. Often they result from thoughtlessness. "I was in a hurry and just didn't think," is a common comment.

Bed siderails help to prevent patients from falling out of bed. Many health agencies have policies that state siderails must be up at all times for certain patients except when care is being given. Examples include elderly or unconscious patients, babies and young children, and restless or confused patients. Patients will sometimes complain of siderails and ask that they be removed. In such instances, often an explanation of why they are there will satisfy the patient. If the patient continues to refuse to have siderails raised on his bed, many health agencies require that he sign a release form which frees the hospital and health practitioners of responsibility should an accident occur. Figure 6-3 illustrates such a release form.

Sometimes, visitors ask to have siderails down and say they will watch the patient. The nurse must remember that she, not the visitor, is responsible for the patient's safety. Therefore, she must use extreme caution before leaving siderails down, and consult with her supervising nurse when the slightest doubt exists.

At times, patients are so restless that they must be restrained in bed

RELEASE OF SIDE RAILS

Having been informed by _Pine Memorial Hospital_ that protective side rails should be placed on my bed and raised for my personal protection, I hereby instruct the hospital and its employees not to place or raise protective side rails on my bed and hereby assume all risks in connection therewith and fully release the said hospital, its employees and my physician from any and all liability for any injury or damage to me by reason of its failure to place or raise protective side rails on my bed.

Signature _Helen Jones_

Room No. _420_

Witness _Nancy Smith, L.P.N._

Witness _Helen Wixon, R.N._

Date _July 17, 1974_ Hour _2_ P. M.

RELEASE OF SIDE RAILS

Fig. 6-3 An example of a form used to release the hospital and its employees of responsibility when the patient refuses to have siderails raised on the bed.

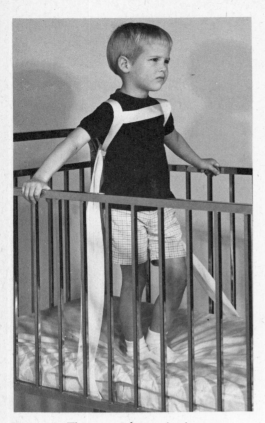

Fig. 6-4 This type of restraint is commonly used for youngsters to prevent them from falling from a crib. The straps are crisscrossed in back and then secured to the side of the crib. (Photograph courtesy of the Posey Company)

for their own protection. For example, they may be able to crawl over siderails and fall, or they may remove dressings or tubes used in their treatment. Protective restraints in such cases serve a good purpose. However, they must be used with good judgment and placed on the patient so that they will not bruise the skin, cut off circulation, or permit the patient to become tangled in them. Chapter 2 pointed out that a patient can sue claiming false imprisonment when, in his opinion, protective restraints were used unwisely. Therefore, it is best to consult with your supervising nurse if there can be any doubts about using them. Figures 6-4 through 6-7 illustrate various types of restraints.

Some miscellaneous precautions that will help prevent falls are as follows:

- Use tub and shower stools and sturdy handrails in bathrooms. Figure 6-8 illustrates a piece of equipment attached to the side of a bathtub that helps the patient in and out of the tub.
- Use nonskid mats in tubs and showers.
- Use sturdy stepstools when you need items out of easy reach.
- Use equipment and supplies for their intended purpose. Chairs are dangerous stepstools!
- Place adjustable beds in the low position when patients are getting in

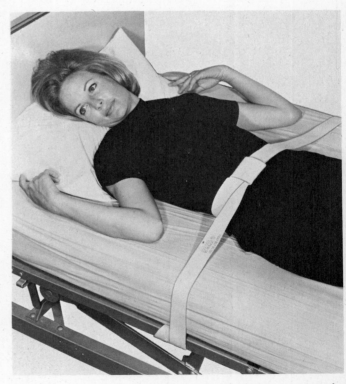

Fig. 6-5 This type of restrain prevents the patient from falling from a bed while still allowing her to turn from side to side and to sit up in bed. (Photograph courtesy of the Posey Company)

　　　　　　　　　　The patient's environment

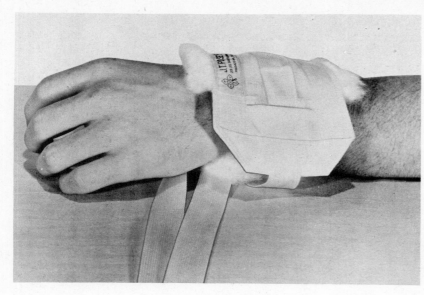

Fig. 6-6 This restraint may be used for the ankle or wrist. It is padded to prevent irritating the patient's skin. (Photograph courtesy of the Posey Company)

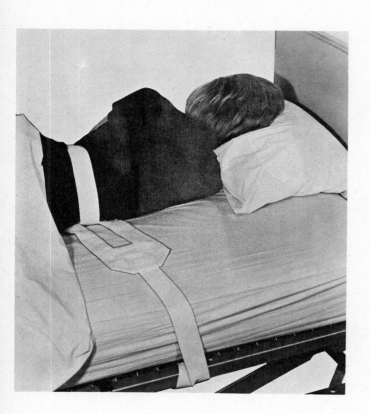

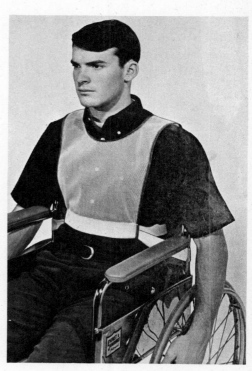

Fig. 6-7 A restraining vest prevents the patient from leaving the wheelchair and helps support him in place. The waist belt on the restraint illustrated is adjustable. (Photograph courtesy of the Posey Company)

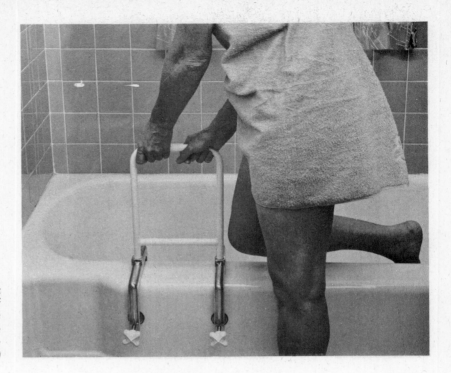

Fig. 6-8 This aid helps the patient get in and out of the bathtub. Supports of this type are also convenient in the home, and are available in many medical-surgical supply stores. (Bollen Products Company, East Cleveland, Ohio)

and out of bed. Have a patient use a sturdy stepstool when the bed is high and not adjustable.

- Mop up spilled liquids promptly. Post signs and warn patients and visitors when floors are wet after scrubbing them. Wet floors are slippery!
- See that patients wear good shoes with low heels for walking. Floppy, high-heeled, soft, and loose-fitting shoes often cause falls.
- Keep the floor and stairways free of litter, such as books, magazines, toys, handicraft items, clothing, shoes, and so on.
- Do not use rugs that are torn, curled, or slippery.
- Stay with patients who are unsteady when they walk and give them firm support. Assisting patients to walk is discussed further in Chapter 12.
- Have patients in wheelchairs use wide doorways, ramps, and elevators so that they are not tempted to try to walk stairways.

Helping to Prevent Electrical Shocks. Health agencies as well as homes contain much electrical equipment and so the danger of accidents from electrical shock is ever-present. One important way to prevent accidents is to keep all electrical equipment in good working order and in good repair. Another important measure is to use equipment for its intended purpose. A hot plate, for example, is a poor way to warm a chilly room.

The following are additional measures that will help to prevent accidents caused by electrical shocks:

- Do not use frayed or broken electrical cords.
- Remove plugs from wall sockets by grasping the plug. Pulling on the cord to remove the plug may damage both the plug and the wire.

The patient's environment

- Do not kink cords. The fine electrical wires inside the cord may break.
- Do not overload a wall outlet.
- Do not use an appliance that overheats, produces a shock, or gives off an odor while being used.
- Use plugs and outlets with a ground when possible. These plugs have three prongs and will fit only into outlets with three-prong receivers.
- Water conducts electricity well. Do not stand in water or on a wet floor or wear wet shoes and then handle electrical equipment. Keep AC-DC radios away from bathtubs and sinks.
- Test electrical equipment before use. Never use faulty pieces of equipment.

Helping to Prevent Poisoning. There are many housekeeping supplies that are poisonous. Therefore, they should be put away immediately after use and stored someplace where children and confused patients cannot get at them. Anything that is poisonous should be conspicuously labeled. Be sure you know where emergency instructions on how to handle poisoning are posted in the health agency where you study or work. Having such instructions handy in the home is also important.

Chapter 17 will discuss methods used to help prevent accidents with drugs in homes and health agencies.

Helping to Prevent Fires. Despite fire regulations and the use of much fire-retardant material, fires still occur. Most health agencies have regular fire drills so that all health practitioners, students included, know exactly what to do in case of fire.

Here are some steps that can be taken to prevent fires:

- Be sure smoking regulations are enforced. When patients and visitors are allowed to smoke, provide safe ashtrays, preferably ones from which a burning cigarette cannot fall. Many fires have started when wastebaskets were used for ashtrays.
- It is best that the confused, sleepy, or drugged patient does not smoke. When he does, remain with him and take care of the cigarette for him when he has finished smoking.
- Oxygen supports combustion. The smallest flame or a live cigarette can become a torch in the presence of concentrated oxygen. When a patient is receiving oxygen as part of his treatment, be sure the patient, his visitors, and his roommates know of the fire dangers. Post signs to show that oxygen is in use and that smoking is prohibited.
- Know where there are emergency exits. Know where fire extinguishers are kept and how to use them.
- Do not store materials saturated with solutions that could lead to spontaneous combustion unless they are in an airtight metal container. Certain cleaning solutions are among offenders in this regard.

Helping to Prevent Scalds and Burns. Hot-water bottles and heating pads are common sources of burns. The use of heat in the care of patients and measures to prevent burns are discussed in Chapter 18.

A good safety measure is to check the temperature of water being used by patients in tubs and showers. This is especially important if there is any doubt whatsoever about whether the patient can safely regulate or test the temperature of the water.

Place hot liquids, such as coffee and tea, in a place that is convenient for the patient. The nurse will wish to help the patient if he is unable to handle liquids safely on his own.

Helping to Prevent Asphyxiation and Drowning. Asphyxiation means suffocation because of lack of oxygen. It may occur, for example, when people choke on food or liquids. When feeding patients, offer small bite sizes of food and give the patient sufficient time between mouthfuls to chew it well.

A problem among children is choking on small items, such as marbles, small balls, and so on, or on broken pieces from toys. Any small item should be kept out of a child's reach.

To prevent accidents in water, remain with the patient while he is in the tub if there is any possible danger of drowning. Never leave a child alone in a bathtub!

Helping to Prevent the Spread of Infections. Chapters 4, 15, and 22 discuss ways to prevent the spread of microorganisms. Observing practices presented in those chapters will mean a safer environment for patients.

Helping to Prevent Accidents Through Safety Education. Chapter 1 pointed out that nurses are teachers. The alert nurse will find many times when she can teach her patients how to prevent accidents and she will wish to take advantage of such opportunities. Remember, the nurse also teaches through her own actions. When the care she gives shows that she is concerned and interested in safety measures, her patients will learn from her. Also, the patient is often very quick to realize when a nurse is not observing safety measures and will soon lose confidence in her.

When accidents occur

Despite efforts to prevent accidents, unfortunately, they still occur. The first step to take is to call for help. If the patient falls, he is made as comfortable as possible and moved only after it is considered safe to do so. If a bone has been broken, moving the patient without proper support may cause further injury to the bone and surrounding tissues. Try to comfort and reassure the patient by explaining that help is available and on the way.

The well-prepared nurse is ready to give first aid when accidents occur. Since first aid care is discussed in other nursing courses, no discussion will be included in this text.

After the patient is properly cared for, an **incident** or **accident report** is prepared which becomes a part of his record. All information related to the accident is entered on a form and it is signed by those persons completing the form. The same form is used when there is an error in the patient's care. Figure 6-9 illustrates an incident report; record keeping is described in Chapter 7.

Making the unoccupied bed

The nurse who is preparing a room to receive the patient will want to have a bed ready for his use. Hospital procedure will state the type of

The patient's environment

Confidential Information

INCIDENT REPORT

(Patient or Visitor)   Not a Part of Patient's Permanent Chart

1. Date of Admission July 25, 1974

2. Diagnosis C V A

3. Date of Incident July 27, 1974 Time 8⁴⁵ p.m.

Room No., Name, Age, Sex, Hospital Number, Attending Physician

4. Were Bed Rails up? YES (YES OR NO)

5. Hi Lo Bed Position DOWN (UP OR DOWN)

6. Was Safety Belt or Restraints in use? No

DESIGNATE SPECIFICALLY

7. Activity (Complete Bed Rest, Bathroom Privileges, Etc.) BRP c̄ HELP

8. Sedatives NONE Dose Time M

9. Narcotics NONE Dose Time M

10. Tranquilizers VALIUM Dose 5mg 'o' Time 4⁰⁰ p.m. M

{ Given within 12 hours previous to incident

11. Nurse's Account of Incident (State incident, where discovered, condition of patient, etc.)

I HEARD A NOISE AND ENTERED ROOM TO CHECK. I DISCOVERED MRS. BROWN SITTING ON THE FLOOR NEXT TO THE BED. SHE WAS ALERT. HER SKIN WAS WARM AND DRY, PULSE 78. I NOTED A SMALL LACERATION ON HER LEFT SHOULDER. MRS. BROWN WAS ABLE TO STAND WITH HELP AND MISS SMITH AND I HELPED HER SIT ON THE ROLL-A-MODE.

12. History of Incident as related by Patient "I HAD TO GO TO THE BATHROOM AND THOUGHT I COULD MAKE IT BY MYSELF, BUT MY LEFT SIDE IS WEAK AND GAVE OUT ON ME. I SLID TO THE FLOOR. AS I SAT DOWN, I BUMPED MY SHOULDER ON THE BED."

13. List Witnesses or Persons Familiar with Details of Incident (Include roommate's name and hospital number.)

Name Jane Doe, L.P.N. Address 256 EAST MAIN

Name Mary Smith Address 9841 NORTH OAK ST.

Name Nancy Jones Address 3692 NORTH MAPLE AVE.

14. Time Doctor was called AM 8⁵⁰ PM

15. Time Doctor Responded AM 8⁵⁵ PM

16. Time Supervisor called AM 8⁵⁰ PM

17. Date of Report July 27, 1974

18. Jane Doe L.P.N.
SIGNATURE OF PERSON REPORTING

19. Rebecca Black, R.N.
SIGNATURE OF DEPARTMENT SUPERVISOR

20. Helen Green, R.N.
SIGNATURE OF DEPARTMENT HEAD

Complete **IMMEDIATELY** for **EVERY** incident and send to Administrator via Department Head.

Fig. 6-9 An example of an incident or accident report form. The reverse side (not shown) provides for the physician's statement about the accident or error.

linen to use and how certain items, such as the mattress and pillows, are to be protected.

Procedures for making an unoccupied bed will vary among health agencies. For example, some agencies require that linens be secured on the mattress with square corners while others require mitered corners. The description in Chart 6-1 will serve as a guide, even though details may vary from place to place.

Conclusion

The nurse will wish to do whatever she can in order to insure the patient a safe, comfortable, and attractive environment. Thoughtfulness and ingenuity will help to provide the same type of environment in home

Chart 6-1 Making an unoccupied open or closed bed

The purpose is to prepare a comfortable and clean bed with economy of the nurse's time and energy

Suggested Action	Reason for Action	Figure to Illustrate
Bring necessary linens to bedside.	Having linens on hand saves nursing time by unnecessary trips to linen storage area.	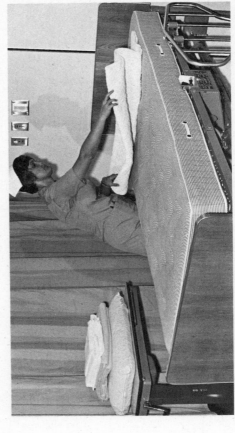 Fig. 6-10 The mattress pad is placed on the bed in the position in which it will be unfolded. Note that the nurse has linens on hand and has placed them in the order of their use. She faces her working area.
Place linens on chair or bedside stand in same order in which they will be placed on bed, as illustrated in Figure 6-10.	Having linens in order in which they will be used saves nursing time.	
Place adjustable bed in high position, as illustrated in Figure 6-10.	Having bed in high position reduces strain on nurse's back muscles.	
Face in direction of work and move with work rather than twisting body and over-reaching, as illustrated in Figures 6-10 through 6-16.	Facing in direction of work and moving with work prevent straining and twisting muscles.	
Place mattress pad on bed and in position so that as it is unfolded, it will be in proper place. Do same with remaining bottom linens.	Opening linens by shaking them causes movement of air. Air currents can carry dust and microorganisms about room. Holding linens overhead to open them causes strain on nurse's arms.	

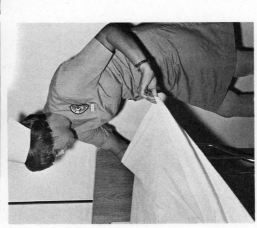
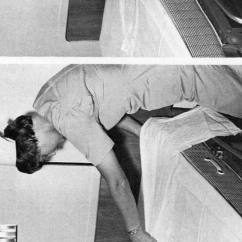
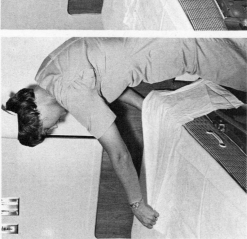

Tuck all bottom linens on one side of bed into place securely, making corners according to agency procedure. Do same on other side of bed, being sure to secure bottom linens tightly.

When tucking linens under mattress, separate feet slightly and flex knees.

Having bottom linens free of wrinkles results in comfortable bed. Making bed on one side and then completing bed on other side save nursing time.

Longest and strongest muscles in nurse's legs and back are at work in this position.

Fig. 6-11 (Upper left) To make a mitered corner, the nurse folds the sheet back on the bed and holds her right hand to form the corner. (Upper right) She tucks the bottom of the sheet forming the corner under the mattress. (Bottom) She places her hand at the side of the mattress to hold the corner in place, and with her other hand brings the sheet down over the corner. She is then ready to tuck the entire length of the sheet under the mattress.

Chart 6-1 continued

Suggested Action	Reason for Action	Figure to Illustrate
When pulling bottom sheet tightly, hold hands with palms downward so that pull is produced by arms and shoulder muscles; spread feet as though to walk backward and rock back so that weight of body helps produce force needed.	Longest and strongest muscles in nurse's arms are at work in this position. Rocking backward uses body's weight as a force and reduces work of nurse's body muscles.	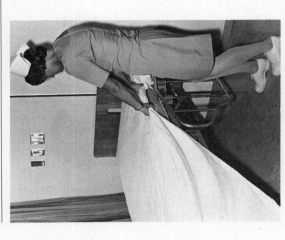
Place top sheet on bed so that as it is unfolded, it will be in proper position.	Opening linens by shaking them causes movement of air. Air currents can carry dust and microorganisms about room. Holding linens overhead to open them causes strain on nurse's arms.	Fig. 6-12 The bottom sheet on the opposite side of the bed is already tucked in securely. Note position of the nurse as she pulls the sheet tightly before tucking it under the mattress: her feet are separated; her knees are flexed; and she grasps the sheet in her hands with palms downward.

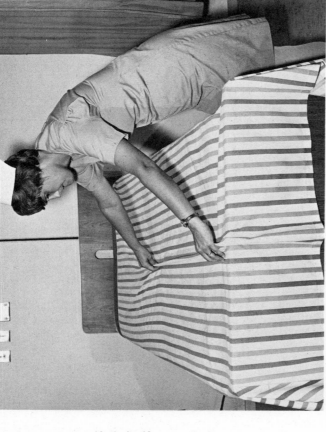

Fig. 6-13 A vertical toe pleat. For a diagonal toe pleat, the nurse would fold the top sheet so that the pleat would lie across the bottom of the bed rather than on the vertical plane.

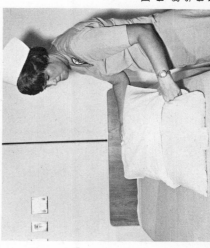

Fig. 6-14 The nurse places protectors and cases on a pillow by gathering them first and then sliding them one at a time over the pillow which rests on the bed.

Make toe pleat by making small diagonal or vertical fold in top sheet near the bottom of the bed. Or, slightly gather linen before tucking under mattress. Place blanket and spread in same manner as top sheet.

Providing room for patient's feet prevents top linens from forcing patient's feet into uncomfortable position.

Tuck top linen securely on one side of bed, making corners according to agency procedure. Complete bed on other side.

Securing bed linens well, but without placing pressure on patient's feet and toes, results in comfortable bed. Making bed completely on one side and then finishing by making bed on other side saves nursing time.

Turn spread down from top and fold it under top edge of blanket.

Protecting blanket with spread prevents blanket from touching and irritating patient's skin.

Place pillows on bed. Open each pillow protector in same manner as when unfolding other linens. Gather pillow protector in same way as one puts on hosiery. Do same for pillow case. Place pillows in place.

Opening linens by shaking them causes movement of air. Air currents can carry dust and microorganisms about room. Covering pillow while resting pillow on bed reduces strain on nurse's arms.

This completes a closed bed.

Chart 6-1 continued

Suggested Action	Reason for Action	Figure to Illustrate
If bed is to be opened to receive a patient, fan-fold or pie-fold top linens.	Having linens opened makes it more convenient for patient to get into bed.	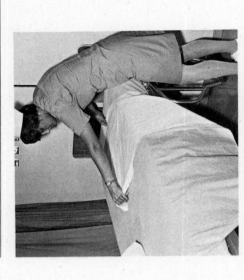 Fig. 6-15 The nurse pie-folds the top linen so that the bed is convenient to receive the patient.
Secure signal device on bed according to agency procedure. Adjust bed to low position.	Having signal device handy for patient makes it possible for him to call for assistance as necessary. Having bed in low position makes it easier and safer for patient to get into bed.	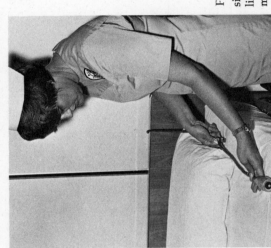 Fig. 6-16 The nurse attaches the signal device to the bottom bed linen so that the device will remain in place and be handy for the patient's use.

situations. Efforts are well worthwhile since such an environment will contribute to the patient's well-being.

References

Allekian, Constance I., "Intrusions of Territory and Personal Space: An Anxiety-Inducing Factor for Hospitalized Persons—An Exploratory Study," *Nursing Research*, 22:236–241, May–June 1973.

Althouse, Harold L., "How OSHA Affects Hospitals and Nursing Homes," *American Journal of Nursing*, 75:450–453, March 1975.

Bartholet, Mary Nigg, "Effects of Color on the Dynamics of Patient Care," *Nursing Outlook*, 16:51–53, October 1968.

Budgett, Anna Belle, "My Unforgettable Nursing Experience: Fire!", *The Journal of Practical Nursing*, 21:27,36, April 1971.

Cogliano, Janet F., "Providing Safety for the Aged: A Complex Issue," *Nursing Care*, 8:29–31, April 1975.

Feyock, Joanne M. Webber, "Doing It Better: A Do-It-Yourself Restraint That Works!" *Nursing '75*, 5:18, January 1975.

Rosenhouse, Leo, "Noise," *Nursing Care*, 7:26–28, November 1974.

Trought, Elizabeth A., "Equipment Hazards," *American Journal of Nursing*, 73:858–862, May 1973.

Walker, Patricia H., "Detecting Electrical Hazards in the Hospital," *Nursing Care-Bedside Nurse*, 6:11–14, March 1973.

Weaver, Peter, "How Safe Is *Your* Home?" *Today's Health*, 52:40–43, October 1974.

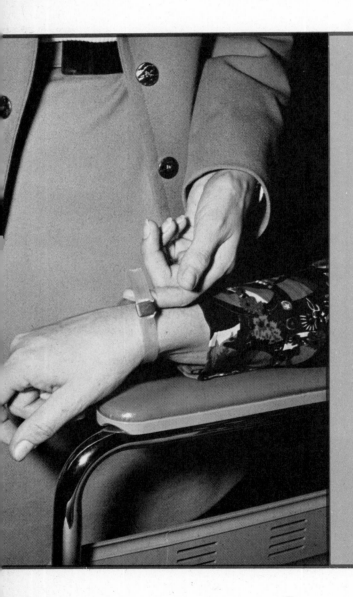

7 admitting, discharging, and transferring the patient; the patient's record and nursing care plan

behavioral objectives

When mastery of content in this chapter is reached, the student will be able to

Define terms appearing in the glossary.

Describe the legal problems that could arise if a patient claims he lost personal items while he was a patient; if he claims he was given care without his consent; if he claims he was uncovered and left exposed while being admitted to the health agency.

Describe how each of the above problems can be avoided.

List four purposes of the patient's record.

List six rules that are followed when writing on the patient's record in the health agency where the nurse gives care.

Demonstrate how an error on the patient's record is handled in the health agency where the nurse gives care.

Describe how clothing and valuables are handled in the health agency where the nurse gives care.

Describe how to collect a urine specimen when the patient can use a bedpan or urinal in the bathroom.

Identify abbreviations commonly used when adding information to the patient's record.

List three purposes of a nursing care plan.

List five ways in which members of the nursing and the health teams exchange information about the patients to whom they are giving care.

List ten forms that are commonly used in a patient's record and state the primary purpose of each.

Explain how transferring a patient is like admitting and discharging a patient.

Explain how a referral helps to provide the patient with continuity of care.

Write a paragraph or two describing how the nurse can help a good nurse-patient relationship to develop and grow as she admits, discharges, and transfers patients.

Discuss briefly how to admit, discharge, and transfer a patient and describe how to record these procedures.

glossary

Chart The sum total of forms that contain information about the patient. Synonym for record.

Nursing Care Plan A guide for nursing care.

Nursing Order A directive that tells what nursing care is to be done.

Record The sum total of forms that contain information about the patient.

Referral The process of sending or guiding someone to another place for help.

Urinalysis The laboratory examination of a urine specimen.

introduction

Each health agency has a procedure and follows certain policies when patients are admitted, discharged, or transferred. Each agency also has its own method of record keeping and uses a variety of forms on which health practitioners enter information concerning the patient. The duties of the nurse for admitting, discharging, and transferring patients and for record keeping will depend on the agency. This chapter will discuss duties that are common, but it is recommended that you refer to the policies and procedures of your health agency for specific details.

Nursing care plans are also discussed in this chapter. They are started when patients are admitted and are used until patients are discharged. As the discussion will indicate, nursing care plans are an important part of each patient's care.

Preparing the patient's room for admission

Chapter 6 discussed the patient's room. When the nurse learns that a patient is arriving, she will wish to check the room and stock it properly when there are missing items, using Chapter 6 and the health agency's procedures as guides. If the patient is known to be in need of any special equipment, for example, equipment necessary for a blood transfusion, it is helpful to have it at the bedside and ready for the patient.

When the bed is made but closed, the nurse will open it for the patient's convenience. She places the bed in its low position or has a footstool at the bedside if the bed is not adjustable. If the patient is to arrive by stretcher, she places the bed in the high position. Moving patients who are helpless is described in Chapter 12. The patient will need a gown; or many agencies permit him to use his own if he so desires.

Admitting the patient and starting his care

Upon admission, the first procedure usually is to place an identification bracelet on the patient. These bracelets generally cannot be removed without breaking the band. It is imprinted with the patient's name and certain other identifying information, such as the agency's identification

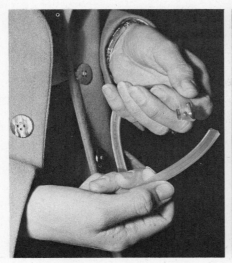 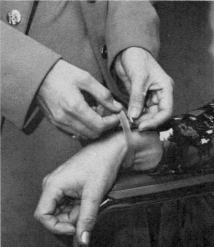 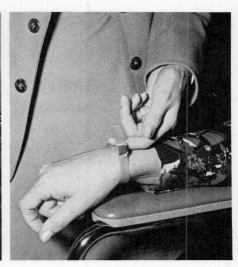

Fig. 7-1 (Left) A type of identification bracelet used in many hospitals. (Center) The clerk in the admission suite applies the bracelet to the patient's wrist. (Right) After the clasp is secured, the bracelet cannot be removed without cutting the band. Checking the patient's bracelet before giving any nursing care is important to assure proper patient identification.

number, the name of the physician caring for the patient, and the patient's room number. Figure 7-1 illustrates one type of identification bracelet being attached to the patient's wrist. It is helpful to have the patient's name on his bed, but this in itself is not considered sufficiently safe for accurate identification.

The identification bracelet is usually applied by someone in the admission suite or from the agency's business office. At the same time, the patient's record is generally started. The patient is then escorted to the unit where he will be housed.

Chart 7-1 describes a suggested method for admitting a patient to a health agency's unit. More specific details will depend largely on the patient's condition and agency policies and procedures. For example, if the patient is not acutely ill, he may be allowed to remain in his street clothes until after his relatives leave.

If the nurse is responsible for handling the patient's clothing and valuables, she must *be sure to observe the agency's policies carefully.* Losing personal items belonging to the patient can have serious legal implications for both the nurse and the health agency. The patient could sue, claiming they were lost or stolen because they were handled carelessly. The nurse will also wish to note any supplies or equipment the patient brings with him, such as medications, a heating pad, glasses, crutches, a wheelchair, and so on. Figure 7-2 illustrates one type of clothing and valuables check list commonly used by many health agencies (see p. 97).

Chapter 3 pointed out that the nurse-patient relationship begins with the first contact the patient has with his nurse. Therefore the nurse will

Chart 7-1 Admitting a patient to a health agency

The purpose is to admit the patient in a manner consistent with the agency's procedures and policies, to welcome the patient, and to start his care

Suggested Action	Reason for Action
Check patient's identification band to be sure of his name. Greet patient and relatives. Introduce yourself to patient and patient to his roommate(s).	Calling patient by name, extending common courtesies, and welcoming patient and relatives often help them to feel at ease and less frightened.
Provide for privacy. Ask relatives to leave unless they will assist with undressing patient.	Providing privacy shows respect and interest in patient as a person. Invading patient's privacy can lead to serious legal problems.
Help patient to undress and assist him into comfortable position in bed.	Assisting patient to undress and into bed conserves his strength, helps prevent accidents, as falling, and prepares patient for receiving care.
Take care of patient's clothing and valuables. Follow agency procedure.	Losing items is upsetting to the patient and can result in serious legal problems.
Explain use of bathroom and of agency equipment, such as call system, adjustable bed, television, telephone, and so on. Explain agency routines, such as meal times, visiting hours, and so on.	Explaining agency routines and how to use equipment helps put patient at ease. Knowing how to use equipment helps prevent accidents.
Place signal device and other equipment so they will be convenient for patient to use.	Being unable to call for help is unsafe and can result in accidents. When equipment is handy for patients, accidents, as falling, are less likely to occur.
Obtain patient's temperature, pulse and respiratory rates, and blood pressure. Obtain urine specimen at time that is convenient during admission procedure.	Obtaining these signs and specimen is an important part of patient's admission physical examination and it is the nurse's responsibility to obtain them.
Indicate to relatives that they may return to patient's bedside.	Relatives have worries and fears too and usually feel better when they know the patient is admitted, settled, and comfortable.
Do necessary recording on patient's record, following agency policy.	The information is an important part of the patient's permanent record and is used to begin the patient's care.

wish to begin to work at developing good relationships at the time the patient is admitted. Until you feel very much at ease when admitting patients, it may be wise to review the content in Chapter 3 regularly.

At the time of admission, the patient's physical examination begins. For example, the nurse will obtain the patient's temperature, pulse and respiratory rates, and blood pressure. Obtaining these signs and recording them are described in Chapter 8.

CLOTHING LIST:
(Please check articles of clothing with patient and describe.)

Dress	*1 - BLUE & WHITE*	Pants	
Slip	*1 - WHITE (½ SLIP)*	Shirt	
Bra	*1 - WHITE*	Undershirt	
Panties	*1 - WHITE*	Undershorts	
Hose		Socks	
Girdle		Tie	
Slippers	*1 - PINK*	Shoes	*1 - WHITE*
Nightgown	*1 - BLUE, 1 - PINK*	Pajamas	
Suit		Robe	
Sweater		Coat	
Slacks		Truss	
Blouse		Backsupport	
Shorts		Belt	
Skirt		Hat	

Other items not listed:

_____

Check valuables below and describe if necessary:

Watch _____   Earrings _____
Medals _____   Rings - Type & Number *1 - YELLOW METAL, PLAIN BAND*

Other Jewelry _____

Dentures - Yes ✓ No _____   Prosthesis - Yes _____ No ✓
Contact Lenses - Yes _____ No ✓   Glasses - Yes ✓ No _____
Removed - Yes _____ No _____   Hearing Aid - Yes _____ No ✓

Wallet ✓ Color *RED* With Pt. ✓ In Safe _____ To Family or Friend _____
Purse ✓ Color *WHITE* With Pt. ✓ In Safe _____ To Family or Friend _____
Cash *$25.00* With Pt. _____ In Safe ✓ To Family or Friend _____
Checks/Check Book _____ With Pt. _____ In Safe _____ To Family or Friend _____

The above list is correct:

Patient's signature *Helen Jones*   Witness *Nancy Smith, L.P.N.*

Clothing taken home by _____

Relationship _____

Witness _____

Received by on Nursing Unit _____

CLOTHING AND VALUABLES LIST

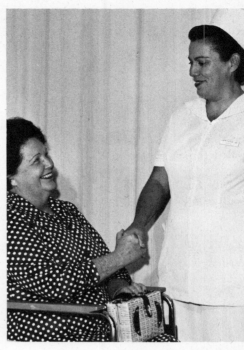

Fig. 7-3 Admitting the patient sincerely and with courtesy helps her to feel welcomed and at ease.

Fig. 7-2 A type of form for listing the patient's clothing and valuables that is commonly used in health agencies. It is completed at the time the patient is admitted to the health agency.

The nurse may also be required to collect a urine specimen. Laboratory study of a urine specimen is called **urinalysis.** If the patient is up and about, he may be allowed to use a bedpan or urinal in the bathroom. He is instructed to discard toilet tissue in the toilet rather than in the bedpan. Tissue in the specimen makes it more difficult to study. The nurse observes the appearance of the urine, places a sample in a container, labels it properly, and sends it to the laboratory for examination, according to agency procedure. Chapter 10 includes a discussion on how to offer and remove a bedpan when the patient is not able to use the bathroom. Chapter 16 will give suggestions on how to describe the appearance of urine. Special procedures, such as obtaining a catheterized specimen, are also discussed in Chapter 16.

Assisting the Patient to Undress. There will be times when the patient is unable to undress without the nurse's help. If he cannot cooperate, it may be necessary to ask another person to assist. Relatives of the patient may be able to help. For instance, they are often especially helpful when admitting a child.

If the patient is weak and tired, have him sit on the edge of the bed which has already been lowered, or assist him to step on a stool to get into bed if the bed is not adjustable. Remove his shoes. Assist him to turn on the bed and help him to the lying position. After fasteners are opened, such as zippers and buttons, slip off his clothing in a manner least disturbing to him. For example, fold or gather a garment in your hands as you work it up the body. Have the patient lift his hips, if he can, to slide clothes up or down. Remove arms from sleeves. Lift the head as you slide the garment over the head. Roll the patient from side to side to remove clothes that fasten up the front or back, after removing arms from sleeves. Gather a stocking as you slide it down the leg and over the foot. After the patient is undressed, put on his gown. To prevent exposing the patient unnecessarily, cover him with a bath blanket, after removing the outer clothing, as you work.

Recording the Procedure. After the nurse has admitted the patient, she is expected to enter certain information on his record. It includes the time of admission, how the patient arrived (wheelchair, stretcher, walking), his temperature, pulse and respiratory rates, and blood pressure, whether a urine specimen was obtained, what equipment and supplies he brought with him, and his general condition. Suggestions that will help to describe the patient's condition are included in Chapter 9.

The patient's record

There is a variety of printed forms that health agencies use for keeping records. These include nurses' notes; physicians' order sheets; graphic sheets for temperature, pulse and respiratory rates, and blood pressure; medication sheets; history and physical examination sheets; progress sheets; laboratory report forms; consultation forms; and consent forms. A few examples are illustrated in Figure 7-4; others have been or will be illustrated elsewhere, as appropriate. Health agencies place forms used for each patient in a folder or binder and all of this material makes up the patient's **record.** In some agencies, the word **chart** is used instead. The process of making entries on the patient's record or chart is called recording or charting.

The patient's record is used for several purposes. It is a way to exchange information among health practitioners. For example, the physician learns about the patient's nursing care when he reads the nurses' notes; the nurse learns about the patient's past health problems from the history sheet, and so on.

Records are used to plan the patient's care. For instance, the physician may plan a change in the patient's medical care when he notes on the graphic sheet that the patient's blood pressure is slowly inching upward each day. Nurses may use a form completed by the physical therapist to plan nursing care that will exercise certain of the patient's muscles.

Records are often used for research purposes. For example, nurses have used patients' records when studying how large numbers of patients responded to a particular kind of nursing care. In the same

NURSES ADMISSION NOTES

DATE TIME	

DATE: MONDAY, JULY 15, 1974   TIME OF ARRIVAL: 3:00 P.M.
ADMITTED TO: 2-A   ROOM NO.: 297   FROM: E.R.   HOW ARRIVED: STRETCHER
ACCOMPANIED BY: MARY BROWN   RELATIONSHIP: SISTER
HEIGHT: 5'2"   WEIGHT: 134#   T. 102⁶ (R) P. 108   R 26   B/P 136/84
PROSTHESIS: NO   DENTURES: YES   ARTIFICIAL EYE: NO   CONTACT LENS: NO
ARTIFICIAL LIMB: NO   GLASSES: YES   HEARING AID: NO
VALUABLES: $25.00 - 1 PLAIN YELLOW METAL RING ENVELOPE NO.: O9683
ADMITTED BY: JANE DOE, L.P.N.

ALLERGIES (List and Describe Reaction):
PENICILLIN - RASH
CODEINE - NAUSEA & VOMITTING

MEDICATIONS TAKEN AT HOME AND REASON FOR USE (Underline those brought to hospital):
LANOXIN - FOR HEART
DIUPRES - FOR BLOOD PRESSURE

DISPOSITION OF MEDICATIONS (Home or Med. Box)   LEFT AT HOME

EVER BEEN ON CORTISONE?   NO   IF YES, WHEN AND WHY?

PHYSICAL AND PSYCHOLOGICAL STATUS OF PATIENT ON FIRST OBSERVATION:
APPEARS LETHARGIC. SKIN HOT TO TOUCH, APPEARS FLUSHED.
NO REDDENED OR BROKEN AREAS NOTED ON SKIN, STATES
SHE ACHES ALL OVER.   Jane Doe, L.P.N.

NURSES ADMISSION NOTES

PERSONAL HISTORY

Final Diagnosis: To be recorded when determined C.O.P.D.
Femoral-popliteal occlusive disease
Age 68 Sex F Race W S/M/W. yrs. Adm. 7/15/74 His.
Occupation Housewife

Family History	Age	Health, if living, or cause of death. Note especially Hereditary or Infectious diseases
Father	D	Cancer
Mother	D	C.V.A.
Brothers		None
Sisters		

Chief Complaint: Date and mode of onset, probable cause, course
68 yr. old white ♀ was awakened
from sleep 2 days PTA ē pain
in ® lower leg & foot. Pain sharp
and unrelated to external stimuli,
rest, ē it is a coldness of the
foot. She has no history of
claudication. No hx of C.V.A.,
diabetes. Has history of C.O.P.D.

Past History: Diseases from childhood to date, habits, Menstrual history, social data
No previous hospitalization.
History of COPD, but no known
allergies. Smokes 1 pkg. of
cigarettes per day. Drinks
up to 1 qt. of vodka daily.

Former or Subsequent admissions to this or other hospitals

	Date	Case No.	Diagnosis
1			
2			
3			

Signed H. Jones, M.D.

PERSONAL HISTORY

NURSES NOTES

DATE TIME	

JULY 18, 1974

13³⁰ PT. C/O OF SEVERE, CRUSHING TYPE CHEST PAIN, BP 90/60
P. 122 - IRREGULAR, DR. JONES NOTIFIED. O₂ STARTED @
5L/MIN. MEDICATION GIVEN FOR PAIN.

14⁴⁵ EKG. DONE. 1000 cc 5% D/W STARTED IV IN LT. ARM BY
DR. JONES. BP 8/42 P. 140 - IRREGULAR. SKIN FEELS
COLD, & CLAMMY TO TOUCH.

15⁰⁵ FAMILY NOTIFIED.

15⁰⁰ TRANSFERRED TO CORONARY CARE UNIT. PER BED. CLOTHING
DENTURES, EYEGLASSES & YELLOW METAL RING ACCOMPANIED
PATIENT.   J. Doe L.P.N.

15⁵⁵ RECEIVED IN C.C.U. & IV RUNNING HOOKED TO MONITOR.
H. Wixon, R.N.

NURSES NOTES

PHYSICIAN'S ORDERS

Date	Time	Nurse	Orders
8/9/74			1. Ambulate in hall B.I.D.
			2. Irrigate wound with H₂O₂ and apply wet to dry betadine dressings q 8 h.
			3. D.C. foley catheter.
			4. Furadantin 50 mg gid
			J. Brown, M.D.

PHYSICIAN'S ORDERS

Fig. 7-4 Some forms commonly used in health agencies.

manner, a physician may use records to see how certain kinds of medical care influenced patients who have been ill with a particular disease.

The patient's record is an important legal document and may be used in courts of law. This will be discussed below.

Each health agency follows certain policies and procedures in relation to record keeping. The following are some examples: the personnel who are responsible for writing on each form; the order in which forms appear in the record; the frequency with which information is recorded; whether routine nursing care is recorded; the manner in which health practitioners identify themselves at the end of the entry; and which types of abbreviations are acceptable. Many agencies now microfilm records. Certain colors of ink, such as blue, cannot be used when they do not photograph well. The nurse will wish to become familiar with and to observe her own agency's policies.

The following are some general guides for recording that many health agencies use:

- Record only after care has been given. For example, it is not recommended that the nurse write, cleansing enema to be given.
- Record how a patient tolerates a particular procedure, such as a lumbar (spinal) puncture.
- Record anything abnormal or out of the ordinary.
- Use a pen—not a pencil—when recording.
- Record times when the patient leaves a unit for any reason, when he returns, and where he has been.
- Record times of admission, discharge, and transfer.
- Do not use ditto marks.
- Use commonly accepted abbreviations only or those specified by the agency in which care is given. Table 7-1 on page 107 lists some commonly used abbreviations. Abbreviations commonly used for medications are given in Chapter 17.
- Do not erase. Rather, draw a single line through the mistake; put the word, error, near it, and continue the recording with the correct information, as in the following illustration:

1:30 P.M. ~~Pt. refused digitalis.~~* (error)   *R. Smith, R.N.*
1:30 P.M. Digitalis omitted.
Pulse rate —46—
Dr. Brown notified. *R. Smith, R.N.*

It is important to record accurately, clearly, and as briefly as possible. More specific suggestions will be given as nursing care is described in this book.

The patient's record as a legal document

Patients' records have been used as evidence in law courts in this country. Therefore, it is important that the record be accurate and

*Digitalis is a medication often given to patients with certain heart diseases. When the pulse rate is very slow, usual procedure is to omit the medication and notify the physician promptly.

complete. Also, only information that is related to the patient's health problems and care should be recorded. Inappropriate information can be considered an invasion of the patient's privacy and can lead to legal problems.

Chapter 2 pointed out that giving certain kinds of care without the patient's consent can be considered assault and battery. Therefore, it is very important that the patient sign the proper consent form. If he cannot, a person legally responsible for him signs the form. For example, parents sign for their children's care. Usually, a consent form is signed at the time of the patient's admission. However, it is wise to check to see that the form is present in the record and properly signed. An example of a properly executed consent form to perform surgery is illustrated in Chapter 21 on page 439.

Opinion differs about the legal standing of nurses' notes. In some agencies, the notes are kept as a permanent part of the patient's record; other agencies may destroy them after a certain period of time. State laws often guide health agencies on this point.

Legal problems have occurred in the past when nurses took verbal orders from physicians about which misunderstandings arose. Therefore, safe practice is to follow only written orders. In fact, many health agencies allow verbal orders only under certain emergency situations and then only by authorized people.

Nursing care plan

A **nursing care plan** is a guide to the patient's nursing care. Plans are generally made up by the team leader who often consults other team members as she prepares the plans. They are used by all members of the nursing team. One plan is developed for each patient. It is changed as the patient's needs for nursing care change. Each agency has its own form for a nursing care plan. Figure 7-5 gives an example.

A nursing care plan includes **nursing orders,** that is, directives that tell what nursing care is to be done. Two examples of nursing orders are: have patient walk length of hall three times daily; give patient bed bath

NURSING CARE PLAN

DATE	NEEDS AND/OR PROBLEMS	APPROACH
7/20/74	1. Prevent skin breaking down.	1. Turn & position q 2H. on even hrs. Rub back & shoulders each time turned. Inspect heels, elbows, etc.
	2. Enc. independence in personal care.	2. Enc. him to shave, brush teeth, comb hair, wash face, eat, etc. c̄ Lt. hand. Set up equipment so he can handle it. Assist as needed and allow him plenty of time.
	3. Prevent foot drop.	3. Keep feet against foot board.
		IMMEDIATE GOAL
		Prevent contractures and skin break down. Teach him to assist in moving and in his own care.

DIAGNOSIS: C.V.A (Rt.)   OPERATION:
DIET: 0.5 Gm Na, Soft.   ALLERGIES: Morphine
CONDITION: Fair   NEXT OF KIN: Mary Jones, Wife   PHONE: 483-2601
DATE OF ADM.: 7/19/74   TIME: 1:15 PM   RELIGION: Prot.   S.Ⓜ W. D. SEP.   SEX: M   AGE: 64
ROOM: 2912   NAME: Jones, John   HOSP. NO.: 29-068-125   DR. D. Henry

Fig. 7-5 One of a variety of forms used by health agencies for describing nursing care.

daily. Figure 7-5 illustrates additional nursing orders, under the section entitled APPROACH.

Nursing care plans are a way to exchange information among nursing team members. For instance, the team leader communicates the overall nursing care for a patient to other members of the team. The plan helps new members with the nursing care needs of the patient. In other words, the nurse, after studying the plan, does not have to go from person to person to find out what care the patient needs. Such a practice would result in incomplete care and is wasteful of time as well. Asking the patient directly what care he needs usually does little to inspire his confidence in the nurse.

Nursing care plans are prepared so that each patient will receive total nursing care. Without a plan, one nurse may not know what another nurse is planning. As a result, there may be either gaps or overlaps in the care the patient receives.

A nursing care plan helps the nurse to give the patient individualized care. Each patient has his own plan since no two patients have identical needs. It has been observed that care is more likely to meet individual needs when nursing care plans are used.

Nursing care plans and nurses' notes are very different. Nurses' notes describe care given and observations the nurse makes during and after giving care. A good guide in preparing them is to ask the question, "What information is needed by people who will read and use what I enter in the nurses' notes?" On the other hand, the nursing care plan answers the question, "What nursing care does this patient need?"

The one who eventually benefits most from a nursing care plan is the patient. It serves as a necessary bridge between knowing what the patient's nursing care needs are and carrying out the specific care that meets those needs.

Ways in which information is exchanged among health practitioners

In addition to the nursing care plan and the patient's record, there are several other ways that are commonly used for exchanging information among team members and that assist the nurse with the care of her patients.

Telephone. Using the telephone is a helpful way for exchanging information when it is inconvenient for two people to meet together. For example, the nurse may call various departments in a health agency, such as the laboratory, x-ray department, and the operating room, concerning appointments for patients. Using the telephone often saves much time.

There are common courtesies that the nurse will wish to remember when using the telephone. She should identify herself and the unit from which she is calling and state the reason for her call in a businesslike way. She should identify the patient carefully. When receiving a call, she also identifies herself and the unit where the call is being received. Calls are kept as short as possible in order not to tie up the telephone and waste people's time. Business telephones are not used for personal matters.

Conferences. Various types of conferences are commonly used for exchanging information. For example, two nurses may meet to discuss a particular patient's care. A physician will often confer with a nurse about a patient's condition. Other health practitioners, such as dietitians and physical therapists, may meet with the nurse to discuss care.

Team conferences are used to exchange information about patients for whom the team is caring. Nursing team conferences include all members except possibly clerical assistants and volunteers. These conferences offer the nurse an excellent time to learn to know her patients better, and also to learn about new equipment, new kinds of treatment, and other current developments.

Nurses meet together regularly at change-of-shift times. Information about the patient's condition and new nursing and medical orders are

NURSING ASSIGNMENT SHEET

TEAM MEMBER _JANE DOE L.P.N._   BREAK _9:15 A.M._   CONFERENCE _10:30 A.M._   LUNCH _12:00 N._   DATE: _7/23/74_

TEAM LEADER _MARY BLACK RN_   ASSIGNMENT _Filling and distributing water carafes on the Northwing_

ROOM	PATIENT	BATH	ACTIVITY	DIET	FLUIDS	TO BE CHECKED	TREATMENTS	SPECIMEN	COMMENTS
296¹	FLORA BROWN DUODENAL ULCER	BED / SELF * / SHOWER / (TUB) / SITZ	BED / DANGLE / B R P / B R P . HELP / AMB . HELP / WALKER / CRUTCHES / W C	REGULAR / SOFT / SURG. LIQ. / FULL LIQ / SPECIAL Bland / FASTING / TUBE FEEDING	FORCE / N P O / LIMIT / SIPS WATER / ICE CHIPS / I V / DIST WATER	BLOOD PRESSURE 8A / T P R 8A / TEST URINE A.C. & HS / SLIDING SCALE / I & O / LEVIN TUBE / CHEST TUBE / FOLEY / OXYGEN	ENEMA / DOUCHE / PERI CARE . LIGHT / WEIGH / ORAL HYGIENE / SPECIAL BACK CARE / PREPARE FOR SURG. / O T . P T . E C T	STOOL ✓ / URINE / SPUTUM / BLOOD / CULTURE / TISSUE	
296²	MARY GREEN CORONARY	(BED) / SELF * / SHOWER / TUB / SITZ	(BED) / DANGLE / B R P / B R P . HELP / AMB / AMB . HELP / WALKER / CRUTCHES / W C	REGULAR / SOFT / SURG. LIQ. / FULL LIQ / SPECIAL 2Gm Na / FASTING / TUBE FEEDING	FORCE / N P O / LIMIT / SIPS WATER / ICE CHIPS / I V / DIST WATER	BLOOD PRESSURE 12 / T P R 8-12 / TEST URINE A.C. & HS / SLIDING SCALE / I & O / LEVIN TUBE / CHEST TUBE / FOLEY 44/M - 1hr pc / OXYGEN 4/M & 115	ENEMA / DOUCHE / PERI CARE . LIGHT / WEIGH 8A / ORAL HYGIENE / SPECIAL BACK CARE / PREPARE FOR SURG. / O T . P T . E C T	STOOL / URINE / SPUTUM / BLOOD / CULTURE / TISSUE	
298¹	JOHN SNAPP C.O.P.D.	BED / (SELF *) / SHOWER / TUB / SITZ	BED / DANGLE / B R P / B R P . HELP / AMB c O₂ / AMB . HELP / WALKER / CRUTCHES / W C	REGULAR / (SOFT) / SURG. LIQ / FULL LIQ / SPECIAL / FASTING / TUBE FEEDING	(FORCE) / N P O / LIMIT / SIPS WATER / ICE CHIPS / I V / DIST WATER	BLOOD PRESSURE / T P R / TEST URINE A.C. & HS / SLIDING SCALE / I & O / LEVIN TUBE / CHEST TUBE / FOLEY / OXYGEN 1 4/M CONT.	(ENEMA) FLEETS / DOUCHE / PERI CARE . LIGHT / WEIGH / ORAL HYGIENE / SPECIAL BACK CARE / PREPARE FOR X-RAY / O T . P T . E C T	STOOL / URINE / (SPUTUM) / BLOOD / CULTURE / TISSUE	1000cc 5% D/W c̄ 500mg Aminophyllin @ 100cc/hr CONT.
298²	TOM HENRY C.H.F.	BED / SELF * / SHOWER / TUB / SITZ	(BED) / DANGLE / B R P / B R P . HELP / AMB / AMB . HELP / WALKER / CRUTCHES / W C	REGULAR / SOFT / SURG. LIQ / FULL LIQ / SPECIAL 2Gm Na / FASTING / TUBE FEEDING	FORCE / N P O / (LIMIT) - 300/8h / SIPS WATER / ICE CHIPS / I V / DIST WATER	BLOOD PRESSURE q2hr / T P R q2hr / TEST URINE A.C. & HS / SLIDING SCALE / I & O / LEVIN TUBE / CHEST TUBE / (FOLEY) / OXYGEN 4L/M Cont.	ENEMA / DOUCHE / PERI CARE . LIGHT / WEIGH 8-12 / ORAL HYGIENE 8-12 / SPECIAL BACK CARE / PREPARE FOR SURG. / O T . P T . E C T	STOOL / URINE / SPUTUM / BLOOD / CULTURE / TISSUE	CHANGE POSITION q 2hr.
299	JIM SMITH DIABETES MELLITUS	BED / SELF * / (SHOWER) / TUB / SITZ	BED / DANGLE / B R P / B R P . HELP / (AMB) / AMB . HELP / WALKER / CRUTCHES / W C	REGULAR / SOFT / SURG. LIQ / FULL LIQ / SPECIAL 1800cal Diabetic / FASTING / TUBE FEEDING	FORCE / N P O / LIMIT / SIPS WATER / ICE CHIPS / I V / DIST WATER	BLOOD PRESSURE / T P R / (TEST URINE A.C. & HS) / (SLIDING SCALE) / I & O / LEVIN TUBE / CHEST TUBE / FOLEY / OXYGEN	ENEMA / DOUCHE / PERI CARE . LIGHT / WEIGH / ORAL HYGIENE / SPECIAL BACK CARE / PREPARE FOR SURG. / O T . P T . E C T	STOOL / URINE / SPUTUM / BLOOD / CULTURE / TISSUE	
		BED / SELF * / SHOWER / TUB / SITZ	BED / DANGLE / B R P / B R P . HELP / AMB / AMB . HELP / WALKER / CRUTCHES / W C	REGULAR / SOFT / SURG LIQ / FULL LIQ / SPECIAL / FASTING / TUBE FEEDING	FORCE / N P O / LIMIT / SIPS WATER / ICE CHIPS / I V / DIST WATER	BLOOD PRESSURE / T P R / TEST URINE A.C. & HS / SLIDING SCALE / I & O / LEVIN TUBE / CHEST TUBE / FOLEY / OXYGEN	ENEMA / DOUCHE / PERI CARE . LIGHT / WEIGH / ORAL HYGIENE / SPECIAL BACK CARE / PREPARE FOR SURG. / O T . P T . E C T	STOOL / URINE / SPUTUM / BLOOD / CULTURE / TISSUE	
		BED / SELF * / SHOWER / TUB / SITZ	BED / DANGLE / B R P / B R P . HELP / AMB / AMB . HELP / WALKER / CRUTCHES / W C	REGULAR / SOFT / SURG LIQ / FULL LIQ / SPECIAL / FASTING / TUBE FEEDING	FORCE / N P O / LIMIT / SIPS WATER / ICE CHIPS / I V / DIST WATER	BLOOD PRESSURE / T P R / TEST URINE A.C. & HS / SLIDING SCALE / I & O / LEVIN TUBE / CHEST TUBE / FOLEY / OXYGEN	ENEMA / DOUCHE / PERI CARE . LIGHT / WEIGH / ORAL HYGIENE / SPECIAL BACK CARE / PREPARE FOR SURG. / O T . P T . E C T	STOOL / URINE / SPUTUM / BLOOD / CULTURE / TISSUE	
		BED / SELF * / SHOWER / TUB / SITZ	BED / DANGLE / B R P / B R P . HELP / AMB / AMB . HELP / WALKER / CRUTCHES / W C	REGULAR / SOFT / SURG LIQ / FULL LIQ / SPECIAL / FASTING / TUBE FEEDING	FORCE / N P O / LIMIT / SIPS WATER / ICE CHIPS / I V / DIST WATER	BLOOD PRESSURE / T P R / TEST URINE A.C. & HS / SLIDING SCALE / I & O / LEVIN TUBE / CHEST TUBE / FOLEY / OXYGEN	ENEMA / DOUCHE / PERI CARE . LIGHT / WEIGH / ORAL HYGIENE / SPECIAL BACK CARE / PREPARE FOR SURG. / O T . P T . E C T	STOOL / URINE / SPUTUM / BLOOD / CULTURE / TISSUE	

CODE * — YOU WASH BACK AND LEGS   W C — WHEELCHAIR   E.C.T. — ELECTRICAL CONVULSIVE THERAPY
B R P — BATHROOM PRIVILEGES   B P — BLOOD PRESSURE   O.T. — OCCUPATIONAL THERAPY
AMB — AMBULATORY   N P O — NOTHING BY MOUTH   P.T. — PHYSICAL THERAPY
I & O — INTAKE AND OUTPUT   DIST — DISTILLED WATER

Fig. 7-6 A nursing assignment sheet describing the team member's responsibility for the day. Note the definition of abbreviations at the bottom of the form. This practice eliminates the dangers of misunderstandings when abbreviations are used.

discussed so that responsibility for the patient's care continues smoothly and without omissions. Change-of-shift conferences may or may not include all nursing team members.

Rounds. Nursing and health teams use rounds to exchange information. The members visit patients' bedsides in a group. The patient may be asked to participate as his care is discussed. Attending nursing and medical rounds is usually a very educational experience and the nurse will wish to attend whenever she has the opportunity.

Assignment Sheets. Assignment sheets are used to give people a description of the work they are to do. The nursing team leader prepares them for each member of the team. For example, the assignment sheet will tell you which patients you are to care for, special duties you have (e.g., assisting a patient to eat while his nurse is at lunch), what times you may leave for meals, and so on. An example of a nursing assignment sheet is illustrated in Figure 7-6 on page 103.

Discharging the patient

Preparing the patient for discharge begins when he is admitted to the health agency. The purpose of his stay is to help him reach a state of high-level wellness, and this begins at the time of admission.

As is true when the patient is admitted, there are certain policies that are carefully observed when he is discharged. Chart 7-2 describes discharging the patient from a health agency, and Figure 7-7 illustrates a discharge conference.

There are times when a patient leaves a health agency against medical advice, usually abbreviated AMA. In such instances, he signs a special form which states that he is leaving against his physician's orders and he will hold no one responsible for anything that may happen to him as a result of his leaving. Figure 7-8 illustrates a form used when a patient leaves against advice (see p. 106).

Transferring patients within the same agency

There are times when patients are moved from one unit to another in the same agency. For example, because of a change in the patient's condition, he may be moved to a special care unit, as an intensive care unit, a surgical unit, a cardiac care unit, or a unit for patients recovering and able to care for their own hygienic needs.

A transfer is similar to an admission and discharge. The patient is prepared for transfer in the same manner as for discharge, except that financial arrangements are not included. Also, he usually does not dress in street clothes. The nurse records the transfer in the same manner as she would record a discharge.

A patient is received on the new unit in much the same manner as was used for his admission. The surroundings are new for the patient and he may be fearful and worried, even though he is in the same agency. He should be introduced to those who will be caring for him as well as to his new roommates. He will need help to learn about equip-

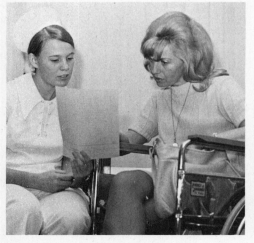

Fig. 7-7 Before this patient is discharged, the nurse has a final conference with her to be sure that she has understood teaching in relation to the diet she will follow at home.

Chart 7-2 Discharging the patient from a health agency

The purpose is to discharge a patient in a manner consistent with the health agency's procedures and policies and to help patient feel that there is concern for his welfare

Suggested Action	Reason for Action
Check to see that patient has discharge order.	It is the physician's responsibility to discharge patient.
If patient is leaving without physician's consent, check to see that proper form has been completed.	Patient cannot legally be held in an agency against his wishes. Having him sign proper form relieves agency and physician from responsibilities should problems arise because patient refused further care.
Check to see that patient or relative has had discharge instructions, as for example, instructions concerning his diet.	The patient or relative will be able to continue with necessary care after discharge when properly instructed.
Check to see that all necessary equipment and supplies are in readiness for patient to take with him, such as medications, dressings, and so on. Obtain missing items as necessary.	Having equipment and supplies ready saves time and annoyance of having to wait for them when patient is ready to leave.
Check to see that proper financial arrangements have been made by patient or relative. Obtain patient's clothing and valuables. Observe agency policies.	These actions help to avoid legal problems.
Assist patient to dress and pack belongings. See to it that he has all of his belongings.	Assisting patient conserves his strength. Time and trouble are saved when patient leaves with all of his belongings.
Transport patient and belongings to car and assist him into car as necessary.	Assisting patient conserves his strength. Such assistance is courteous and helps patient feel that personnel are interested in his welfare.
Do necessary recording on patient's record.	The information is important to complete patient's permanent record.

ment and routines if they are different. The nurse records receiving the patient in the same manner as she described his admission to the health agency.

It is a courteous and thoughtful gesture when the nurse caring for the patient on one unit visits him from time to time on the unit to which he was transferred. Patients generally appreciate such visits.

Referrals and transfers to other agencies

A **referral** means sending or guiding someone to another place for assistance. A referral is commonly used among health agencies. For example, a patient may be referred by a hospital to a visiting nursing service for assistance with home care. A school nurse may refer a student to his physician or to a hospital emergency room. A woman may be

LEAVING HOSPITAL AGAINST ADVICE

Date JULY 13, 1974

This is to certify that HELEN JONES,

a patient in Pine Memorial Hospital is leaving the hospital against the advice of the attending physician and the hospital administration. I acknowledge that I have been informed of the risk involved and hereby release the attending physician, and the hospital, from all responsibility and any ill effects which may result from this action.

Helen Jones
Patient

____
Other Person Responsible

____
Relationship

Witness Nancy Smith, L.P.N.

Witness Helen Wren, R.N.

Leaving Hospital Against Advice

Fig. 7-8 An example of a form commonly used when a patient leaves a hospital against advice.

referred by a clinic which cares for her before she has her baby to a clinic that will care for her after she has delivered. An example of a referral form when a patient was transferred from a hospital to a nursing home appears in Figure 7-9.

Referrals and transfers to other agencies are especially important in order to help patients receive continuity of care, as described in Chapter 1.

Conclusion

Nurses are interested in giving patients safe, total, and continuous care that meets each patient's individual needs in a thoughtful and courteous manner. Hopefully, content in this chapter will help you to give that kind

PATIENT TRANSFER FORM

Name
Hosp. No.
Birthdate
Sex
Pay Code
Medicare No.

(imprint)

Date of Transfer _AUGUST 2, 1974_

Transferred to _BED ROSE CONVALESCENT HOME_

Address _358 WEST YORKTOWN_

Relative or Guardian _JOHN BROWN_ _HUSBAND_ (RELATION)

Relative or Guardian's Address _1964 NORTH OAK_ Tel. _468-3921_

Next of Kin _SAME AS ABOVE_

Next of Kin's Address _____ Tel. _____ (RELATION)

Religion _PROTESTANT_

Soc Sec. # _986-06-5332_

Physician in Charge at Time of Transfer _SAMUEL HARRIS_ M.D.

Physician in Charge Following Transfer _SAME_ M.D.

Clinic Appt. _AUGUST 30, 1974_ _8:00 A.M._ (DATE) (TIME)

II. MAJOR DIAGNOSES

C.V.A.

(Check if present)

Disabilities
Amputation
Paralysis
Contracture
Decub. Ulcer

Impairments
Mentality
Speech
Hearing
Vision
Sensation

Incontinence
Bladder — CATHETER
Bowel
Saliva

Activity Tolerance Limitations
None (Moderate) Severe

Patient knows diagnosis?
YES

DIET, DRUGS, AND OTHER THERAPY
at Time of Discharge

1. 1200 CALORIE & 0.5 Gm Na SOFT DIET
2. FURADANTIN 50 mg qid.
3. LANOXIN 0.25 mg DAILY.
4. DIUPRES - 250 T BID.
5. IRRIGATE FOLEY CATHETER & 4% ACETIC ACID BID. CHANGE q 10 DAYS - DONE 8/1/74

IMPORTANT MEDICAL INFORMATION
(State allergies if any)
ALLERGIC TO PENICILLIN - RASH
CODEINE - NAUSEA & VOMITTING

(Physician, please sign below)

	date	result
Chest X-ray	7/25/74	NEG.
C.B.C.	7/25/74	W.N.L.
Serology	7/25/74	NON-REACTIVE
Urinalysis	8/1/74	Occ. W.B.C. Albumint

SUGGESTIONS FOR ACTIVE CARE

BED
Position in good body alignment and change position every _2_ hrs.
Avoid _____ position
Prone position _____ times/day as tolerated.

SIT IN CHAIR
_2_ hrs. _3_ times/day.

WEIGHT BEARING
Full _____ Partial ✓ None _____ on _RIGHT_ leg

LOCOMOTION
Walk _2 WALKER_ 2 times/day.

EXERCISES
Range of motion _3_ times/day to _BT. ARM & LEG_

by patient _____ nurse ✓ family _____
Other as outlined below _____
Stand _____ Min. _____ times/day.

SOCIAL ACTIVITIES
Encourage group _____ individual ✓
within _____ outside _____ home.
Transport: Ambulance ✓ Car _____
Car for handicapped _____ Bus _____

SUGGESTIONS FOR COMPLETING FORM
1. The purpose of this form is to insure continuity of care in transfer from hospital to home or home to hospital.
2. The form is not intended to supply information of long-term nature.
3. Original should accompany patient with transfer. Carbon retained in patient's record.

Signature of Physician or Nurse _Jane Doe L.D.N._ Date _8/2/74_

Fig. 7-9 A form used when patients are transferred from one health agency to another which illustrates the type of information the receiving agency needs in order to make continuity of care possible. On the reverse side (not shown), there is space for additional information, such as the patient's self-care status, his general behavior patterns, his diet, special equipment he uses, social information, and so on.

of care when admitting, discharging, and transferring patients, when using nursing care plans, and when taking care to record accurately and completely.

Table 7-1   Commonly used abbreviations

Abbreviation	Meaning
Abd.	Abdomen
AM	Morning
AMA	Against medical advice
Amb.	Ambulatory (able to walk about)
Amt.	Amount
Approx.	Approximately
BM	Bowel movement
BP or Bl.Pr.	Blood pressure
BPR	Bathroom privileges
$\bar{c}$	With
CCU	Cardiac care unit

Conclusion

107

Table 7-1 continued

Abbreviation	Meaning
CD	Communicable disease
c/o	Complains of
DC	Discontinue
ER	Emergency room
Exam.	Examination
GI	Gastrointestinal, meaning stomach and small and large intestines
GU	Genitourinary, meaning genital and urinary organs
Hi-vit	High vitamin
Hi-cal	High caloric
H_2O	Water
ICU	Intensive care unit
Invol.	Involuntary
Lab.	Laboratory
Lb.	Pound
Min.	Minute
NKA	No known allergy
No.	Number
Noc.	Night
NPO	Nothing by mouth
NS	Normal saline
O_2	Oxygen
OB	Obstetrics
OD	Right eye
OOB	Out of bed
OR	Operating room
OS	Left eye
OT	Occupational therapy
OU	Both eyes
Ped. or Peds.	Pediatrics
Per	By or through
PO or Os	By mouth
Postop.	Postoperative, meaning after having surgery
Preop.	Preoperative, meaning before surgery
Pt.	Patient
PT	Physical therapy
s̄	Without
TPR	Temperature and pulse and respiratory rates
Via	By way of
WC	Wheelchair
WNL	Within normal limits
Wt.	Weight

References

Atwood, Judith, et al, "The POR: A System for Communication," *The Nursing Clinics of North America*, 9:229–234, June 1974.

Beaumont, Estelle and Wiley, Loy, eds., "Thinking About Discharge on Admission Day," *Nursing '74*, 4:17, March 1974.

Crawford, Christine F. and Palm, Mary Louise, " 'Can I Take My Teddy Bear?' " *American Journal of Nursing*, 73:286–287, February 1973.

Fuller, Dorothy and Rosenaur, Janet Allan, "A Patient Assessment Guide," *Nursing Outlook*, 22:460–462, July 1974.

Keller, Nancy S., "Care Without Coordination: A True Story," *Nursing Forum*, 6:280–323, Number 3, 1967.

Kerr, Avice H., "'Nurses' Notes' 'That's Where the Goodies Are!'" *Nursing '75*, 5:34–41, February 1975.

Little, Dolores E. and Carnevali, Doris L., *Nursing Care Planning*, J. B. Lippincott Company, Philadelphia, Pennsylvania, 1969, 245 p.

Mead, Jackie, "The Lemonade Party," *Nursing Outlook*, 21:104–105, February 1973.

Moreland, Helen J. and Schmitt, Virginia C., "Making Referrals Is Everybody's Business," *American Journal of Nursing*, 74:96–97, January 1974.

Niland, Maureen B. and Bentz, Patricia M., "A Problem-Oriented Approach to Planning Nursing Care," *The Nursing Clinics of North America*, 9:235–245, June 1974.

Stephens, Kathleen Schmidt, "A Toddler's Separation Anxiety," *American Journal of Nursing*, 73:1553–1555, September 1973.

Woody, Mary and Mallison, Mary, "The Problem-Oriented System for Patient-Centered Care," *American Journal of Nursing*, 73:1168–1175, July 1973.

8 obtaining the vital signs

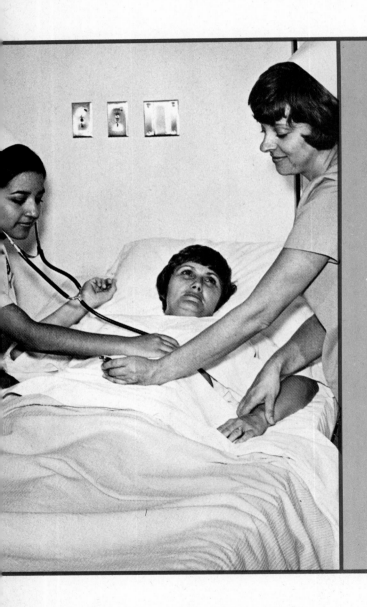

behavioral objectives

When mastery of content in this chapter is reached, the student will be able to

Define terms appearing in the glossary.

List average normal ranges for adults for pulse and respiratory rates and blood pressure.

List six factors that normally tend to influence body temperature, pulse and respiratory rates, and blood pressure; describe in what way these factors influence vital signs.

Describe the difference between an oral and a rectal thermometer and explain why an oral thermometer should not be used to obtain a rectal temperature.

Describe how a mercury thermometer, a sphygmomanometer, and a stethoscope work.

Describe the usual general appearance of a person with an elevated temperature; with a subnormal temperature; with difficult and labored breathing; and with cyanosis.

List five situations when obtaining body temperature orally should be avoided or delayed.

List two situations when obtaining body temperature rectally should be avoided.

Describe how to clean a glass mercury thermometer.

List six sites on the body where the pulse rate can be obtained with relative ease.

Describe why a person cannot purposely hold his breath indefinitely.

Describe briefly how the vital signs are obtained and recorded.

Describe the primary purpose of an EKG (ECG).

glossary

Anoxia Low oxygen content in the body. Synonym for hypoxia.

Apical Pulse Rate The pulse rate obtained by placing a stethoscope over the apex of the heart on the chest wall.

Apical-Radial Pulse Rate The pulse rate obtained by two persons when one obtains the radial pulse rate while the other obtains the apical pulse rate.

Apnea The absence of breathing.

Arrhythmia Irregular pulse rhythm.

Axilla Armpit.

Axillary Temperature A measure of body heat obtained by placing the thermometer in the axilla.

Bounding Pulse A pulse that feels full and strong to the touch.

Bradycardia Abnormally slow heartbeat.

Cardinal Signs Measurements of body temperature, pulse and respiratory rates, and blood pressure. Synonym for vital signs.

Celsius Scale The original scale used in the centigrade thermometer.

Celsius Thermometer An instrument having zero for the temperature at which water freezes and 100 degrees for the temperature at which water boils. Synonym for centigrade thermometer.

Centigrade Thermometer An instrument having zero for the temperature at which water freezes and 100 degrees for the temperature at which water boils. Synonym for Celsius thermometer.

Cheyne-Stokes Respiration A gradual increase and then gradual decrease in depth of respirations followed by a period of apnea.

Continued Temperature A temperature that remains consistently elevated and fluctuates very little.

Crisis A rapid drop of body temperature to normal.

Cyanosis A bluish coloring of skin and mucous membrane.

Diastole The period when the least amount of pressure is exerted on the walls of the arteries during heartbeat.

Dyspnea Difficult breathing.

Electrocardiogram The graphic record produced by the electrocardiograph. Abbreviated EKG or ECG.

Exhalation The act of breathing out. Synonym for expiration.

Expiration The act of breathing out. Synonym for exhalation.

Fahrenheit Thermometer An instrument having 32 degrees for the temperature at which water freezes and 212 degrees for the temperature at which water boils.

Feeble, Weak, or Thready Pulse Pulse that feels weak to the touch.

Fever Above normal body temperature. Synonym for pyrexia.

Hypernea Increased depth of respiration.

Hypertension Abnormally high blood pressure.

Hypotension Abnormally low blood pressure.

Hypothermia Body temperature that is below average normal range.

Hypoxia Low oxygen content in the body. Synonym for anoxia.

Inspiration The act of breathing in. Synonym for inhalation.

Intermittent Pulse Periods of normal pulse rhythm broken by periods of irregular rhythm.

Intermittent Temperature Periods of normal temperature broken by periods of elevated temperature.

Invasion or Onset of Temperature The period when pyrexia begins.

Lysis The gradual return of body temperature to normal.

Meniscus The curved surface at the top of a column of liquid in a tube.

Oral Temperature A measure of body heat obtained by placing the thermometer in the mouth under the tongue.

Orthopnea The condition in which breathing is easier when the patient is in the sitting or standing position.

Polypnea The respiratory rate above average normal range.

Pulse A wave set up in the walls of the arteries with each beat of the heart.

Pyrexia Above normal body temperature. Synonym for fever.

glossary cont.

Radial Pulse Rate The pulse rate obtained by placing the fingertips on the radial artery at the wrist.

Rectal Temperature A measure of body heat obtained by placing the thermometer in the rectum.

Remittent Temperature Above normal fluctuating temperature.

Respiration The act of breathing.

Sphygmomanometer An instrument to measure blood pressure.

Stertorous Respiration Noisy breathing.

Stethoscope An instrument that carries sounds from the body to the ear of the examiner.

Subsiding Stage of Fever The period when the temperature returns to normal.

Systole The period when maximum pressure is exerted on the arterial walls during heartbeat.

Tachycardia Rapid heartbeat.

Thermometer An instrument used to measure body temperature.

Vital Signs Measurements of body temperature, pulse and respiratory rates, and blood pressure. Synonym for cardinal signs.

introduction

Changes in the way the body is functioning are often reflected in the body temperature, pulse and respiratory rates, and the blood pressure. The mechanisms in the body regulating them are very sensitive and that is why they are frequently referred to as **vital signs** or **cardinal signs.** When it is seen that the vital signs are not normal, it means that the patient needs to be observed carefully and the abnormal signs should be reported promptly.

The use of monitoring machines in many health agencies has made it possible to keep patients' vital signs under constant watch. These devices have been a life-saving measure for many patients. They are generally used in special units where the very ill are cared for, such as in the intensive care unit of a hospital.

Obtaining a patient's vital signs is a part of most admission procedures. Health agencies have policies concerning how often vital signs are to be obtained after admission. For example, if a patient has a body temperature above normal, usual policy is that his vital signs are to be checked every four hours, with the possible exception of blood pressure. For patients who have had surgery, most hospitals require that the vital signs be checked every four hours for a period of time. Policies may require daily or even less frequent checking of vital signs for patients who care for themselves or who are chronically or mentally ill. Blood pressure often is measured more frequently when a heart or blood vessel disease is present.

Body temperature

Body temperature remains within a fairly constant range through a balance between heat production and heat loss. Heat is produced primarily by exercise and by the body's ability to burn and use food (metabolism). Heat is lost from the body primarily through the skin, the

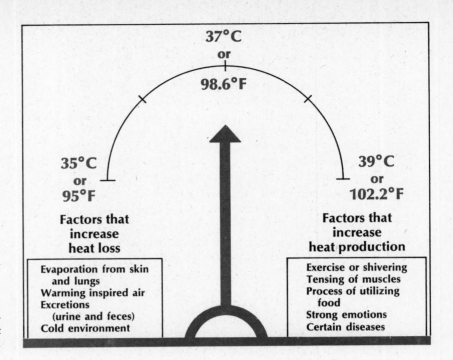

37°C
or
98.6°F

35°C
or
95°F

39°C
or
102.2°F

Factors that increase heat loss

Evaporation from skin and lungs
Warming inspired air
Excretions (urine and feces)
Cold environment

Factors that increase heat production

Exercise or shivering
Tensing of muscles
Process of utilizing food
Strong emotions
Certain diseases

Fig. 8-1 A diagram illustrating the balance between factors that increase heat loss and heat production.

lungs, and the body's waste products. When more heat is produced than is lost, the body's temperature will be above normal, or elevated. Conversely, when more heat is lost than produced, the body's temperature will be below normal, or subnormal. Figure 8-1 illustrates how heat loss and heat production determine the body's temperature.

Signs of elevated or subnormal temperature are usually fairly easy to see. When the temperature is elevated, the skin will appear pink/reddish and feel warm or hot to the touch; the patient is often restless and thirsty. The skin ordinarily will feel cool and appear pale when the temperature is subnormal.

Body temperature is recorded either in degrees of centigrade, abbreviated °C., or degrees of Fahrenheit, abbreviated °F. The **Celsius scale** was the original scale used in the centigrade thermometer. It was named after the man who devised it. Centigrade means consisting of 100 degrees or equal parts. The **Celsius thermometer** or **centigrade thermometer** has a scale at which zero is the temperature at which water freezes and 100 degrees is the temperature at which water boils. The Fahrenheit scale is used in the **Fahrenheit thermometer;** water freezes at 32°F. and boils at 212°F. Table 8-1 gives comparable centigrade and Fahrenheit temperatures and explains how temperatures can be converted from one system to another.

Thermometer. The instrument used to measure the heat of the body is the **thermometer.** The thermometer is placed in the mouth to obtain an **oral temperature.** Studies have shown that there are two areas where maximum mouth temperature can be obtained. They lie under the tongue where the tongue and the floor of the mouth join on *either* side of the frenum lingulae, which is the fold of mucous membrane on the underside of the tongue. These pockets have a rich supply of arterial

Obtaining the vital signs

Table 8-1:   Equivalent centigrade and Fahrenheit
temperatures and directions for converting
temperatures from one measure to another*

Centigrade	Fahrenheit	Centigrade	Fahrenheit
34.0	93.2	38.5	101.3
35.0	95.0	39.0	102.2
36.0	96.8	40.0	104.0
36.5	97.7	41.0	105.8
37.0	98.6	42.0	107.6
37.5	99.5	43.0	109.4
38.0	100.4	44.0	111.2

*To convert centigrade to Fahrenheit, multiply by $\frac{9}{5}$ and add 32. To change Fahrenheit to centigrade, subtract 32 and multiply by $\frac{5}{9}$.

blood. Therefore, it is important to place the thermometer in either of these pockets just described for greatest accuracy. Other areas under the tongue and in the mouth have been found to be from approximately $\frac{1}{2}$ to $1\frac{1}{2}$°F. cooler.

The thermometer is placed in the anal canal, approximately $1\frac{1}{2}$ inches, to obtain a **rectal temperature.** It is placed well into the **axilla,** or armpit, to obtain the **axillary temperature.**

The glass thermometer most commonly used to measure body temperature contains mercury and has two parts: the bulb and the stem. Mercury is a liquid metal and will expand in size when exposed to heat, thus causing it to rise in the stem of the thermometer. The stem is marked in degrees and tenths of a degree. The range is from about 34°C. or 93°F. to about 42.2°C. or 108°F. Fractions of a degree are recorded in even numbers, as 0.2, 0.4, 0.6, and 0.8. If the mercury appears to be a bit more or less than an even tenth of a degree, it is usual practice to report the temperature to the nearest tenth.

Usually, oral thermometers have a long slender mercury bulb which gives the largest possible surface for contact with tissues under the tongue or in the axilla. The blunt bulb thermometer is used to obtain a rectal temperature; the shape of the bulb helps to prevent injuring or puncturing tissue when it is being inserted. When using a thermometer in the home or in a different agency, check to see whether it is oral or rectal. Some thermometers have this printed on them, but others do not. It is dangerous to use a long slender oral thermometer for obtaining rectal temperatures! Figure 8-2 illustrates glass thermometers.

There are electric (or electronic) thermometers on the market that measure body temperature in a matter of seconds. These have two temperature sensors, one for oral and one for rectal use. They are generally equipped with disposable covers, a feature that helps to eliminate chances of spreading infections and that decreases cleaning chores. Reports in the literature indicate that these thermometers have great accuracy and their use saves considerable nursing time. Figure 8-3 illustrates an electric thermometer (see p. 117).

Normal Body Temperature. The average normal oral temperature for adults is considered to be 37°C. (98.6°F.); the average normal rectal temperature is 37.5°C. (99.5°F.); and the average normal axillary temperature is 36.7°C. (98°F.).

Variations in body temperature occur in each person and a range of

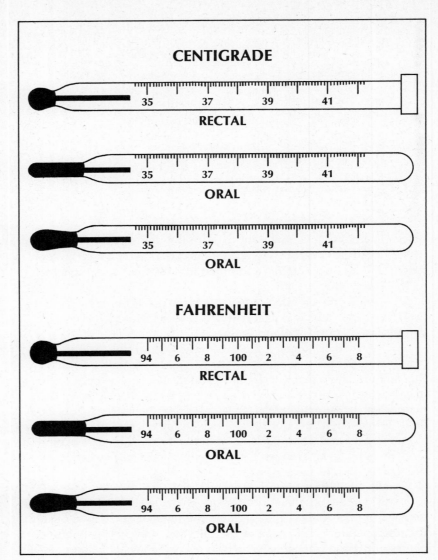

CENTIGRADE

35   37   39   41
RECTAL

35   37   39   41
ORAL

35   37   39   41
ORAL

FAHRENHEIT

94   6   8   100   2   4   6   8
RECTAL

94   6   8   100   2   4   6   8
ORAL

94   6   8   100   2   4   6   8
ORAL

Fig. 8-2 Clinical glass thermometers. The three on the top use the centigrade scale to measure temperature; the three on the bottom use the Fahrenheit scale. Note the blunt mercury bulb on the rectal thermometers.

0.3 to 0.6°C. (0.5 to 1.0°F.) from the average normal temperature is usually considered to be within normal limits. The body temperature has been observed to be lowest during the early morning hours and highest during the late afternoon and early evening hours. Exercise, lifestyle, amount and kind of food, and cold or hot weather may influence body temperature. Body temperature rises as much as 1°F. approximately midway between menstrual periods and drops again just prior to menstruation. Newborn babies and young children normally have a higher body temperature than adults. Older persons tend to run a lower than average temperature.

Elevated Body Temperature. An elevation above normal body temperature is called **pyrexia,** or **fever.** A patient is considered in danger when the temperature reaches and passes 41°C. (105.8°F.) and rarely survives when it reaches 43°C. (109.4°F.).

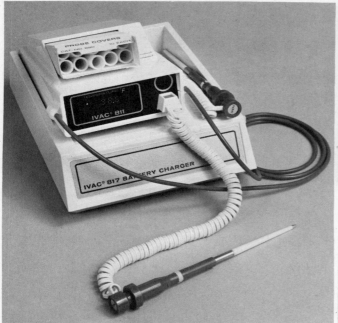
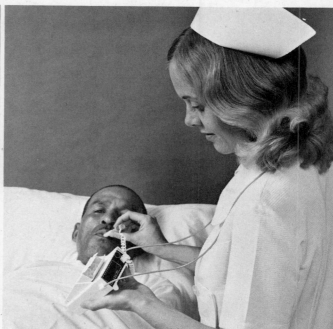

Fig. 8-3 (Left) An electric thermometer. There are interchangeable oral and rectal probes. The cylindrical items near the top of this model are disposable plastic probe covers. (Right) The nurse reads the thermometer on the clocklike face when the thermometer signals that peak temperature has been reached. (Photographs courtesy of the IVAC Corporation)

Fever may take a variety of courses. The **onset,** or **invasion,** is the period when fever begins; it may be sudden or gradual in nature. When the temperature alternates regularly between a period of fever and a period of normal or subnormal temperature, it is called an **intermittent temperature.** A **remittent temperature** is one that fluctuates several degrees above normal but does not reach normal between fluctuations. A **continued temperature** is one that remains consistently elevated and fluctuates very little. The **subsiding stage** is that time when the temperature returns to normal. When pyrexia ends suddenly, the drop to normal is called a **crisis;** a gradual return to normal temperature is called **lysis.** Most of the terms just defined are illustrated in Figure 8-4.

Occasionally, when body temperature has returned to normal following fever, a patient may have a temporary return of an elevated temperature. This may be due to increased activity or exertion, in which case there is usually little cause for alarm. However, a recurring temperature may also be a sign of relapse or complications, and, therefore, the temperature should be reported promptly and will need frequent checking.

When body temperature is elevated, the pulse and respiratory rates usually will be above normal also.

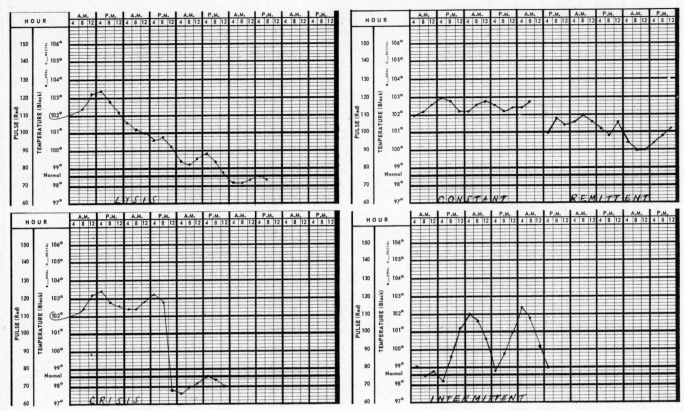

Fig. 8-4 Several types of fevers and methods by which an elevated temperature may return to normal.

Subnormal Body Temperature. A body temperature below the average normal range is called **hypothermia.** Death usually occurs when the temperature falls below approximately 34°C. (93.2°F.). However, cases of survival have been reported when body temperature has fallen considerably lower. There are some illnesses in which the patient typically has a subnormal temperature. Therefore, it is important to observe a patient closely when body temperature falls below normal average ranges.

Selecting a Site for Obtaining Body Temperature. Most agency policies specify the site to be used for obtaining the temperature. However, the nurse must use her judgment, especially when caring for patients in their homes where there is no set policy.

Oral temperatures are not recommended for unconscious and irrational patients and for infants and young children because of the danger of breaking the thermometer in the mouth. They are also not used for patients who breathe through their mouths, those with diseases or surgery of the nose or mouth, and those receiving oxygen through nasal tubes.

If the patient has had hot or cold foods or fluids, it is generally

Obtaining the vital signs

recommended that one should wait approximately 30 minutes before obtaining an oral temperature to allow time for the tissues in the mouth to return to normal temperature. It is also recommended that an oral temperature not be obtained while or directly after the patient has been smoking or chewing gum.

A rectal temperature is more accurate than an oral or axillary temperature. Some hospitals require rectal temperatures on all patients having an elevated temperature. It is usual procedure to obtain rectal temperatures for infants and small children, and for unconscious or mentally disturbed patients. If a patient's oral temperature shows a sudden change, it is a good idea to double check it by taking a rectal temperature. Rectal temperatures cannot be used when the patient has had rectal surgery, or is suffering from diarrhea or other diseases involving the rectum. Some health agencies do not recommend obtaining rectal temperatures on patients who have had a myocardial infarction (heart attack) because the thermometer may stimulate a nerve that affects the rate of heartbeat.

An axillary temperature is used only when both oral and rectal temperatures cannot be obtained. It is the least accurate way to obtain body temperature. Unless the patient is able to cooperate, the nurse will need to remain with him to hold the thermometer in place. If the axillary area has just been washed, taking the temperature should be delayed since the temperature of the water and the friction created by drying the skin may influence the temperature.

Chart 8-1 describes how to obtain an oral, a rectal, and an axillary temperature. Figures 8-5 through 8-7 illustrate how these temperatures are obtained.

Cleansing Glass Thermometers. In most health agencies, nurses are no longer required to clean and disinfect thermometers. Usually, thermometers are issued from a central supply unit. After being used, one thermometer for each patient, they are returned to the supply unit for cleaning and disinfection. In other agencies, thermometers are issued to patients upon admission, charged to the patients, and then sent home with them at the time of discharge. However, there are times when nurses are expected to clean and disinfect thermometers, especially when caring for patients in their homes. Chart 8-2 was prepared to help you with the procedure.

Heat sufficient to kill microorganisms will ruin thermometers by causing the mercury to expand beyond the column within the thermometer. Therefore, thermometers are disinfected with a chemical solution, as described in Chart 8-2 on page 124.

Pulse

The heart is a remarkable organ. In the average person's life, it beats millions of times. It rests for only a part of a second between each beat, and, except when certain heart diseases are present, it rarely misses a beat. Over a gallon of blood is estimated to be pumped from the heart every minute.

Chart 8-1 Obtaining body temperature

The purpose is to measure body temperature by three different methods

Oral Method

Suggested Action	Reason for Action	Figure to Illustrate
If thermometer has been stored in a chemical solution, rinse with water and wipe dry with a firm twisting motion, using clean soft tissue.	Chemical solution may irritate mucous membrane and have an objectionable odor or taste. Soft tissue and twisting motion help to contact entire surface of thermometer.	
Wipe once from bulb toward fingers with each tissue.	Wiping from an area where there are few or no organisms to an area where organisms may be present minimizes spread of organisms to cleaner areas.	
Grasp thermometer firmly with thumb and forefinger, and with snapping wrist movement, shake thermometer until mercury reaches lowest marking.	A constriction in the mercury line near bulb of thermometer prevents mercury from dropping below previous temperature reading unless thermometer is shaken forcefully.	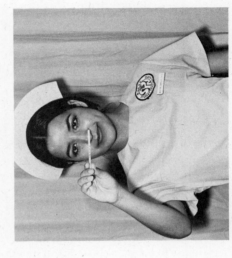
Read thermometer by holding it horizontally near eye level and turn it slowly between fingers until mercury line can be seen clearly.	Holding thermometer near eye level makes reading it easier. Turning thermometer will help to place mercury line in position where it can be read best.	Fig. 8-5 The nurse reads the thermometer by holding it near eye level and rotating it until mercury line is clearly seen.

Place the mercury bulb of thermometer under patient's tongue and in the right or left posterior pocket at the base of the tongue.

When bulb rests against surface blood vessels under tongue and mouth is closed, a measurement of body temperature can be obtained.

Leave thermometer in place seven to ten minutes.

Allowing sufficient time for oral thermometer to reach maximum temperature results in a more accurate measurement of body temperature. Pulse and respiratory rates are obtained while thermometer is in place.

Remove thermometer and wipe it once from fingers down to mercury bulb, using a firm twisting motion.

Mucus on thermometer may make it difficult to read. Cleansing from an area where there are few organisms to area where organisms may be present minimizes spread of organisms to cleaner areas. Friction from twisting motion helps loosen matter, such as mucus.

Read thermometer and shake it down as described above.

Dispose of tissue in receptacle used for contaminated items.

Confining contaminated articles helps to reduce spread of organisms.

Follow agency policy for handling thermometer after use.

Rectal Method

Rinse, wipe, and shake rectal thermometer as suggested in procedure for obtaining oral temperature.

Place lubricant on paper wipe and lubricate mercury bulb and an area about 1 inch above bulb.

Placing lubricant on wipe prevents contaminating lubricant supply. Lubricant reduces friction and thereby helps insert thermometer and minimizes irritation of mucous membrane of anal canal.

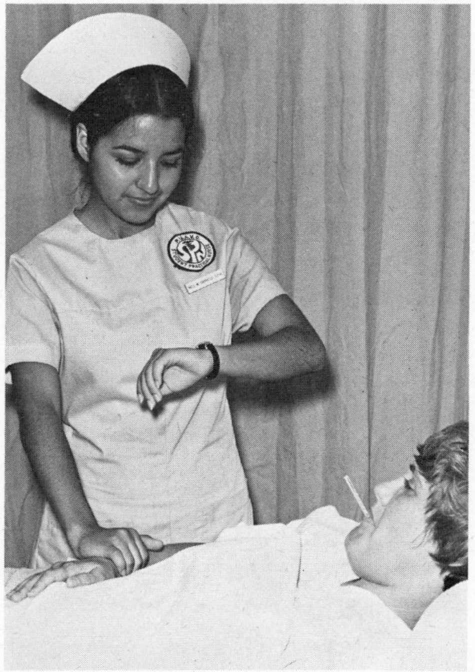

Fig. 8-6 While the thermometer is in place, the nurse counts the patient's pulse rate. She will then count the respiratory rate while still keeping her fingertips on the radial artery so that the patient is less likely to alter respirations voluntarily.

Chart 8-1 continued

Suggested Action	Reason for Action	Figure to Illustrate
With patient on his side, fold back bed linen and separate buttocks so that anal opening is seen clearly. Insert thermometer about 1½ inches. Permit buttocks to fall in place.	If thermometer is not placed directly into anal opening, bulb may injure tissue at opening, or hemorrhoids if present. Separating buttocks well makes anal opening easier to see.	
Leave thermometer in place for two to three minutes. Hold thermometer in place if patient is confused or restless or if patient is a child or infant.	Allowing sufficient time for thermometer to register results is a more accurate measurement of body temperature. Holding thermometer in place prevents accidents and prevents thermometer from sliding out of place.	
Remove thermometer and wipe it once from fingers to mercury bulb, using firm twisting motion.	Fecal matter on thermometer makes it difficult to read. Cleansing from an area where there are few organisms to area where organisms are numerous minimizes spread of organisms to cleaner area. Friction from twisting motion helps loosen matter, such as fecal material.	
Read and shake thermometer and dispose of wipe in receptacle for contaminated items.		
Follow agency policy for handling thermometer after use.		

Axillary Method

Rinse, wipe, and shake thermometer as for obtaining oral temperature.

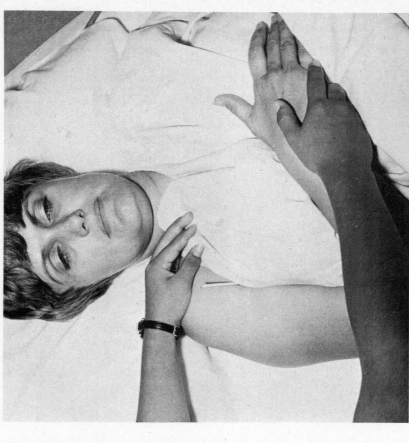

Fig. 8-7 Note the position of the thermometer, well down into the axillary space and pointing toward the patient's head. Bringing the patient's arm across her chest helps keep axillary tissue in good contact with the thermometer.

Place thermometer well into axilla with bulb directed toward patient's head. Bring patient's arm down close to his body and place his forearm over his chest.

When bulb rests against superficial blood vessels in axilla and skin surfaces are brought closely together to reduce air surrounding bulb, a reasonably accurate measurement of body temperature can be obtained.

Leave thermometer in place ten minutes or more.

Allowing sufficient time for thermometer to reach its highest temperature results in a reasonably accurate measurement of body temperature.

Remove thermometer and wipe it clean of perspiration in manner as described above. Read it and shake it down. Dispose of wipe in receptacle for contaminated items.

Follow agency policy for handling thermometer after use.

Chart 8-2 Cleansing and disinfecting the glass thermometer
The purpose is to cleanse and disinfect a glass thermometer that has been
used for obtaining a patient's temperature

Suggested Action	Reason for Action
Use a soft, clean tissue for wiping thermometer.	Material on thermometer interferes with disinfection. Soft tissue comes into close contact with all surfaces of thermometer.
Hold tissue at part of thermometer near fingers and wipe down toward bulb, using a twisting motion.	Cleansing an area where there are few microorganisms to an area where there are numerous microorganisms minimizes the spread of microorganisms to cleaner area. Friction helps to loosen material on thermometer.
Cleanse thermometer with soap or detergent solution, again using friction.	A soap or detergent solution and friction loosens material on thermometer.
Rinse thermometer under cold running water.	Cold water prevents breaking thermometer. Rinsing helps remove material loosened by washing. Certain chemical solutions are not effective in presence of soap—benzalkonium chloride (Zephiran Chloride) being an example.
Dry thermometer after rinsing it with water.	The strength of chemical solution is decreased when water is added to solution.
Place thermometer in chemical solution, as specified.	Chemical solutions must be used in proper strength for proper length of time to be effective.
Rinse thermometer with water after disinfection and before reuse.	Chemical solutions may irritate mucous membrane of mouth or rectum or skin in axillary area. Solutions may have an objectionable taste or odor.
Return thermometer to storage receptacle.	

Each time the heart beats, it forces blood into the arteries which causes the arterial walls to expand or distend. This creates a wave through the arterial walls which can be felt as a light tap by the fingertips. The sensation of this tap is called the **pulse.**

Usually, the artery on the inner side of the wrist is used for obtaining the pulse rate. This is the radial artery, and, therefore, the pulse rate obtained at the wrist is called the **radial pulse rate.** The radial artery is used most often because it is easy to reach and generally disturbs the patient the least. If it is not possible to obtain the pulse at the wrist, other arteries that also lie near the surface of the skin may be used. Figure 8-8 shows places where the pulse can be obtained with relative ease; it also shows a nurse counting the pulse rate at these different sites. Whichever site is used for obtaining the pulse rate, the nurse will wish to use one

Obtaining the vital signs

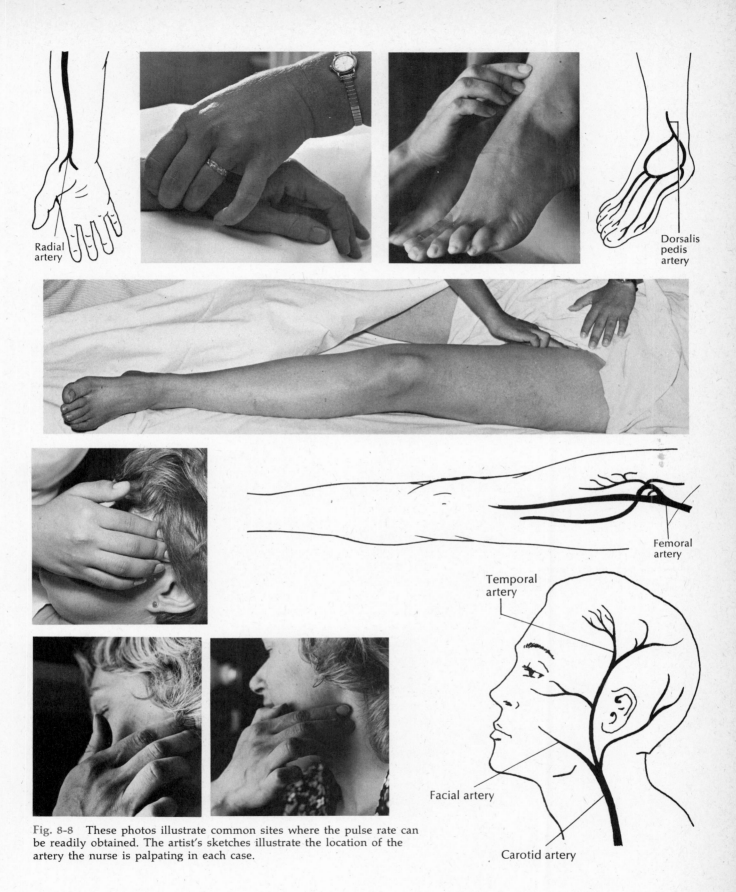

Fig. 8-8 These photos illustrate common sites where the pulse rate can be readily obtained. The artist's sketches illustrate the location of the artery the nurse is palpating in each case.

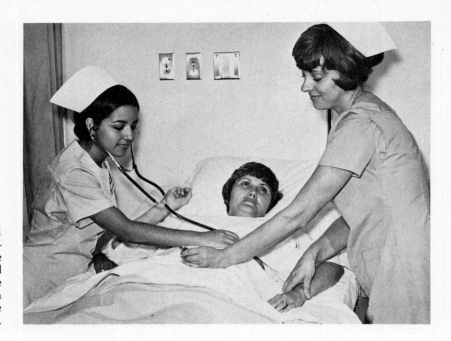

Fig. 8-9   To obtain an apical-radial pulse rate, one nurse, using a stethoscope, obtains the patient's apical pulse rate at the same time that a second nurse obtains the patient's radial pulse rate. Note that one nurse holds a watch which both nurses use for counting the pulse rates simultaneously.

that will disturb the patient as little as possible in order that the pulse rate will not be altered by the patient's moving or being uncomfortable.

There are times when it is difficult to count the pulse rate at the wrist, and when using other places on the body may be no more helpful. In such instances, the nurse may wish to place a stethoscope slightly below the level of the nipple on the chest to the left of the breastbone and over the tip, or apex, of the heart. A pulse rate obtained in this manner is called an **apical pulse rate.**

On occasion, the **apical-radial pulse rate** may be taken; that is, the apical and the radial pulse rate are taken at the same time. This requires two persons, one of whom listens over the tip of the heart while the other feels the pulse at the patient's wrist. They use one watch placed conveniently between them, decide on a specific time to start counting, and count for a full minute. If a difference is noted in the two pulse rates, the findings should be reported promptly. Figure 8-9 shows two nurses obtaining an apical-radial pulse rate.

Pulse Rate. On awakening in the morning, the pulse rate of the average healthy male is approximately 60 to 65 beats per minute. The rate for women is slightly faster—about seven to eight beats per minute more than for men. Pulse rates vary with age, gradually diminishing from birth to adulthood and then tending to increase somewhat in old age. It has been noted also that body size and build may affect pulse rate. Tall, slender persons often have a slower rate than short, stout ones. Wide variations in pulse rates have been noted in normal healthy adults. The American Heart Association accepts as normal for adults a pulse rate of between 50 and 100 beats per minute.

There are numerous causes for changes in pulse rate, for example, exercise, states of emotion (such as anger and fear), pain, and body temperature. In each of these examples, the rate tends to increase.

Diseases of the heart also usually influence pulse rate, as do some drugs and moderate to large losses of blood.

When the pulse rate is over 100 beats per minute, the condition is referred to as **tachycardia.** The term used to describe the pulse rate when it falls below 50 beats per minute is **bradycardia.** A slow pulse rate is less common during illness than a rapid pulse rate, but when either is present, the nurse will want to report the sign promptly.

Rhythm of the Pulse. Normally, the pulse rhythm is regular; that is, the time interval between heartbeats is equal. The force of the normal pulse, or the force of the tap felt on the fingertips, is also equal with each

Chart 8-3 Obtaining the radial pulse rate

The purpose is to count the number of times the heart beats each minute and to obtain an estimate of the quality of the heart's action

Suggested Action	Reason for Action
In lying position, have patient rest his arm alongside his body with wrist extended and palm of hand downward. In sitting position, have forearm at about a 90° angle to his body, rest arm on a support with wrist extended and palm of hand downward, as illustrated in Figure 8-8 on page 125.	These positions are ordinarily comfortable for patient and convenient for nurse. An uncomfortable position for patient may influence heart rate.
Place first, second, and third fingers along radial artery and press gently against bone at wrist (radius). Rest thumb on back of patient's wrist, as illustrated in Figure 8-8 on page 125.	Fingertips are sensitive to touch and will feel pulsation of patient's radial artery. If thumb is used for feeling patient's pulse, nurse may feel her own pulse.
Apply only enough pressure so that patient's pulsating artery can be felt distinctly.	Moderate pressure allows nurse to feel superficial radial artery expand and contract with each heartbeat. Too much pressure will shut off pulse. If too little pressure is applied, pulse will not be felt.
Using a watch with a second hand, count number of pulsations felt on patient's artery for minimum of one-half minute. Multiply this number by two to obtain rate for one minute.	Sufficient time is necessary to study rate, volume, and quality of pulse.
If pulse is abnormal in any way, count pulse rate for full minute. Repeat counting if necessary to determine accurate rate, quality, and volume.	When pulse is abnormal in any way, minimum of full minute countings are necessary to study rate, quality, and volume of pulse.

beat. Irregular pulse rhythm is called **arrhythmia.** An **intermittent pulse** is one that has a period of normal rhythm broken by periods of irregular rhythm. An intermittent rhythm may be a serious sign, such as in certain heart diseases, or it may be a simple condition due to being upset or frightened. An intermittent pulse rate and arrhythmia should be reported promptly.

Volume of the Pulse. Under normal conditions, the amount of blood pumped with each heartbeat remains constant. It should be relatively easy to stop the feel of the pulse wave by placing mild pressure on the artery with the fingertips. When this is not particularly easy to do, the pulse is called **bounding.** If the volume of blood is small and it is very easy to stop the feel of the pulse wave with pressure from the fingertips, the pulse is called **feeble, weak,** or **thready.** A patient with a thready pulse usually also has a rapid pulse. A feeble or bounding pulse should be reported promptly. Chart 8-3 describes how to obtain the radial pulse rate.

Respiration

Respiration is the act of breathing. **Inhalation,** or **inspiration,** is the act of breathing in, and **exhalation,** or **expiration,** is the act of breathing out. One act of respiration consists of one inhalation and one exhalation. Through the act of respiration, the body takes the oxygen it needs from the air and gets rid of carbon dioxide, a waste product of the body.

The respiratory center in the brain, which is very sensitive to the amount of carbon dioxide in the blood, controls respirations without our having to think about breathing. Nevertheless, we can also voluntarily control breathing to a certain extent. For example, a person automatically controls his breathing when talking, singing, laughing, crying, eating, and so on. He can also purposely take deep or shallow breaths. There are limitations, however, on how long a person can voluntarily hold his breath. When the body becomes desperate for lack of oxygen or for getting rid of carbon dioxide, the person will have to breathe sooner or later. A new mother, not realizing this, may panic when her child has a temper tantrum and holds his breath. The child will eventually breathe, whether he wants to or not.

Respiratory Rate. Normally, healthy adults breathe approximately 16 to 20 times a minute, although wider variations have been seen in well people. The respiratory rate is more rapid in infants and young children. It has been noted that the relationship between the pulse rate and the respiratory rate is fairly consistent in normal persons. The ratio is one respiration to approximately four heartbeats. An increased rate of respiration is often called **polypnea.**

During illness, the respiratory rate may vary from normal. For example, when body temperature is elevated, the respiratory rate tends to increase as the body tries to get rid of excess heat. There are certain illnesses, many of which you will be studying later in your nursing courses, that usually are associated with either rapid or slow breathing. Certain drugs influence the respiratory rate also. A respiratory rate of

Obtaining the vital signs

less than 8 or one of above 40 per minute is cause for alarm and should be reported promptly.

Respiratory Depth. Normally, the depth of each respiration is approximately the same for each person. The amount of air exchanged with each respiration, however, varies widely among different people. The depth of respiration is referred to as shallow or deep, depending on whether the volume of air taken is below or above normal for that person. Increased depth of respirations is often called **hyperpnea.**

Nature of Respiration. Ordinarily, breathing is automatic, and respirations are noiseless, regular, even, and without effort. Between each respiration, there is a short resting period.

Difficult breathing is called **dyspnea.** Dyspneic patients usually appear to be anxious and worried, and their faces are often drawn from the work of breathing. The nostrils will flare (widen) as the patient fights for his breath. The abdominal muscles may be used to assist in the act of breathing.

Dyspneic patients frequently find it easier to breathe when they stand or when they sit up in bed. This condition is called **orthopnea.** Some patients with dyspnea find the position illustrated in Figure 6-2 on page 75 comfortable. Others may prefer Fowler's position which is illustrated in Figure 12-19 on page 228.

Cheyne-Stokes respirations refer to breathing that consists of a gradual increase in the depth of respirations followed by a gradual decrease in the depth of respirations and then a period of no breathing, or **apnea.** Dyspnea is also usually present. Cheyne-Stokes respirations are a serious symptom and often occur as death approaches.

Breathing that is unusually noisy is referred to as **stertorous respirations.** A snoring sound is common.

Observation of the Patient. While the respiratory rate is being obtained, the color of the patient and his act of breathing should be noted. **Hypoxia** is present when the patient is not receiving an adequate supply of oxygen. **Anoxia** is commonly used as a synonym for hypoxia.

As a result of poor oxygen supply, the skin and the mucous membranes will appear bluish and the patient is said to be cyanotic. **Cyanosis** is defined as a bluish coloring of the skin and mucous membranes. It is more marked on the body where numerous small blood vessels lie close to the skin surface, as the nailbeds, the lips, the lobes of the ears, and the cheeks. When cyanosis is not marked, these may be the only areas appearing cyanotic. When cyanosis is marked, all areas of the body may appear bluish. In persons with dark skin, the color of the mucous membranes of the mouth and under the tongue should be examined. They will appear dusky when cyanosis is present. Chart 8-4 describes how to obtain the respiratory rate.

Blood pressure

Blood pressure measures a force. The force results when the heart beats and the blood vessels offer resistance to the blood being pushed out of

Chart 8-4 Obtaining the respiratory rate

The purpose is to obtain the respiratory rate per minute and
an estimate of the patient's respiratory status

Suggested Action	Reason for Action
While fingertips are still in place after counting pulse rate, observe patient's respirations.	Counting the respiratory rate while presumably still counting pulse keeps patient from becoming conscious of his breathing and possibly altering respiratory rate.
Note rise and fall of patient's chest with each inspiration and expiration.	A complete respiration consists of one inspiration and one expiration.
Using a watch with a second hand, count number of respirations for minimum of one-half minute. Multiply this number by two to obtain rate for one minute.	Sufficient time is necessary to observe rate, depth, and other characteristics of patient's respirations.
If respirations are abnormal in any way, count respiratory rate for full minute. Repeat if necessary to determine accurate rate and characteristics of respirations.	When respirations are abnormal in any way, minimum of full minute countings are necessary to make accurate observations of respiratory rate and quality.

the heart. If the vessels offered no resistance, the blood would leave the heart as water leaves the spout of a pump.

The most force or pressure on the arterial walls occurs when the heart pushes blood into the large artery leaving the heart. This vessel is called the aorta. The highest point of pressure in the arteries is called the **systolic pressure,** or **systole.** The lowest point, or the amount of pressure which is constantly present on the arterial walls, is called the **diastolic pressure,** or **diastole.**

Blood pressure is measured in millimeters of mercury, abbreviated mm. Hg. and recorded as follows: 120/80, 120 being the systolic pressure and 80 being the diastolic pressure.

Normal Blood Pressure. Studies of healthy persons show that blood pressure can be within a wide range and still be normal. Since individual differences can be considerable, it is important to know what the normal blood pressure for a particular person is. If there is a rise or fall of 20 to 30 mm. Hg. in a person's pressure, it is significant, even if it is well within the generally accepted range for normal.

The normal newborn infant has a systolic pressure of approximately 20 to 60 mm. Hg. Blood pressure increases gradually until adolescence when a more sudden rise occurs. At about 17 or 18 years of age, blood pressure reaches adult level. At age 20 a man's average, normal blood pressure is usually given as 120/80 mm. Hg. A steady but not great rise continues from then to old age in healthy individuals. For a young adult, a systolic pressure of 140 may be considered high, but for a person of 60 years of age, it may not arouse great concern. Having a consistently low blood pressure, for example, a systolic pressure of 90 to 105 mm. Hg. in

Obtaining the vital signs

an adult, seems to cause no harm. Rather, a lower than average blood pressure is usually associated with long life.

It has been found that nearly all persons will show normal changes within the course of a day. The blood pressure is usually lowest early in the morning before breakfast and before activity starts. The blood pressure has been noted to rise as much as 5 to 10 mm. Hg. by late afternoon, and it will gradually fall again during the sleeping hours.

Several factors may influence blood pressure. Age has already been mentioned. The sex of the person also influences blood pressure, with women usually having a lower blood pressure than men of the same age. Blood pressure tends to rise after eating and also during a period of exercise. Emotions, such as anger and fear, generally cause a rise in blood pressure. A person who is lying down will have a lower blood pressure as a rule than when he is sitting or standing, although the difference in most people may be insignificant. Pain and a full urinary bladder have also been seen to increase blood pressure.

Hypertension refers to an abnormally high blood pressure. **Hypotension** is abnormally low blood pressure.

Measuring Blood Pressure. A sphygmomanometer and a stethoscope are necessary to measure blood pressure. A **sphygmomanometer** is the instrument that measures the pressure. The **stethoscope** is an instrument that carries sounds from the body to the ear of the examiner.

The sphygmomanometer has a cuff that consists of an airtight, flat rubber bladder covered with cloth which extends beyond the bladder to various lengths. There are two tubes attached to the bag. One is connected to a manometer which registers the pressure, and the other is attached to a bulb that is used to inflate the bladder with air. A needle valve on the bulb allows the nurse to permit air to escape while pressure is being measured.

The cuff should be of a size that is appropriate for the patient. Otherwise, blood pressure may be inaccurately obtained. Cuffs of various sizes are available. For the average adult, a width of 12 to 14 cm., or approximately $4\frac{1}{2}$ to $5\frac{1}{2}$ inches, is usually satisfactory. Smaller ones are used for people with small arms and for children; larger ones are used for people with large arms or for use on the upper leg.

There are two types of manometers in common use, both of which are illustrated in Figure 8-10. One is a mercury gravity manometer which has a mercury-lined tube marked in millimeters. It is the type being used by the nurse in Figure 8-13. When the mercury rises in the tube, the upper or top surface of the mercury is slightly curved upward. The topmost point on the curved surface is called the **meniscus.** When determining blood pressure on the mercury manometer, the meniscus indicates the pressure. The meniscus of the mercury is read at eye level. If the meniscus is above eye level, the pressure reading will appear higher than it really is. Conversely, if the meniscus is below eye level, the pressure reading will appear lower than it really is. Figure 8-11 illustrates the meniscus.

The stethoscope is used to listen to the sound directly over the artery as the pressure in the cuff is released and the blood is permitted to flow through the vessel. The disc- or conelike construction in the tip of the

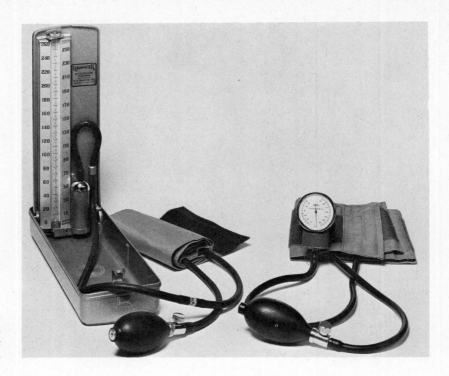

Fig. 8-10 (Left) A mercury manometer. (Right) An aneroid manometer. The cuffs on both are self-securing.

stethoscope magnifies the sounds in the artery, like a microphone. These sounds are transmitted by means of the tubing to the ear of the nurse. By listening to the sounds and watching the mercury column or dial, she obtains the blood pressure reading.

The nurse listens for a series of sounds when she obtains the patient's blood pressure. The first clear tapping sound when the blood first is able to flow through the compressed artery as air is released in the cuff is the systolic pressure. The sound then normally becomes louder. The next sound is muffled. The onset of the muffled sound is regarded as the best

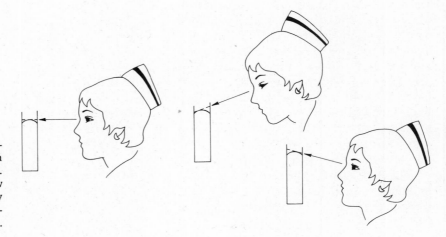

Fig. 8-11 The sketch on the left illustrates meniscus, the point at which a reading of pressure should be made. The remaining sketches illustrate how blood pressure readings could vary when the eye is at different levels in relation to the meniscus.

132   Obtaining the vital signs

Chart 8-5 Obtaining the blood pressure with a mercury manometer
The purpose is to measure the patient's systolic and diastolic blood pressure

Suggested Action	Reason for Action	Figure to Illustrate
Have patient in a comfortable lying or sitting position with the forearm supported and the palm upward, as illustrated in Figures 8-12 and 8-13.	This position places the brachial artery on the inner aspect of the elbow so that a stethoscope can rest on it conveniently.	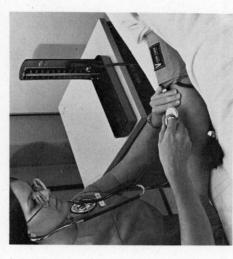
Place self so that meniscus of mercury can be read at eye level, and no more than 3 feet away.	If eye level is above or below meniscus, inaccurate readings occur. A distance of more than 3 feet will result in inaccurate reading.	
Place cuff so that inflatable bag is centered over brachial artery, approximately midway on arm so that lower edge of cuff is about 1 or 2 inches above anterior part of elbow as illustrated in Figures 8-12 and 8-13.	Pressure in cuff applied directly to artery will give most accurate readings. If cuff gets in way of stethoscope on anterior of elbow, readings are likely to be inaccurate.	Fig. 8-12 When obtaining the patient's blood pressure, the nurse feels for pulsation over the artery and then places the disc of the stethoscope directly over the area.

Chart 8-5 continued

Suggested Action	Reason for Action	Figure to Illustrate
Wrap cuff around arm smoothly, fasten securely or tuck end of cuff well under preceding wrapping.	A smooth cuff and wrapping produces equal pressure and thus an accurate reading.	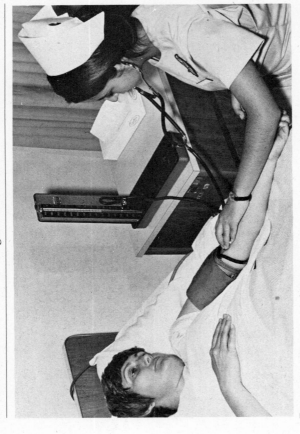
With fingertips, feel for pulse beat over artery. Place stethoscope cone or disc over artery where beat was felt, as illustrated in Figures 8-12 and 8-13.	Having stethoscope directly over artery makes more accurate readings possible.	
Pump bulb of manometer until mercury rises approximately 20 to 30 mm. Hg. above point where it is expected that systolic pressure will be. (Lack of blood in patient's arm may cause temporary tingling and numb sensation.)	Pressure in cuff now prevents blood from flowing through artery.	Fig. 8-13 The nurse obtains blood pressure after making sure that the patient is comfortable. The nurse sits comfortably and keeps her eyes on the mercury manometer as she listens for the characteristic sounds of systole and diastole.

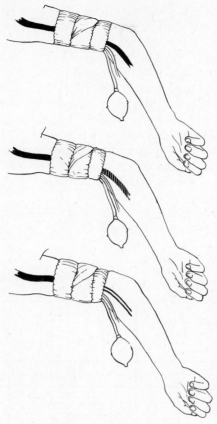

Fig. 8-14 (Left) When the cuff has been inflated sufficiently, it will prevent the flow of blood into the forearm. No sound will be heard through the stethoscope at this time. (Center) When pressure in the cuff is reduced sufficiently for the blood to begin flowing through the brachial artery, the first sound is recorded as the systolic pressure. (Right) As the pressure in the cuff continues to be released, the muffled sound heard through the stethoscope is the diastolic pressure. At this time blood flows through the brachial artery freely.

Using valve on bulb, release air 2 to 3 mm. Hg. per heartbeat and note on manometer point at which first sound is heard. Record this figure as systolic pressure.

Continue to release air in cuff evenly and gradually. Note reading on manometer when muffling sound is heard. Record this figure as diastolic pressure.

Allow remaining air to escape quickly, remove cuff, and cleanse and store equipment according to agency policy.

Systolic pressure is that point at which blood in artery is first able to force its way through vessel against pressure exerted by cuff of manometer.

Diastolic pressure is that point at which blood flows easily in brachial artery and is approximately equivalent to amount of pressure normally present on walls of arteries when heart is at rest.

index of diastolic pressure, according to the American Heart Association. The last phase occurs when sounds can no longer be heard. At this point, the blood flows freely through the blood vessels.

Chart 8-5 describes how to obtain the blood pressure, using the arm and a mercury manometer. Figure 8-14 illustrates the effect of the pressure cuff on the artery in the arm (see pp. 133–135).

Blood pressure may also be obtained in the thigh by using a larger cuff. The patient lies on his abdomen and the cuff is applied with the compression bag over the back side of the middle of thigh. The stethoscope is placed over the artery in back of the knee, called the popliteal space. The systolic pressure usually is a little higher when measured in the thigh than when measured in the arm, but the diastolic pressure is about the same.

The technique for obtaining blood pressure in children and infants is like that used for adults. If an infant is crying, the systolic pressure may

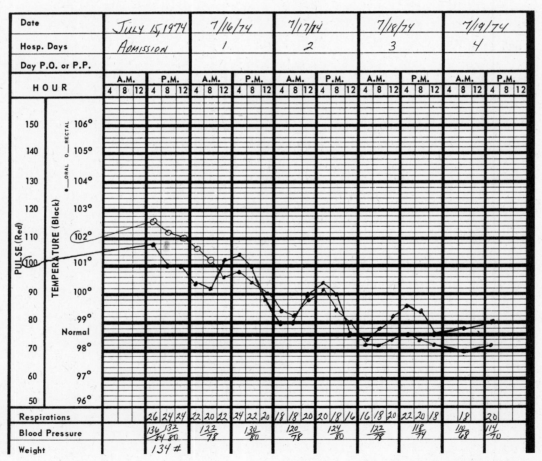

Fig. 8-15   An illustration of how the vital signs are usually recorded.

Obtaining the vital signs

be elevated. In such instances, it may be necessary to obtain the blood pressure reading when the child is asleep. It is important to use an appropriate-sized cuff for children and infants. The chief source of error is using a poorly-sized cuff.

If it becomes necessary to repeat the procedure in order to be sure an accurate blood pressure reading is obtained, the nurse allows all of the air to escape from the cuff and waits a few minutes before inflating the cuff again. This permits circulation to return to normal.

If a patient is to have frequent blood pressure readings and the cuff is left in place, it is necessary to check to see that it has not rotated out of position before taking the next reading. It is important to make certain that the cuff cannot be inflated accidently between readings.

There are electronic instruments now available for measuring blood pressure. According to the manufacturers, accurate blood pressure readings are available in a matter of seconds.

Recording the vital signs

The manner in which vital signs are recorded depends on the health agency's policies. Different agencies use different forms and the nurse will use what is provided. Figure 8-15 is an example of a form used to record vital signs.

If anything unusual is observed while the nurse obtains the vital signs, she will wish to report this and record according to policy. For example, she may describe her observations in the nurses' notes. Many terms used to describe the vital signs were defined in this chapter. While it is important to be familiar with these terms, it is recommended in some hospitals that a particular observation be described, rather than summarized in a term. This tends to avoid confusion, should the nurse or the person reading the nurses' notes not be familiar with a particular term. For example, if the patient is breathing very deeply, the nurse would record the fact as such rather than noting that the patient has hyperpnea.

Electrocardiography

The **electrocardiograph** is an instrument that measures and records the actions of the heart. The record produced by the electrocardiograph is called the **electrocardiogram.** It is abbreviated EKG or ECG. Obtaining and reading the electrocardiogram requires skill and practice. It is an invaluable tool to study the heart. For nurses working with patients having heart diseases and with patients in intensive care and coronary care units, considerable study and practice are necessary. Figure 8-16 illustrates a normal electrocardiogram. The horizontal lines represent the measurement of voltage while the vertical lines measure time.

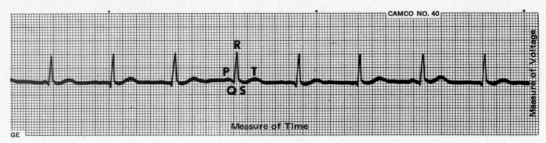

Fig. 8-16 A normal electrocardiogram. (From Sharp, L. N. and Rabin, B., *Nursing in the Coronary Care Unit.* Philadelphia, J. B. Lippincott Company, 1970)

Conclusion

The vital signs are important in helping to study the patient's condition. Nurses are almost always responsible for obtaining the vital signs and are expected to be highly skilled in obtaining and recording them accurately.

References

Beaumont, Estelle, "Blood Pressure Equipment," *Nursing '75,* 5:56–62, January 1975.

Blainey, Carol Gohrke, "Site Selection in Taking Body Temperature," *American Journal of Nursing,* 74:1859–1861, October 1974.

"Caffeine and Fever," *Time,* 100:56, October 2, 1972.

"Electronic Sphygmomanometer," *American Journal of Nursing,* 72:131, January 1972.

"Equipment Review: Electronic Thermometers," *Nursing Update,* 5:1, 3–9, November 1974.

Foley, Mary F., "Variations in Blood Pressure in the Lateral Recumbent Position," *Nursing Research,* 20:64–69, January-February 1971.

Graas, Suzanne, "Thermometer Sites and Oxygen," *American Journal of Nursing,* 74:1862–1863, October 1974.

Lee, Richard V. and Atkins, Elisha, "Spurious Fever," *American Journal of Nursing,* 72:1094–1095, June 1972.

Meehan, Marjorie, "EKG Primer," (Programmed Instruction) *American Journal of Nursing,* 71:2195–2202, November 1971.

Nichols, Glennadee A., "Taking Adult Temperatures: Rectal Measurements," *American Journal of Nursing,* 72:1092–1093, June 1972.

———— and Kucha, Deloros H., "Taking Adult Temperatures: Oral Measurements," *American Journal of Nursing,* 72:1090–1093, June 1972.

Schmidt, Alice J., "TPR's: An Old Habit or a Significant Routine?" *Hospitals, Journal of the American Hospital Association*, 46:57–60, December 16, 1972.

Sparks, Colleen, "Peripheral Pulses," *American Journal of Nursing*, 75:1132–1133, July 1975.

Tate, Gayle V., et al, "Correct Use of Electric Thermometers," *American Journal of Nursing*, 70:1898–1899, September 1970.

Warren, Freda M., "Doing It Better: Blood Pressure Readings: Getting Them Quickly on an Infant," *Nursing 75*, 5:13, April 1975.

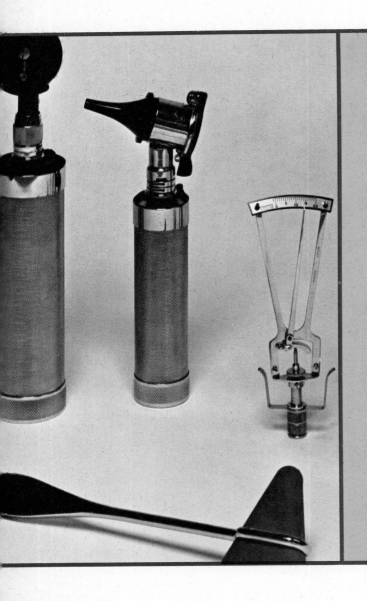

9 the physical examination

behavioral objectives

When mastery of content in this chapter is reached, the student will be able to

Define terms appearing in the glossary.

List four purposes of the physical examination.

Describe information commonly found in the patient's health history.

List two examples of each of the following kinds of symptoms: objective; subjective; prodromal; constitutional; and local.

List common equipment and supplies used during a physical examination.

Identify instruments commonly used during the physical examination and demonstrate how each one operates.

Describe how a patient is prepared for a physical examination and how he is cared for after the examination.

Demonstrate how to place and drape a patient in each of these positions: prone; erect; dorsal recumbent; lithotomy; left and right Sims'; and knee-chest, or genupectoral.

List one or two common normal and abnormal findings of each part of the body that can be observed during a physical examination.

State common responsibilities of the nurse when she assists the physician during a physical examination.

Demonstrate how to record information concerning a physical examination according to policy in the agency where the nurse gives care.

glossary

Audiometer An instrument to gauge and record the power of hearing.

Auscultation Listening to sounds within the body.

Cardiovascular Pertaining to the heart and blood vessels.

Constitutional Symptoms Symptoms produced by the effect of a disease on the whole body.

Dehydration The lack of a normal

glossary cont.

amount of body fluid causing the skin to be loose and wrinkled and to feel dry.

Diaphoresis Excessive perspiration.

Disoriented Being unaware of time, place, and one's surroundings.

Distention Swelling or expansion of a part.

Dorsal Recumbent Position The patient is on his back; his legs are separated; the soles of his feet are flat on the bed; and his knees are bent.

Ecchymosis The collection of blood in tissues causing the skin to have a purplish color.

Edema The retention of fluid in tissues.

Emotion A strong feeling, such as love, hate, or fear.

Erect Position The normal standing position.

Expectoration Sputum.

Flatus Gas in the stomach and intestines.

Flush Redness of the skin, as in a blush.

Genupectoral Position The patient rests on his knees and chest with his body bent at approximately a 90° angle. Synonym for knee-chest position.

Head Mirror A mirror worn on the examiner's head to direct light into an area.

Horizontal Recumbent Position The patient lies flat in bed on his back.

Incoherent Disconnected thought or speech.

Inspection Using the eyes to observe.

Jaundice Yellowness of the skin.

Knee-Chest Position The patient rests on his knees and chest with his body bent at approximately a 90° angle. Synonym for genupectoral position.

Lithotomy Position Same as the dorsal recumbent position except that the feet are supported in stirrups.

Local Symptom A symptom limited to a particular part of the body.

Mucus A watery secretion produced by mucuous membranes.

Neurological Pertaining to the nervous system.

Objective Symptom A symptom pre-sented by one person that can be observed by another person.

Ophthalmoscope An instrument used for observing the interior of the eye.

Oriented Being aware of time, place, and one's surroundings.

Otoscope An instrument used for observing the eardrum and external ear canal.

Palpation Feeling or pressing on a part of the body.

Pap Test An examination of secretions from the uterus and cervix to determine whether cancer cells are present. The word Pap is from Papanicolaou, the name of the physician who devised the test.

Percussion Striking or tapping an area of the body.

Prodromal Symptom A symptom appearing before a disease develops.

Prosthesis An artificial part used in place of a natural part of the body which has been removed.

Purulent Drainage A discharge containing pus.

Quadrant One-fourth of a whole.

Rash An eruption on the skin.

Responsive Able to answer with a word and/or a gesture.

Sanguineous Drainage A discharge containing blood.

Serosanguineous Drainage A discharge containing both serum and blood.

Serous Drainage A discharge containing the clear portion of the blood, or serum.

Serum The clear portion of blood.

Sims' Position, Right or Left The patient is on his right or left side; his top knee is sharply bent onto his abdomen; his lower knee is less sharply bent.

Speculum An instrument used for opening a cavity so that it can be examined.

Sputum A substance from the mouth containing saliva and mucus.

Stirrups Foot supports used when the patient is in the lithotomy position.

The physical examination

Subjective Symptom A symptom that can be felt and described by one person but cannot be directly observed by another person.

Tonometer An instrument used to measure pressure within the eyeball.

Umbilicus Navel.

Unconscious Lacking the ability to respond to one's surroundings.

Unresponsive Unable to answer when spoken to.

Wound A break in the skin.

introduction

Many people now recognize that a regular physical examination is an important part of health care. Most authorities recommend having at least one every year. The physical examination serves various purposes. It is an excellent way to help people stay well, for it is a time when health practitioners can teach patients the importance of following healthful living habits. The physician may include in the physical examination protection of the patient from certain diseases. For example, a physical examination will often include giving the patient a vaccine to prevent poliomyelitis if he has not already been protected. Having regular examinations helps to find early signs of illness which can usually be treated with greater ease and effectiveness. Also, findings of the examination assist in guiding care that the patient may need.

There is no one correct way for doing a physical examination. Most health agencies have a physical examination form which serves as a guide and also is used for recording findings.

The patient's health history

Before doing a physical examination, most physicians will have taken the patient's health history. If the patient is in a hospital, the history usually has been taken before admission. If it has not, the patient's physician or an intern on the hospital staff will take it, usually shortly after admission. A nurse is ordinarily not present when the health history is taken. However, if the physician does not mind and when time permits, attending the health history interview is a good way for the nurse to learn to know the patient better.

The health history ordinarily includes a description of the patient's present complaints and illness, his past illnesses and how they were cared for, and the health history of the patient's parents. A member of the nursing team, usually its leader, may also interview the patient. She is interested in learning present and past problems so that she can plan better nursing care for the patient.

Physicians rely on information from the patient's health history, as well as from the physical examination, to diagnose and to prescribe treatment. Nurses also use this information to plan care. With this kind of knowledge, both physicians and nurses can plan medical and nursing care to meet each patient's individual needs.

Methods to gather information during the physical examination

There are various ways to gather information during the physical examination. **Inspection,** that is, using the eyes to observe, is most commonly used. Chapter 3 discussed observation. It was pointed out that when a nurse and patient are together, observing the patient for signs, symptoms, and nonverbal communication is important.

Percussion means striking or tapping a particular part of the body, either with the fingertips or with a rubber hammer. The examiner listens to the sound when using percussion. For instance, if fluid or a mass is present in the chest, the sound will be dull. Normally, a hollow sound will be heard when the examiner strikes the chest wall.

Palpation uses the sense of touch. The examiner feels or presses on the body. For example, palpation is used when the abdomen is examined to feel the various abdominal organs, and the breasts are palpated to learn whether lumps are present.

Auscultation uses the sense of hearing. Using the stethoscope, the examiner is able to listen to sounds within the body, such as heart sounds.

Many different instruments are used to assist with the physical examination. The stethoscope and percussion hammer have already been mentioned. The thermometer and the scale are also used. There are still more, many of which will be described and illustrated later in this and other chapters.

Chapter 3 discussed the importance of listening carefully to what patients have to say. Listening is an important part of the physical examination as well as of the patient's health history.

There are common terms used to describe signs and symptoms the patient has. A **subjective symptom** is one that is felt and described by the patient. It cannot be observed directly by another person. Pain is a subjective symptom which can be felt and described only by the person who has it.

An **objective symptom** is one that can be seen by another person. A skin rash and a swelling someplace on the body, such as at the ankles, are objective symptoms.

A **constitutional symptom** is one that is produced by the effect of a disease on the whole body. Fever is a typical constitutional symptom of most infectious diseases, as for example, measles, mumps, and chicken pox.

A **prodromal symptom** is one that is noticed before illness develops. Common prodromal symptoms of the flu include feeling achy and out of sorts.

A **local symptom** is one limited to a particular part of the body. A swollen jaw, or redness and swelling around a sprained ankle are local symptoms.

The study of specimens contributes a great deal to the physical examination, as do x-rays and electrocardiograms. The nurse's duties in relation to collecting specimens will be discussed later in this book, wherever appropriate, as will her responsibilities when certain x-rays are to be taken. The electrocardiogram was discussed in Chapter 8 on page 137.

Preparation for a physical examination

The physical examination is often done in an examining room. Or, if the patient is at home or in a hospital, it may be done in the patient's room. Most health agencies have a tray or basket for equipment ordinarily used during a physical examination. Although there are differences among agencies, the items listed below are usually kept in readiness. Some of them are illustrated in Figure 9-1.

Ophthalmoscope An instrument used for observing the interior of the eye.

Otoscope An instrument for observing the eardrum and external ear canal.

Speculum An instrument used for opening a cavity so that it may be more easily examined. A nose and a vaginal speculum are necessary.

Tonometer An instrument used to measure the pressure within the eyeball. A mild anesthetic solution applied directly to the surface of the eye with an eyedropper is used before examining with a tonometer.

Head mirror The mirror worn on the examiner's head to direct light into an area, such as into the throat.

The following items may also be used:

Sphygmomanometer	Stethoscope
Flashlight	Tongue depressors
Tape measure	Tuning forks
Skin pencil	Tissues and waste container
Sterile or clean gloves	Lubricant
Paper towels	Waste container for
Percussion hammer	soiled instruments
Material for draping	Patient's gown
Disposable pad	Lightweight blanket

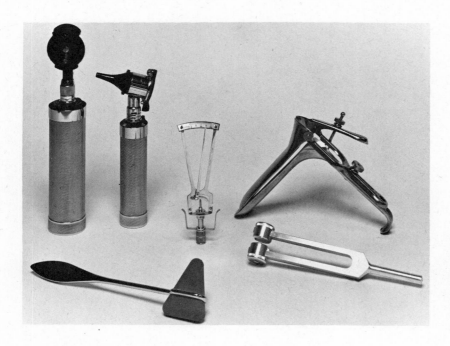

Fig. 9-1 These are instruments often used during the physical examination. From left to right, top: ophthalmoscope, otoscope with speculum attached, tonometer, vaginal speculum. Lower left: percussion hammer. Lower right: tuning fork. Tuning forks are made in various sizes.

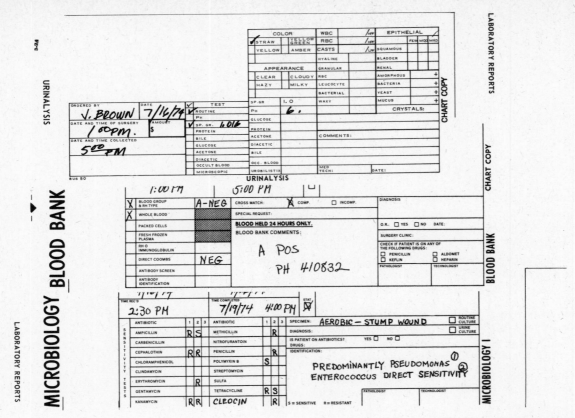

Fig. 9-2 An example of a form used for laboratory reports. Each specimen has its own color-coded slip on which laboratory findings are entered. The slips are then attached to the report form, thus eliminating copying laboratory findings onto the record.

Containers and slides for specimens, as indicated Pins, cotton, test tubes for hot and cold water, and various materials having different odors are included if a neurological examination is to be done.

As part of a physical examination, several laboratory tests usually are done. Each agency has its own policies concerning such items as the type of container for the specimen; how the specimen is to be labeled; the laboratory to which the specimen is sent; and so on. The nurse's duties in relation to specimen collection will vary. She will wish to have containers and slides available as necessary. The collection of certain specimens and common laboratory findings are discussed later in this text. Laboratory test results become a part of the patient's record. Figure 9-2 illustrates an example of laboratory reports.

The nurse will wish to have material available for draping the patient.

Some agencies use disposable paper drapes. However, a bath blanket, a drawsheet, or a bed sheet can be used. The purpose for draping is to avoid exposing the patient except for the part being examined. A lightweight blanket is handy should the patient become chilly. This is particularly necessary when the patient is very ill or elderly.

The patient should wear a hospital gown that opens up the back, if possible, because it is easier to examine him in this type of gown.

Before a physical examination, the patient is given an opportunity to go to the bathroom. A urine specimen is collected at this time if necessary, as was described in Chapter 7. If the patient needs a urinal in bed or a bedpan, the procedure described in Chapter 10 is followed. It is difficult to palpate the abdomen when the urinary bladder is full, or to do a rectal examination if the patient needs to have a bowel movement. Also, using the bathroom before the examination generally helps the patient feel more at ease.

Positioning and draping the patient

There are several common positions used when a physical examination is done. These are illustrated in Figure 9-3.

The **erect position** is the normal standing position. The patient wears slippers, or the floor is protected with paper towels. The draping is arranged so that the body outlines, posture, muscles, and extremities can be inspected conveniently.

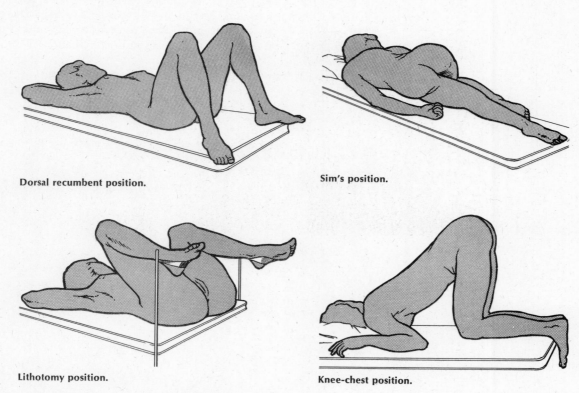

Dorsal recumbent position.

Sim's position.

Lithotomy position.

Knee-chest position.

Fig. 9-3 Commonly used examining positions.

In the **horizontal recumbent position,** the patient lies flat on his back with his legs together, in bed or on the examining table. His head is supported with a small pillow, and his legs may be bent slightly to help relax muscles in the abdomen. He is covered with a drape. Parts of the drape are folded back to expose the area being examined. This position is used most commonly for examination of the abdomen, anterior chest, breasts, reflexes, extremities, head, neck, eyes, ears, nose, and throat.

In the **dorsal recumbent position,** the patient is brought close to the edge of the bed while lying on his back with his legs separated and knees bent. Or, he may be in the center of the bed. The patient's buttocks may tend to sink into the mattress, making examination difficult. This is more likely to happen when the patient is heavy. A simple solution for elevating the hips is to place a bedpan, upside down and back to front, under the patient. The bedpan is protected with an appropriate cover. The soles of the feet rest flat on the bed or table. One pillow may be placed under the head. A drape is placed diagonally over the patient. Opposite corners protect the legs and are wrapped around the feet so that the drape will stay in place. The third corner is placed between the legs. A disposable pad may be placed under the patient's buttocks to avoid soiling linen. The corner of the drape between the patient's legs is raised and folded back on the abdomen to expose the part being examined. This draping is illustrated in Figure 9-4.

The **lithotomy position** is the same as the dorsal recumbent position except that the patient is on a table equipped with foot supports, called **stirrups.** The patient's buttocks are brought to the edge of the table. The knees are bent and the feet are supported in the stirrups. A disposable pad may be placed under the patient's buttocks. Draping is the same as for the dorsal recumbent position. The lithotomy and the dorsal recumbent positions are used most commonly for examination of the rectum and vagina.

In the left **Sims' position,** the patient lies on his left side and rests his left arm behind his body. The right arm is forward with the elbow bent,

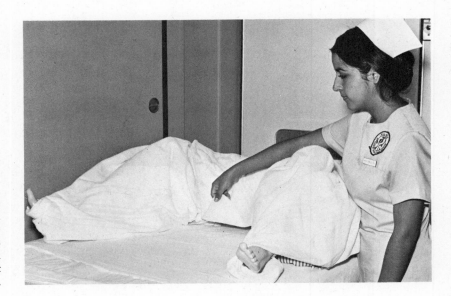

Fig. 9-4   The mannequin, placed in the dorsal recumbent position, is draped with a bath blanket. The corner of the blanket between the mannequin's legs is raised and placed over the abdomen when the examiner is ready to inspect the exposed area.

The physical examination

and the arm resting on a pillow placed under the patient's head. The patient's body is bent slightly forward. The knees are bent, the right one sharply on the abdomen and the left one less sharply. In the right Sims' position, the patient lies on his right side. A disposable pad may be used under the buttocks. One corner of the drape is folded back on the patient's hip to expose the area being examined. This position usually is used for examination of the rectum or vagina.

In the **knee-chest** or **genupectoral position,** the patient rests on his knees and chest with his body bent approximately 90°, or in a right angle, at the hips. The head, turned to one side, rests on a small pillow. A pillow also may be placed under the chest. The arms are above the head, or, they may be bent at the elbows and rest alongside the patient's head. The drape is placed so that the patient's back, buttocks, and thighs are covered. Only the area to be examined is exposed. The position is commonly used for examining the rectum. It is a very difficult position for most patients, especially for the elderly. Therefore, the nurse should have all equipment in readiness, and she should not assist the patient into position until the examiner is to begin.

Certain examining positions are embarrassing to some patients. The examination can be made easier for the patient if the nurse takes every precaution to prevent exposure and to give careful explanations and directions. Even when a patient is properly draped, there may be concern that someone can see or enter the unit. The nurse should make every attempt to see that this does not happen.

Obtaining the vital signs

Chapter 8 discussed how to obtain the vital signs. Vital signs are an important part of every physical examination. In most instances, it is the nurse's responsibility to obtain the vital signs. Usually, this is done before the patient is made ready for the physical examination.

Observing the patient's general mental state

While observing the patient physically, the nurse will also wish to note his general mental state. Below are some common terms used to describe a patient's mental state.

To be **oriented** means to be aware of time, place, and one's surroundings; to be **disoriented** is the opposite. The word, confusion, is sometimes used to describe a condition of mental bewilderment. A **responsive** patient answers by word, or gesture, or both, while the **unresponsive** patient appears to be unaware of his surroundings and unable to answer when spoken to. The word, **incoherent,** describes disconnected thought or speech. The thoughts are unrelated and the listener is unable to make sense from what is being said. The **unconscious** patient lacks the ability to respond to anything about him. When using such terms, it is helpful to describe what the patient actually says or does, or does not say or do. These are some examples: "Could not answer when asked today's date, and city where he was"; "Answered all questions"; "Spoke of relative who has been dead for years as if he were alive"; or "Speaks in phrases which have no apparent relationship to each other."

An **emotion** is a strong feeling, such as fear, hate, anger, grief, joy, and love. Terms like anxious, frightened, unconcerned, resentful, uncooperative, and so on are often used to describe emotions. However, they may be defined differently among health and nursing team members. Therefore, it is better to record the behavior the nurse observes. Here are examples: "Face and extremity muscles tense, jaw set, hands clenched, perspiring heavily"; "Moves frequently about room, talking rapidly"; or, "Told physician he was sick and tired of examinations."

Measuring the patient's height and weight

It is common practice to measure the patient's height and weight upon admission or as part of the physical examination. Even though he may have been weighed recently at home, it is best to weigh him again. This makes it possible to do weight comparisons while using the same scale. The patient's height is measured at the same time. He should be asked to remove his robe and shoes. It is good medical asepsis to place a paper towel on the scale before the patient stands on it with his bare feet and to use a clean towel for each patient.

The patient is assisted onto the scale. The scale is balanced and then read, and the weight is recorded. To obtain height, the nurse asks the patient to stand straight. The height measuring bar is moved down until it lightly touches the top of the head. The height is then read and recorded.

Measuring the patient's height and weight may be delayed if he is too ill, unless it is necessary to know the weight because of a type of treatment being used. To make weighing easier for very ill patients, some agencies have portable or bed scales. The scale can be rolled to the patient's bedside where he can be assisted or lifted onto it.

Many factors influence what is normal weight, such as age, body build, height, and sex. Therefore, it is difficult to determine where abnormality begins. Many authorities accept a 10 to 15 per cent variation from the average described in weight tables as being within normal limits. Table 9-1 gives desirable weights for adults.

The nurse will wish to be aware of signs or comments that suggest the patient is having unusual weight losses or gains, either of which may be an important diagnostic symptom.

Examining various parts of the body

Examining the Skin, Hair, and Nails. Since the skin covers almost the entire surface of the body, it tells a great deal about a person's state of health. In addition to its general appearance, such as smooth, wrinkled, or dry, the nurse also is interested in signs of injury or lack of good care. Examples include bruises, scratches, cuts, insect bites, and sores. All wounds on a patient are treated with great care in order to

Table 9-1 Desirable weights for adults

	Height with shoes on 1-inch heels		Weight in pounds according to frame in indoor clothing		
	Feet	Inches	Small frame	Medium frame	Large frame
Men of ages 25 and over	5	2	112–120	118–129	126–141
	5	3	115–123	121–133	129–144
	5	4	118–126	124–136	132–148
	5	5	121–129	127–139	135–152
	5	6	124–133	130–143	138–156
	5	7	128–137	134–147	142–161
	5	8	132–141	138–152	147–166
	5	9	136–145	142–156	151–170
	5	10	140–150	146–160	155–174
	5	11	144–154	150–165	159–179
	6	0	148–158	154–170	164–184
	6	1	152–162	158–175	168–189
	6	2	156–167	162–180	173–194
	6	3	160–171	167–185	178–199
	6	4	164–175	172–190	182–204

	Height with shoes on 2-inch heels		Weight in pounds according to frame in indoor clothing		
	Feet	Inches	Small frame	Medium frame	Large frame
Women of ages 25 and over	4	10	92– 98	96–107	104–119
	4	11	94–101	98–110	106–122
	5	0	96–104	101–113	109–125
	5	1	99–107	104–116	112–128
	5	2	102–110	107–119	115–131
	5	3	105–113	110–122	118–134
	5	4	108–116	113–126	121–138
	5	5	111–119	116–130	125–142
	5	6	114–123	120–135	129–146
	5	7	118–127	124–139	133–150
	5	8	122–131	128–143	137–154
	5	9	126–135	132–147	141–158
	5	10	130–140	136–151	145–163
	5	11	134–144	140–155	149–168
	6	0	138–148	144–159	153–173

For women between 18 and 25, subtract 1 pound for each year under 25.
Courtesy of the Metropolitan Life Insurance Company

avoid transfer of infection. Because of the danger of infections, newly admitted patients with open or draining wounds are checked carefully. In many agencies, a specimen of drainage is taken. The patient may be placed on special precautions until the laboratory reports are complete. Such precautionary measures are discussed in Chapter 22.

Fingernails and toenails are also indications of the patient's general condition. Brittle or dry nails may be a clue to the patient's state of nutrition or to a state of illness.

The condition of the hair is also a clue to the person's state of health. It is not uncommon for the hair to lose its gloss and texture or even fall out during periods of illness.

The following are some terms used to describe the skin. **Flush** is a redness of the skin, as in a blush. It is usually present when the temperature is elevated. The face and neck are more likely to be affected than other parts of the body.

Cyanosis was defined and discussed in Chapter 8. The nurse will wish to be aware of it when it is present.

Jaundice is a yellowness of the skin. Often, it affects the entire body but almost always the whites of the eyes are affected.

Dehydration is a lack of normal amounts of fluid in body tissues. The skin appears to be loose and wrinkled and to feel dry. Typically, the lips and tongue are dry and parched.

A **rash** is an eruption of the skin. Rashes are common signs of skin disease which are discussed in other courses in nursing. The nurse should indicate exactly where on the patient's body a rash is noticed and its general appearance.

Ecchymosis is a collection of blood in body tissues. It causes the skin to have a purplish color. The nurse should note the location, size, and coloring of bruises when they are present.

Diaphoresis is an excessive amount of perspiration, as when a person's entire skin is moist and perspiring.

Edema means retaining fluid in the tissues. It will cause swelling, for example, when present in the arms, legs, feet, and hands. It may also occur in body cavities. The skin appears tight over the swollen areas. If the fingers are pressed gently into the areas, an impression may remain after pressure has been released.

A **wound** is a break in the skin. The size, shape, depth, and location of the wound should be described. If drainage is present, it too is described as to amount and character, for example, scant, moderate, or profuse. Common terms for describing its appearance are as follows:

Serous Containing **serum,** or the clear portion of the blood.
Sanguineous Containing a great deal of blood.
Serosanguineous Containing both serum and blood.
Purulent Containing or consisting of pus.

Examining the Head and Neck. The shape of the head is noted. Occasionally, the examiner may wish to measure the size of the head with a tape measure. Facial expressions and the condition of the hair and the scalp are noted. The head and neck are palpated for lumps. The organs in the neck (thyroid gland, larynx, and trachea) are palpated.

Examining the Eyes, Ears, and Nose. Eyelids and eyeballs are inspected, and movements of the eyes are noted. A flashlight may be used to determine how the pupils react to light. The inside of the eyeball is inspected with the aid of an ophthalmoscope. Unless there is reason for a detailed examination of sight, test charts are not used for the routine physical examination.

A tonometer is used to test pressure within the eye. Testing pressure within the eye annually is often recommended for patients over 35 or 40 years of age. However, very often, this part of the examination is performed by an ophthalmologist, that is, a physician specializing in the care and treatment of the eye. An increase in pressure is a symptom of glaucoma. If not treated, it often leads to blindness.

If the patient's sight is limited, this should be noted since it will be important when planning nursing care. For example, the patient may need assistance with eating and with personal care.

The general shape of the ears is inspected. The external canal and the eardrum are observed with the aid of an otoscope; or, an ear speculum and head mirror may be used. The bony area behind the ear is palpated and inspected. Tuning forks are sometimes used to test hearing. The most accurate way to test hearing is with an **audiometer,** an instrument for gauging and recording the power of hearing. Unless there is indication for careful study of hearing, an audiometer is not used for most routine physical examinations. The nurse will wish to note if a patient with limited hearing uses a hearing aid.

When speaking to a person who has difficulty in hearing, it is helpful to speak distinctly, face him, and make certain that what has been said is understood. Shouting is to be avoided unless it is absolutely necessary. Many persons learn to read lips. To avoid disturbing others at night, directing a flashlight on one's face so that the patient may watch mouth and facial expressions is helpful. Another measure that is helpful with some types of hearing loss is to place the eartips of a stethoscope in the patient's ears and to speak into the bell portion.

The nose is inspected and palpated. A flashlight or a head mirror and a nasal speculum are used to inspect the nostrils and the septum. Sense of smell is determined by having the patient smell commonly recognized substances.

Examining the Lips, Mouth, and Throat. Examination of the lips is usually done by inspection. A tongue depressor and a light are used for inspecting the mouth, teeth, gums, tongue, hard and soft palate, tonsils, pharynx, and larynx.

Examining the Breasts. The breasts are examined for shape, position, and size. Palpation is used to determine the presence of lumps. The nipples are examined by inspection and palpation.

Examining the Chest and Respiratory Tract. The size and shape of the chest are inspected. Respiratory movements are noted. Percussion is used to help determine whether fluid or a solid mass is present. Auscultation with a stethoscope is used to hear and evaluate breath sounds. During auscultation of the chest, the patient may be asked to cough. He should be provided with tissue wipes to cover his mouth when so doing.

Most authorities agree that a physical examination is incomplete without a chest x-ray. Some health agencies have a policy that patients have a chest x-ray upon admission. A routine chest x-ray is helpful in finding early signs of cancer, tuberculosis, and other lung diseases. X-rays also aid in determining the shape and the size of other organs in the chest, and of the ribs.

If the patient has a cough, it is described as nonproductive if no discharge from the respiratory tract is produced. If there is discharge, it is called a productive cough. **Mucus** is the watery secretions from mucous membranes. **Sputum** or **expectoration** usually is of greater viscosity and thickness and may have a yellow/greenish color. It may be raised and expectorated (spit out) with or without a cough. If a patient has a cough, the nurse should teach the patient how to protect others by covering his mouth and nose. He should also be taught how to discard tissues properly.

Examining the Abdomen and Back. Inspection will determine the general shape of the abdomen, condition of the skin, and distribution of pubic hair. By palpation, organs or masses are noted. Percussion is used to learn whether fluid is present. Auscultation of the abdomen is used to examine the pregnant woman to count the fetal heart rate.

To describe the location of signs and symptoms of the abdomen,

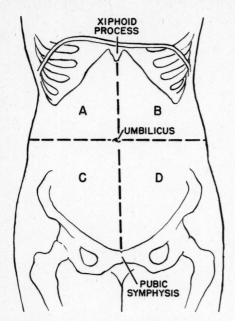

Fig. 9-5 Quadrants of the abdomen: (A) the right upper quadrant—RUQ; (B) the left upper quadrant—LUQ; (C) the right lower quadrant—RLQ; (D) the left lower quadrant—LLQ.

areas of the abdomen have been defined. The most common method is to describe four areas. A line drawn from the tip of the sternum (breastbone) to the pubic bone through the **umbilicus** (navel) and a horizontal line crossing the other at the umbilicus divide the abdomen into four parts. They are called the right and left upper quadrants and the right and left lower quadrants. A **quadrant** is one-fourth of a whole. They are frequently abbreviated RUQ, LUQ, RLQ, and LLQ. Figure 9-5 illustrates these four divisions.

Distention is a swelling or expansion. Abdominal distention often occurs in illness, as for example, when a mass is present in the gastro-intestinal tract or following surgery. It also may occur when a person has eaten foods that are particularly irritating, such as sauerkraut or beans. The distention is caused by gas, called **flatus.** Tapping gently on the area usually will produce a hollow drumlike sound; if a mass is present, there will not be a hollow sound.

The back is inspected and palpated to determine its shape and the position of the spine.

Thorough examinations of the abdomen, pelvis, and back usually include x-ray examinations. However, they are generally used only when these areas seem to have abnormalities.

Observations in relation to nausea and vomiting are discussed in Chapter 11. Observations in relation to gastrointestinal elimination are discussed in Chapter 14.

Examining the Cardiovascular System. The **cardiovascular system** refers to the heart and blood vessels. Inspection, palpation, percussion, auscultation, and x-rays are used to study the size and shape of the heart, abnormal pulse, heart sounds, heart murmurs, and so on. A study of heart function can also be done with the use of an electrocardiograph, as described in Chapter 8. Circulation is checked also by feeling for the type and quality of pulsations in the extremities and at the carotid artery in the neck.

Examining the Musculoskeletal System. Inspection and palpation are used to examine this system. General shape is noted, and joints are inspected. Occasionally, the extremities are measured with a tape measure. X-rays frequently are used as an aid in examining the skeletal system.

The Neurological Examination. This is an examination of the body's nervous system. During the neurological examination, the reflexes and the various senses are examined. Usually, the percussion hammer is used to test reflexes. A skin pencil is employed frequently to mark certain neurological as well as musculoskeletal findings on the patient's body. The senses of touch and pain are examined with cotton and with a pin. Placing test tubes containing hot and cold water on the skin may be used to test heat and cold sensations. The sense of smell is tested by having the patient identify certain common odors.

Examining the Genitalia, Perineum, Anus, and Rectum. These areas are examined by inspection and palpation. Rectal and vaginal examinations rarely are done on children and young adults unless specific complaints are referred to these areas. A vaginal speculum is used to examine the vagina and cervix. Gloves are used for this part of the examination.

It is usually recommended that women over 35 or 40 years of age

The physical examination

have a Papanicolaou test twice a year. The test is named after the physician who first devised it, and is commonly called the **Pap test.** It includes taking a specimen of the secretions from the uterus and cervix to determine whether cancer cells are present.

Physicians usually recommend that men over 40 years of age have a rectal examination at least once a year. The examination aids in finding signs of cancer of the prostate gland.

Observing for Pain. Pain and common terms used to describe it are discussed in Chapter 13.

Noting Physical Limitations. The nurse will wish to observe when the patient has any physical limitations. Observing for limited eyesight and hearing have been discussed earlier. Other examples include patients with various types of amputations; with loss of function in a body part; or with artificial openings into the body, such as a colostomy. The colostomy will be discussed in Chapter 14. Some of these patients may use a **prosthesis,** that is, an artificial part used in place of a natural part of the body which has been removed. Artificial limbs, eyes, or teeth are examples of prostheses. Other patients may use a crutch, a cane, braces, or protective girdles. Still others may use items such as a colostomy belt and bag, elastic hose, or moistureproof underpants. Some patients have heart pacemakers. A scar high on the chest wall is a clue to a pacemaker although most patients having one are likely to tell the nurse about it readily. Any such items suggest possible limitations and the nurse will wish to note their presence and reasons for using them.

It is important to ask the patient if he has any allergies to drugs or other agents. An allergic reaction can be serious. When patients have allergy problems, the information should be clearly and conspicuously stated in the patient's record.

The physical examination for an infant or child

In general, the physical examination for an infant or child is like one for an adult. However, the nurse needs to be prepared if the infant or child is uncooperative or crying. Every effort should be taken to avoid the use of restraints since they often make the problem worse. No one likes being unable to move and youngsters are no exception. Explanations are of little help if the patient is too young to understand. Sometimes holding a small child in your arms or well supported over your shoulder will help win his cooperation. If this is not possible, there are ways to restrain youngsters safely and securely. Such restraints are discussed in courses on the care of children.

Care of the patient after the physical examination

After the physical examination is completed, the nurse assists the patient to return to his room. She helps him back to bed and makes certain that he is comfortably settled. If the patient has visitors, they may be informed when he is ready to receive them.

Recording the findings of
the physical examination

The physician generally writes his findings on the form provided. The agency's policies will tell the nurse what imformation to record in the nurses' notes. Usually, the following items are included: the time when the examination was done; the name of the examiner; the specimens that were obtained and how they were handled; and any observations made by the nurse that help to describe the patient's general condition and that will help plan nursing care.

Many terms used to describe the patient's condition were defined in this chapter. While it is important that you know these terms, it is sometimes better to describe what you observe rather than to use a term that could lead to misunderstandings. The descriptions should be accurate and complete. For example, a patient may say he has a "stomach ache." The nurse should describe the area of the abdomen where the pain is and the nature of the pain. Or, the patient may say he "threw up." The nurse would record when vomiting occurred, what type of material was vomited, and how much there was.

The nurse's role as assistant
to the physician

Agency policy is followed in relation to assisting a physician during the physical examination. Ordinarily, certain parts of the examination are done by the nurse, as for example, obtaining the vital signs and weighing the patient. Other parts are done by the physician. The nurse may be needed to assist the physician, especially if the patient's condition makes this necessary. Also, most agencies require a female nurse to be present when a male physician is examining a female patient. This is done for the comfort of the patient as well as for protection for the physician and the agency.

There are certain responsibilities the nurse usually has when she assists. Her first duty is to prepare the patient physically, as discussed above. Also, she is expected to prepare the patient psychologically, as discussed in Chapter 3.

The nurse will wish to check the room in which the physical examination is done. There should be good artificial lighting available when natural light is insufficient. The room should be comfortable in terms of temperature and ventilation.

The nurse is responsible for draping and positioning the patient. She is expected to help the patient if he cannot assume certain positions by himself. Only those parts of the body being examined are exposed. The legal implications of unnecessary exposure were discussed in Chapter 2.

The nurse will wish to anticipate the physician's needs for equipment and supplies. Items he is likely to use, as listed previously, should be in readiness and in good working order.

An examining table is ordinarily higher than the average bed. If an adjustable bed is used, it will be in a high position to make it easier for the physician to examine the patient. The nurse will wish to take every precaution so that the patient does not fall off the table or out of bed. Offer the patient assistance and have him use a sturdy stepstool when he gets off and onto the table. The best practice is not to leave any patient alone, even though he may seem very cooperative. Never leave a confused or uncooperative patient or a child alone on an examining table because of the danger of falling.

The nurse generally takes responsibility for seeing that the equipment used during a physical examination is properly cleaned, disinfected, or sterilized, as indicated, and returned to its proper place for storage. Supplies for discard are placed in the proper receptacle to prevent the spread of microorganisms. Specimens are handled according to agency policy.

Conclusion

Having a regular physical examination is an essential part of total health care. The nurse will find that she can often teach patients about the importance of physical examinations and why they should be done. She also sets an excellent example when she has regular checkups herself.

References

Alexander, Mary M. and Brown, Marie Scott, "Physical Examination: The Why and How of Examination," *Nursing '73*, 3:25–28, July 1973.

Jackson, Edgar B. Jr., "In the Screening Clinic: Guidelines to the Appraisal of Some Common Problems," *American Journal of Nursing*, 72:1398–1400, August 1972.

Oelbaum, Cynthia Hastings, "Hallmarks of Adult Wellness," *American Journal of Nursing*, 74:1623–1625, September 1974.

Roach, Lora B., "Assessment: Assessing Skin Changes: The Subtle and the Obvious," *Nursing '74*, 4:64–67, March 1974.

Roberts, Sharon L., "Skin Assessment for Color and Temperature," *American Journal of Nursing*, 75:610–613, April 1975.

Schanche, Don A., "What Your Hands Tell A Doctor About Your Health," *Today's Health*, 53:14–19, April 1975.

Traver, Gayle A., "Assessment of Thorax and Lungs," *American Journal of Nursing*, 73:466–471, March 1973.

You and Your Health, Metropolitan Life Insurance Company, New York, 1973, 34 p.

Weinstock, Frank J., "Tonometry Screening," *American Journal of Nursing*, 73:656–657, April 1973.

10 measures to promote personal hygiene

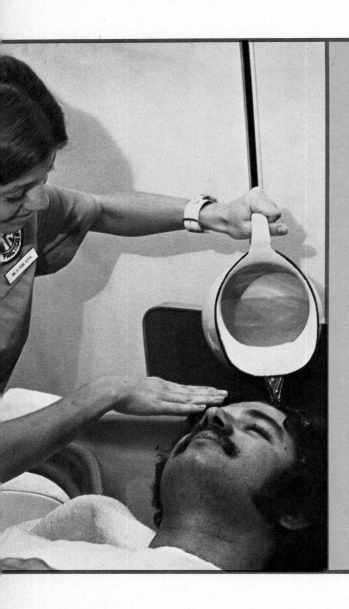

chapter outline

behavioral objectives

When mastery of content in this chapter is reached, the student will be able to

Define terms appearing in the glossary.

List three principles that guide the nurse when caring for the skin and mucous membranes.

List at least ten precautions to observe when selecting and using cosmetics.

List four purposes of the cleansing bath and backrub.

List four or five recommended ways to cut down on caries.

Describe how the mouth and teeth are best kept clean and healthy.

Explain one advantage and one disadvantage of the water spray unit for cleaning the mouth and teeth.

Describe briefly special precautions to observe when cleaning eye glasses; when cleaning dentures; when cleaning the ears and nose; when trimming fingernails and toenails; and when removing a hangnail.

Describe how hangnails can be prevented.

Describe how matting and tangling of long hair may be prevented.

List two symptoms which suggest to the nurse that the patient may have pediculosis.

List two early signs that a decubitus ulcer may develop.

Give the primary causes of a decubitus ulcer.

List six areas where decubitus ulcers commonly develop.

List six practices of nursing care that will help prevent a decubitus ulcer from forming.

Demonstrate or describe the following procedures:

How to offer and remove a bedpan and urinal.

How to measure and record urinary output and how to record a bowel movement.

How to give a complete bed bath and backrub; a partial bath; a tub bath; a

behavioral objectives cont.

shower bath; AM care; and PM or HS care.

How to make an occupied bed.

How to give a patient oral hygiene care.

How to clean a patient's dentures.

How to clean a patient's eye glasses.

How to clean a patient's eyes when there is discharge present.

How to groom a patient's fingernails and toenails.

How to groom a patient's hair.

How to give a patient a shampoo in bed or on a stretcher.

How to give a patient perineal care (external douche).

glossary

Acne A skin eruption due to inflammation and infection of oil glands in the skin.

Antiperspirant A preparation for reducing the amount of perspiration.

Caries The decay of teeth with the formation of cavities.

Commode A chair or wheelchair with an open seat under which a bedpan or other type of receptacle for urine and feces is placed.

Decubitus Ulcer (Plural: Decubiti) A break in the skin with destruction of underlying tissues. Synonym for pressure sore and bedsore.

Defecate To empty the rectum of feces.

Dentures Artificial or false teeth.

Deodorant A preparation to mask or diminish body odors.

Depilatory A preparation to remove unwanted hair.

Feces Waste matter discharged from the bowels.

Follicle A small saclike structure, as for example, in skin from which hair grows.

Genitalia The external organs of reproduction.

Gingivitis Inflammation of the gums.

Hygiene The establishment and preservation of health.

Nits Eggs of lice.

Pediculosis Infestation with lice.

Periodontitis Severe inflammation of the gums and bone tissue around the teeth. Synonym for pyorrhea.

Pressure sore or bedsore A break in the skin with destruction of underlying tissues. Synonym for decubitus ulcer.

Pyorrhea Severe inflammation of the gums and bone tissue around the teeth. Synonym for periodontitis.

Void To empty the urinary bladder.

introduction

Hygiene deals with the establishment and preservation of health. This chapter discusses common practices that promote health through personal care and cleanliness. Good personal hygienic practices help prevent illness and promote general well-being for the patient.

People differ in practices of personal hygiene. For example, some people prefer bathing to showering; some change bed linens weekly and others, more frequently; some shampoo their hair two or three times each week and others shampoo once every week or two; and some people prefer detergents to soap. The important thing is that personal care be carried out conveniently and often enough to promote personal hygiene. The exact way it is done and when it is carried out are less important.

During illness, the nurse helps the patient to continue good hygienic practices. If she notices that the patient is unaware of certain practices or that he uses poor practices, she has an opportunity for teaching. Including family members is important when it is appropriate and especially when patients are being cared for at home. The nurse is often asked about hygienic fads which offers her still another teaching opportunity.

Orders and recording hygienic care

There are differences among health agencies concerning orders for hygienic care. Most agencies do not require a physician's order. Rather, the nursing team leader takes the responsibility for writing nursing orders for hygienic care. These usually will appear on the nursing care plan. In other agencies, some hygienic care requires a physician's order. Examples include the shampoo, and cutting toenails, especially for elderly patients and for those with diabetes. It is recommended that the nurse follow orders on the nursing care plan and consult with her supervising nurse if she has any doubts about what she can or cannot do on her own.

Agency policies also differ concerning what hygienic care is recorded and where. Many agencies no longer require recording routine hygienic care, such as bathing the patient, in the nurses' notes. Others may require that only certain hygienic care, for example, the shampoo, be recorded in the nurses' notes. Still others may record all hygienic care on nursing care plans. The nurse will observe policies concerning recording in the agency where she gives care.

Guides to the care of the skin and mucous membranes

There are certain things we know about the skin and mucous membranes that help guide the nurse when giving care. These guides are principles of nursing care. Principles used as guides was discussed in Chapter 1.

Unbroken and healthy skin and mucous membranes help the body protect itself against harmful agents. For instance, healthy skin can resist organisms that irritated or broken skin cannot. Therefore, while giving care, the nurse will wish to do whatever she can to prevent skin irritation and injury. The following are a few examples of care that help to prevent injury and irritation to the skin and mucous membranes: selecting soaps and makeup that do not irritate the skin; giving mouth care in a way that prevents the mucous membrane from being broken or irritated; smoothing bed linen and tucking it securely under the mattress so that wrinkles do not rub and irritate the skin; and using a cream for a backrub rather than alcohol when the skin is dry.

The skin of some people is more sensitive to injury and irritation

than that of others. There are several conditions that influence a person's skin sensitivity. For example, the skin and mucous membranes of the very young and the elderly are easily injured. The skin and mucous membranes of persons whose diets have been poor or who have not had sufficient fluid intake are easily irritated and injured. Very thin and very fat people tend to have skin and mucous membranes that injure and become irritated easily.

Good blood circulation in the skin and mucous membranes is necessary in order to keep the cells alive and healthy. When circulation is poor, the cells cannot obtain proper nourishment. Irritation and injury will then occur more easily. This fact is especially important to remember when helping to prevent bedsores, as discussion later in this chapter will show.

Commonly used cosmetics

There is a great variety of items used for cosmetic purposes on the market, and most people use at least some of them. Chart 10-1 was prepared to summarize certain information concerning commonly used cosmetics. It will serve as a guide when caring for patients and may be useful when you select your cosmetics. The booklet, *The Look You Like,* listed in the references at the end of this chapter, is recommended for more detailed information about cosmetics and skin care.

Offering and removing the bedpan and urinal

Many patients will wish to use the bedpan or urinal immediately before or after a bath, and also upon awakening and before going to sleep. Chart 10-2 describes how to offer and remove the bedpan or urinal.

To **void** means to empty the urinary bladder. To **defecate** means to empty the rectum of feces. The **feces** is waste matter discharged from the bowels. The feces is frequently referred to as a bowel movement or as the stool.

The male patient confined to bed uses the urinal for voiding and the bedpan for defecating. The female patient uses the bedpan for both voiding and defecating. There are specially designed female urinals that are used in certain situations, for example, when the patient is in a full body cast.

Some bedpans are made of metal and, therefore, feel cold on the patient's skin. They can be warmed before use by rinsing with warm water. Those made of nylon substances or plastics do not usually feel cold to the touch.

A commode is sometimes used instead of a bedpan or urinal when the patient can get out of bed but is unable to go to a bathroom. A **commode** is a chair or wheelchair with an open seat. There is a place under the seat for a bedpan or other receptacle. The same directions given in Chart 10-2 apply when the patient uses a commode, except that the patient is out of bed.

Chart 10-1 Commonly used cosmetics

Cosmetic	Description
Soaps and Detergents	Despite advertising, all soaps and detergents clean about equally well. Perfumes and color may be pleasant but do not improve ability to clean. Laundry-type soaps and detergents may irritate skin. Persons allergic to soaps may use detergents, and vice versa. Detergents are especially helpful when water is cold and/or hard.
Bath Oils	People with dry skin may find bath oils help to prevent chapping. They tend to make tub slippery; use nonskid bath mats to help prevent falling.
Bubble Bath Preparations	These preparations contain perfume and some may help soften water. Mix well in water before getting into tub; in concentrated form, they may irritate skin and mucous membrane in genital area.
Cold, Vanishing, and Dry-Skin Creams and Lotions	All contain essentially the same types of ingredients. They leave film on skin that helps prevent moisture from evaporating, thus decreasing chapping. May be used for cleansing purposes when skin is very dry or sensitive to soaps and detergents.
Skin Nourishing Creams	Skin absorbs very little. It is nourished by bloodstream. Nourishing creams containing, for example, algae, estrogen, and mink and turtle oils, do not prevent skin from normal aging process.
Skin Refreshners and Astringents	These preparations usually contain alcohol, water, and glycerin. Astringents may also contain additional ingredients, such as boric acid or menthol. They make skin feel cool and refreshed but do not seem particularly helpful for shrinking pores.
Deodorants and Antiperspirants	**Deodorants** mask or diminish body odor. **Antiperspirants** contain a chemical to reduce amount of perspiration. Body odors are caused by bacteria normally on skin acting with body secretions. Therefore, the best deodorant is cleanliness. Use deodorants and antiperspirants *after* skin is clean. Use as directed and with care to prevent skin irritation. Do not use when skin is irritated and immediately after shaving. Deodorants used on sanitary pads and in the genital area are intended for external use only; do not use on tampons which are inserted into vagina.
Preparations to Treat Acne	**Acne** is skin eruption due to inflammation and infection of oil glands in skin. At present, acne cannot be cured or prevented but proper care helps to control it. Wash face two to four times daily with soap or detergent and hot water to keep skin free of oils. Shampoo hair frequently to control oiliness. Avoid oily cosmetics. Do not eat foods which tend to make condition worse; common offenders are chocolate and nuts. Use lotions and creams available on market for controlling acne according to directions but do not use them if they irritate skin. Severe cases require medical attention.
Eye Makeup	Ingredients that cause damage to eyes are legally prohibited; therefore, in general, eye makeup is safe if used according to directions. However, eye makeup should be removed with care to avoid irritation to skin around eyes and on eyelids. Do not use eye makeup if skin becomes red, itchy, or swollen.
Nail Polishes and Removers	If used over long period of time, nail polish and polish remover tend to dry nails which then split and break easily. Preparations advertised to reduce splitting nails should be used according to directions; some irritate and dry cuticles and skin around nails.

Chart 10-1   continued

Cosmetic	Description
Depilatories	A **depilatory** is a preparation to remove unwanted hair. Use according to directions and do not use if it irritates skin. Safest and cheapest way to remove unwanted hair is with a razor. Plucking may be used if done with care to avoid injury. Electrolysis removes hair permanently by destroying hair follicle with mild, electric current. Procedure is not generally recommended for home use. One ounce of 6 per cent solution of hydrogen peroxide with 20 drops of ammonia will bleach unwanted hair, thus making it less noticeable.
Wigs	There is no conclusive evidence that hair loss occurs as a result of wearing a wig. Wigs require the same care as normal hair except for less frequent washing since they are not lubricated with scalp oils.
Shampoos and Rinses	Personal preference is best guide but avoid those that irritate scalp or leave hair dry and brittle. Detergents are good when water is hard. Liquid and cream shampoos rinse easier from hair than bar soap. Rinses make hair more manageable by leaving fine film on hair shafts. Dry shampoos are not as effective as regular wet shampoos but are especially convenient for ill patients.
Dandruff Preparations	Preparations for dandruff do not cure condition but may help keep it under control. Brushing hair and frequent shampooing help keep scalp free of dandruff. Severe cases may require medical attention.
Hair Sprays	Hair sprays contain a resin that helps to hold hair in place. Not recommended if they make hair dry and brittle. Some are flammable and therefore, should not be used when smoking or around open flames.
Home Permanent Waves	In general, home permanent waves are safe when used according to directions. Avoid wave lotions that irritate scalp.
Preparations to Stimulate Hair Growth	Despite advertising claims, external treatment to stimulate hair growth is not likely to help. Baldness is believed to be hereditary. Some cases have occured after using certain drugs, having x-ray treatments to head, and having illnesses with high fever. Frequent shampooing does not appear to cause baldness.
Shaving Lotions and Shaving Methods	Preparations used before shaving are intended to soften beard. Preparations used after shaving make skin feel cool and refreshed. Shaving with grain of beard tends to reduce ingrown hairs which are hairs turned back into the skin. Most persons prefer razor blade shaves. Electric razors are especially convenient for the ill and bedridden patient.
Mouthwashes and Breath Freshners	Many find these products pleasant to use but they cannot replace keeping mouth and teeth clean with thorough brushing and flossing. Many odors on breath are being excreted from lungs, alcohol being an example. A breath freshner masks the odor but cannot remove it. Use according to directions. If a preparation intended to be diluted is used in concentrated form, mouth tissues may be injured.
Toothpastes and Powders	Toothpastes and powders make brushing easier and have a pleasant taste. Those containing stannous fluoride help to decrease cavities and are recommended by many dentists. Salt or sodium bicarbonate solutions are good and are far less expensive than toothpastes and powders.

Chart 10-2 Offering and removing a bedpan or urinal
The purpose is to place the bedpan or urinal in the proper position with the least amount of exposure and energy.

Suggested Action	Reason for Action
Assemble equipment, that is, bedpan and/or urinal, toilet tissue, and equipment to wash and dry hands.	Having equipment on hand saves time by avoiding unnecessary trips to storage area.
Elevate head of bed slightly if possible. Place adjustable bed in high position.	This position generally makes it easier for patient to void or defecate and avoids strain on patient's back. Having bed in high position reduces strain on nurse's back as she assists patient onto bedpan.
Place bedpan and/or urinal on chair next to bed or on foot of bed. Pie-fold top linen off patient.	Folding linen back in this manner prevents unnecessary exposure while still allowing nurse to place bedpan or urinal.
If patient needs assistance to move onto bedpan, have him bend his knees and rest some of his weight on his heels. Lift patient by placing one hand under lower back and slip bedpan into place with other hand.	Patient uses less energy as nurse assists by lifting him onto bedpan. Nurse uses less energy when patient can assist by placing some of his weight on his heels.
If patient is entirely helpless, two people may be required to lift him onto bedpan. Or, patient may be placed on his side, bedpan is placed against his buttocks, and patient is rolled back onto bedpan.	Having two people lift helpless patient causes less strain on nurse's back. Rolling patient takes less energy than lifting patient onto bedpan.
When bedpan is in proper place, patient's buttocks rest on rounded shelf of bedpan. Urinal is properly placed between slightly spread legs with bottom of urinal resting on bed.	Having bedpan or urinal in proper place prevents spilling contents into bed and prevents injury to skin from misplaced bedpan.
Replace top bed linen; leave signal device and toilet tissue within easy reach of patient. Leave patient if it is safe to do so. Use siderails as necessary.	Folding linen into place prevents unnecessary exposure. Falls can be prevented when patient does not have to reach for items he needs. Attending patients who are likely to fall helps prevent accidents. Siderails help prevent falls.
Remove bedpan in same manner as it was offered. Cover it and place on chair or on foot of bed. If necessary to assist patient, wrap toilet tissue around hand several times and wipe patient clean, using one stroke from pubic area toward anal area. Discard tissue and use more until patient is clean. Place patient on his side and spread buttocks to clean in anal area.	Cleaning patient after he has used bedpan prevents offensive odors and irritation to skin. Cleaning an area that is less soiled before cleaning an area that is more heavily soiled prevents spreading organisms to cleaner areas.
Do not place toilet tissue in bedpan if specimen is required, in which case have a receptacle handy for discarding tissue.	Toilet tissue mixed with specimen of urine or feces makes laboratory examination more difficult.
Replace top linens in order and offer patient equipment to wash and dry hands, assisting as necessary.	Washing hands after using bedpan or urinal helps prevent spread of organisms.
Collect specimen as necessary, following agency procedure. Empty and clean bedpan and urinal according to agency procedure. Record according to agency procedure.*	

*Observations in relation to feces and urine are described in Chapters 14 and 16. If urine or feces appear abnormal in any way, do not discard contents of bedpan or urinal and report findings promptly.

Measuring and recording the patient's output

There are times when it is important to know how much urine the patient eliminates each day. The findings are used to plan medical and nursing care. Measuring and recording output are important nursing responsibilities.

Health agencies have containers for measuring urine. They are usually calibrated in cubic centimeters or milliliters, abbreviated cc. or ml. respectively. A cubic centimeter or a milliliter is a unit of volume in the metric system. Thirty cc. or ml. are equivalent to approximately one fluid ounce; 1000 cc. or ml. are equivalent to approximately one quart.

Urine is poured into the agency's measuring container from the bedpan or urinal. The container is placed on a flat surface for more accurate reading. After the nurse notes the amount of urine, she discards it into the toilet. Or, if a specimen is needed, she pours the urine into the appropriate specimen container and handles the specimen according to

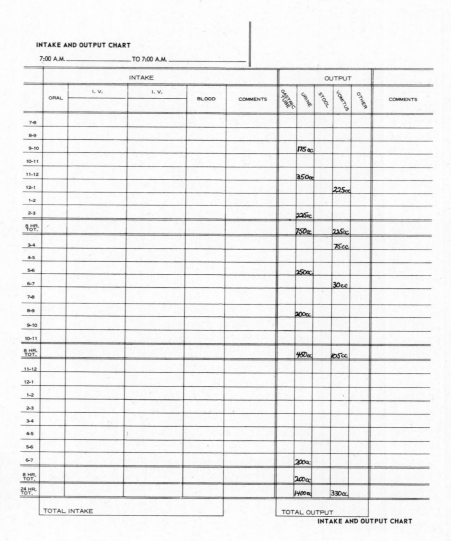

Fig. 10-1 A form used to record the patient's output. Note that there are three 8-hour totals as well as the 24-hour total on his form. Recording the patient's intake is discussed and a form is illustrated in Chapter 11.

agency procedure. She then records the amount of urine the patient has eliminated. Figure 10-1 illustrates an example of one type of form commonly used for recording the patient's urinary output.

If the patient is up and about, he is told when his urinary output is to be measured. In some instances, he may be taught to measure and record his urinary output. Or, he may use a bedpan or urinal. He is then instructed to call the nurse who will measure and record the output.

In home situations, the patient or a member of his family is taught to measure and record output. Any suitably marked container may be used for measuring, but it is aesthetically preferable to use one that can be discarded when it is no longer necessary to measure output.

Patients whose urinary output is to be measured and recorded will almost always need their fluid intake measured and recorded also. This procedure is discussed in Chapter 11.

Elimination from the large intestine is also recorded. Ordinarily, if the patient uses the bathroom, he is asked each day whether he has had a bowel movement. If the patient uses a bedpan, the nurse emptying the bedpan records when the patient has had a bowel movement. The letters, BM, are usually used as an abbreviation for bowel movement; frequency is recorded I, II, III, and so on.

Bathing the patient

For most patients, a bath can be very refreshing, especially when they are warm, restless, and uncomfortable. The feeling of cleanliness and relaxation usually helps people feel better.

The bath has additional benefits for the patient. The friction caused by rubbing when washing and drying the skin and when giving a backrub stimulates blood circulation and muscles. Therefore, a bath can be a good general body conditioner.

The bath can also be valuable for the musculoskeletal system. The activity of the body during bathing is good exercise for most patients. In addition, the nurse can exercise many parts of the body for the patient as she bathes him. This type of exercise and its purposes are discussed in Chapter 12. Usually the respirations are also stimulated, thus helping to reduce secretions that may accumulate in the lungs and improve oxygen intake.

Bathing offers the nurse one of her best opportunities for developing good nurse-patient relationships, for observing the patient, and for health teaching. Health workers have many, usually brief, contacts with patients throughout the day. But the bath offers an important and longer association so that the nurse can carry out other aspects of care.

Health agency procedures vary concerning bathing. For example, some prefer that baths be given during morning hours; others may schedule bathing at other times. Some agencies offer complete baths every day while others schedule them two or three times weekly.

Chart 10-3 describes a suggested way to give a bed bath. However, procedures vary. For example, some agencies recommend that the patient's back be washed after his legs and feet; the **genitalia,** that is, the external organs of reproduction, are then washed as the last part of the bath. Using this procedure, the bath water ordinarily is not changed.

Chart 10-3 Giving a bed bath and backrub

The purpose is to clean the skin and condition the body in a manner that is comfortable and relaxing for the patient and that conserves time and energy

Suggested Action	Reason for Action	Figure to Illustrate
Preparing for bath and mouth care		
Bring articles needed for hygiene and bed-making to bedside and arrange in order of use on bedside table, overbed table, or chair. Bath water should be comfortably warm, about 105 to 110°F. Include equipment for shaving and for care of mouth. If patient uses razor shave, he will need basin of hot water, mirror, and a good light.	Bringing everything to bedside conserves time and energy. Arranging items conveniently and in order of use saves time and helps prevent stretching and twisting nurse's muscles. Warm water is comfortable and relaxing for patient.	
Place adjustable bed in high position. Remove bed siderails.	Having bed in high position prevents strain on nurse's back as she works. Removing bed siderails makes it easier to work without straining muscles.	
Loosen top linen where it is tucked under mattress. Fold spread and blankets individually from top to bottom and in half again (in fourths). Drape over back of chair if items are to be reused. If not, fold again a time or two and place in laundry hamper. Keep linen away from uniform while handling it.	Folding linen in place and as it is removed avoids stretching arms and saves time and energy when used on bed later. Avoiding drafts while handling linen and keeping linen away from uniform help prevent spread of organisms.	
Place fan-folded bath blanket over patient's chest and have patient hold top edge of bath blanket. Grasp bottom of bath blanket and top edge of sheet; pull sheet and bath blanket together to foot of bed. Remove sheet, fold, and place in hamper.	Patient is not exposed unnecessarily as top sheet is removed. Avoiding drafts and keeping linen away from uniform help prevent spread of organisms.	
Assist patient to side of bed where nurse will work. Have him on his back, as illustrated in Figure 10-2.	Having patient positioned near nurse helps prevent unnecessary stretching and twisting of nurse's muscles.	

Assist patient with care of mouth and teeth.

Remove patient's gown by slipping it off under bath blanket. Remove all but one pillow and place bed in flat position.

Expose, wash, and dry each part of body:

Place towel over top part of bath blanket. With no soap on cloth, wipe one eye from inner part of eye near nose to outer part of eye near nose to outer part near forehead. Rinse cloth before washing other eye.

Oral hygiene is important part of helping to keep mouth and teeth comfortable, clean, and healthy.

Keeping bath blanket in place avoids exposure and chilling. Having patient flat in bed with one pillow is comfortable for most patients and convenient for nurse to work.

The following reasons for action apply to bathing body parts:

Exposing, washing, rinsing, and drying one part of body at a time avoid unnecessary exposure and chilling.

Doing one eye and then other prevents spreading organisms from one to other. Soap is irritating to eye.

Keeping bed protected with towel prevents bed from becoming wet.

Washing area where there are fewer organisms to areas where there are likely to be more helps prevent spread of organisms to cleaner areas.

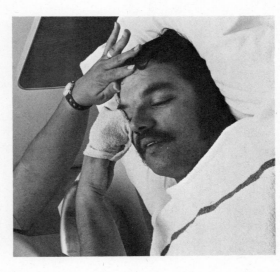

Fig. 10-2 The patient lies near the side of the bed where the nurse works. The nurse washes the patient's eye by moving from the inner aspect of the eye outwardly to the area near the forehead. Note that the washcloth is well tucked into the nurse's hand like a mitt.

Chart 10-3 continued

Suggested Action	Reason for Action	Figure to Illustrate

Face, neck, and ears.

Arms, one furthest from nurse and then other. Place towel under arm while working.

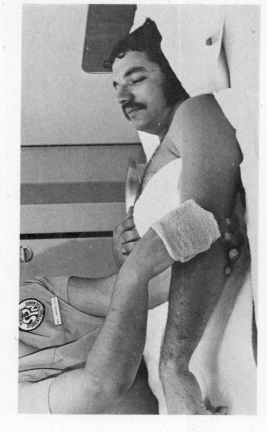

Fig. 10-3   The arm furthest from the nurse is washed before the one nearest her. A towel protects the bed.

Hands. Place basin on towel on bed; place hand in basin.

Chest and axillae. Or, axillae may be done with arms.

Abdomen.

Placing exposed parts in positions convenient for nurse prevents straining muscles.

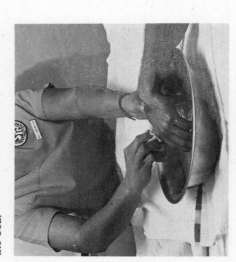

Fig. 10-4   The patient's hand is washed by placing it in a basin of water.

Legs, thighs, and groin areas, one furthest from nurse and then other. Place towel under leg as you work. Front of thighs and groins may be washed with abdomen and back of thighs may be washed with back, if desired.

Supporting legs prevent stretching and twisting patient's muscles. Nurse may accidently drip on clean arm or leg as she reaches across body to other.

Feet. Place basin on towel on bed. Place feet in basin while supporting ankle and heel in hand, and leg on arm. Care for toenails.

Grooming toenails helps keep them clean and comfortable.

Genital area. Leave patient if safe as he cleans this area. Or assist patient as necessary. (See Chart 10-6, p. 188.)

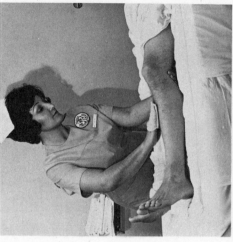

Fig. 10-5 The leg furthest from the nurse is washed before the leg nearest the nurse. A towel protects the bed.

Discard used washcloth, towel, and water. Obtain fresh water. Have patient lying on abdomen if possible. Or, place him on his side, facing away from nurse. Tuck clean towel under length of back. Using clean washcloth and water, wash back of neck, shoulders, back, and buttocks. Expose and do upper back only and then lower back if patient is likely to become chilled.

Discard washcloth, towel, and water after washing genital area since it is considered highly contaminated. By so doing, there is less likelihood of spreading organisms to other parts of body.

(Genital area may be washed after back, thus eliminating need to change washcloth and towel during bathing procedure. Follow agency procedure.)

The following suggestions are observed during entire bathing procedure:

Fold washcloth like mitt or in a manner so that there are no loose ends as in Figures 10-2, 10-3, and 10-5.

Having loose ends of cloth drag across patient's skin is uncomfortable for patient. Loose ends cool quickly and will feel cold to patient.

Chart 10-3 continued

Suggested Action	Reason for Action	Figure to Illustrate
Keep cloth wet enough to wash, lather, and rinse well but not so wet that it drips water.	Dripping water from cloth is uncomfortable for patient and will dampen bed. Too little moisture on cloth makes thorough washing and rinsing difficult.	
Do not leave soap in water.	Soap will become soft and water becomes too soapy for good rinsing.	
Wash, rinse, and dry skin well. Change water as necessary if it becomes dirty or too soapy for thorough washing and rinsing.	Thorough cleaning removes dirt, oil, and many organisms. Soap or moisture left on skin is uncomfortable and may irritate skin.	
Use firm but gentle strokes while washing and drying patient. Use strokes as long as body part allows.	Friction helps remove dirt, oil, and organisms and helps to dry skin well. Friction stimulates circulation and muscles. Too much friction may injure tender skin. Long, firm strokes are relaxing and more comfortable than are short, uneven strokes.	
Pay particular attention to these areas: under breasts; axillae; between fingers and toes; in any folds in skin, as in groin or on abdomen of persons who are fat; behind ears; and umbilicus.	Organisms and dirt that are lodged in areas where skin touches skin, that are not washed, rinsed, and dried well will become irritated and injury to skin will eventually occur.	

Backrub

Suggested Action	Reason for Action	Figure to Illustrate
Give patient backrub using solution or lotion of agency's choice. Alcohol followed by powder are commonly used when skin is not dry. Lotions and creams are better when skin is dry.	Alcohol feels refreshing and tends to toughen skin. Dry skin is easily irritated. Alcohol has drying effect on skin while lotions and creams help prevent drying.	

Rub neck to hair line. Place fingers on one side of spine in neck and thumb on other side of spine. Use circular motion and move fingers and thumb toward hair line.

A backrub stimulates circulation, tones muscles, helps patient relax, and feels comfortable whem firm, smooth, even strokes are used. Short, uneven strokes are uncomfortable. Strokes that are directed in general direction of heart assist circulation to carry blood toward heart and away from extremities.

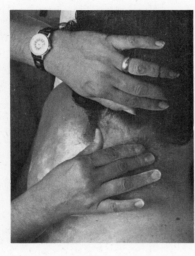

Fig. 10-6   The nurse, with fingers placed on one side of the cervical spine and her thumb on the other side, massages with a circular motion up to the patient's hairline.

Rub area at base of spine with fingers or with heel of hand, using circular motion.

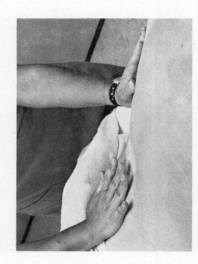

Fig. 10-7   The nurse uses the heel of her hand to massage the area at the base of the patient's spine.

Chart 10-3 continued

Suggested Action	Reason for Action	Figure to Illustrate
Rub length of back, using entire surface of hands. Use long, circular strokes followed by long, vertical strokes. Work outward from spine and up back. Include shoulders.		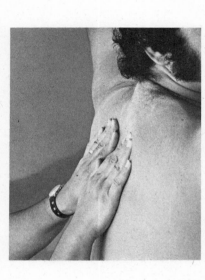
Rub buttocks, using palms of hands and circular motions.		
During entire backrub, use smooth, even, and firm but gentle strokes. In general, stroke toward heart.		**Fig. 10-8** Using the entire surface of her hand, the nurse strokes the length of the patient's back.

Caring for hair and fingernails

Replace patient's gown and cover pillow with towel. Arrange patient's hair. Care for fingernails.	Caring for hair is an important part of helping keep hair and scalp clean, comfortable, and healthy. Grooming fingernails helps keep them clean and comfortable. Grooming helps promote patient's well-being.	
Make bed as described in Chart 10-5.		

Chart 10-4 Modifications of the bath procedure

Type of Care	Suggested Procedure
Tub or Shower Bath	Patient may shave, and care for his mouth, teeth, and hair at the bedside or in bathroom. Offer assistance as necessary.
	Clean tub or shower as necessary. Assemble equipment and supplies near shower or tub. Fill tub approximately half full of warm water (105 to 110°F.). Or, adjust water in shower to appropriate temperature. Assist patient into tub or shower. Support patient by placing your hands in his armpits. Or, place chair next to tub, have patient ease himself from chair to edge of tub, turn him, place feet into tub, and then ease body into tub.
	Guide rails in shower are helpful to prevent falls. Stool may be placed in the shower for patient's comfort and convenience.
	Wash patient's back and any other part of body he cannot reach. Remain with patient if he appears weak or fearful. If it is safe, adult patient may be left but stay close at hand and check patient frequently, every three or four minutes. Nurse may make patient's bed while patient is in tub or shower if patient can be left alone.
	Assist patient out of shower or tub as necessary. Assist with drying and putting on clean gown as necessary and help patient into bed. Give patient a backrub.
	These precautions are necessary in order to prevent accidents and injuries: Ill patients may easily become weak and faint; check patient frequently and do not leave him alone if in doubt.
	Never leave a child or infant alone in water.
	To prevent burning, do not turn on hot water while patient is in tub except with extreme caution and agitate water well while adding hot water.
	Be sure bathroom door is unlocked. Place a DO NOT DISTURB sign on door and assure patient of privacy.
	Have signal device handy for patient's use.
	Tubs and showers may be slippery! Use nonskid bath mats in tubs and showers. A bath towel may be used as a substitute if mat is not available. Have mat on floor also for patient to stand on as he leaves tub or shower.
Bath Taken in Bed	Assemble equipment and supplies at bedside and place within easy reach of patient. Include supplies for shaving and care of mouth, teeth, and hair. Remove top linen and replace with bath blanket. Patient bathes self; assist as necessary.
	Make patient's bed as suggested in Chart 10-5.
Partial Bath	Follow suggested procedure in Chart 10-3, except omit bathing chest, abdomen, legs, thighs, and feet. Tighten bottom linen securely before replacing top linen.

Chart 10-4 continued

Type of Care	Suggested Procedure
Early AM Care carried out before daytime activities begin and breakfast is served.	Offer bedpan or urinal.
	Supply water, soap, washcloth, and towel for patient to wash his hands and face. Assist patient as necessary.
	Give patient equipment and supplies to care for his teeth, mouth, and hair. Assist patient as necessary.
	Straighten bed linens and assist patient to position in bed so that he is ready for breakfast.
PM or HS (Hour of Sleep) Care carried out in preparation for sleep.	Assist patient as necessary with care of teeth, mouth, and hair.
	Offer bedpan or urinal.
	Wash patient's face and hands. Wash patient's back and give him a backrub. Fan-fold top linen to foot of bed if bath blanket is used. Straighten and tighten bed linens.
	Prepare patient for sleep: arrange pillows comfortably; offer extra blanket; lower adjustable bed; put up bed siderails as necessary; and darken room.

Chart 10-3 describes a procedure requiring a change of water. Similarly, the axillae and thighs may be bathed in somewhat different orders, as mentioned in Chart 10-3. Such differences are usually of little significance. The important thing is to accomplish the purposes for which the bath is given. The nurse will be expected to follow the procedures of the agency in which she gives care.

There are several modifications in bathing procedures with which the nurse will wish to be familiar. Common ones are described in Chart 10-4. As was true of the bed bath, the nurse will observe agency procedures concerning these modifications.

It is usual to change linens at the time a patient is bathed. Chart 10-5 describes how to make an occupied bed. Differences in details of bedmaking are less important than the patient's comfort, but agency procedures should be observed.

Care of the teeth and mouth

General good health is as important as cleanliness for keeping the mouth and teeth healthy. Dental disease is common in this country. The American Dental Association estimated recently that Americans have about one billion untreated cavities, with the average person having five. Diseases of the gums are also very common in the adult population.

The decay of teeth with the formation of cavities is called **caries.** There are several commonly recommended ways to help prevent caries: cutting down on sweets, such as soft drinks, candy, gum, pastries, and so on; brushing the teeth often and as soon after eating and snacking as possible; if brushing is not convenient, rinsing the mouth well after

Chart 10-5 Making an occupied bed

The purpose is to make a comfortable and clean bed with economy of time and energy

Suggested Action	Reason for Action	Figure to Illustrate
Note: It is assumed that top linen has been removed and patient has bath blanket protecting him.		
Help patient to his side and to far part of bed where siderail is in position. Loosen bottom linen opposite patient, roll it toward patient and tuck it as close to patient as possible without pushing him so that he may fall out of bed.	With patient on far side of bed, nurse is able to make half of bed (bottom linen only). Rolling linen together with cleaner side of linen to outside helps prevent spreading organisms.	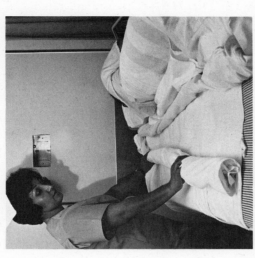
Place bottom sheet on bed; unfold in place. Tuck sheet under mattress securely on side opposite patient, as described in Chart 6-1, page 8b. Fan-fold sheet and place near rolled up linen at patient's back. Unfold draw sheet in place and tuck securely under mattress. Place siderails in position.	Opening linens by shaking them causes drafts that could spread organisms. Having linen free of wrinkles results in a more comfortable bed.	Fig. 10-9 The nurse has the bed siderails in place opposite her work area so that the patient will not accidentally fall from the bed. The soiled linen is then rolled close to the patient. The nurse has secured the bottom linen under the mattress and will roll all of it close to the soiled linen. Before moving to the opposite side of the bed, the nurse raises the siderail for the patient's protection.

Chart 10-5 continued

Suggested Action	Reason for Action	Figure to Illustrate
Assist patient to roll over all linens to that half of bed where bottom linen is in place and secured under mattress.	The nurse is now able to make the second half of bed (bottom linen only).	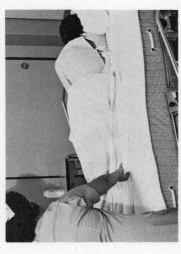
Nurse moves to opposite side of bed and lowers siderails. Loosen soiled linen and continue to roll it together and place in hamper. Keep linen away from uniform.	Avoiding stretching across bed helps prevent straining muscles. Keeping soiled linen rolled together and away from uniform helps prevent spreading organisms.	
Pull bottom sheet into place and tuck under mattress, as described in Chart 6-1. Do same with drawsheet. Be sure linen is pulled and tucked firmly and securely.	Having linens free of wrinkles and well secured under mattress result in a more comfortable bed.	Fig. 10-10 The bed siderail is in place on the side opposite the nurses work area. After assisting the patient over the rolls of clean and soiled linen and removing the soiled linen, the nurse pulls the clean linen toward her and finishes placing all bottom linen securely.
Assist patient to middle of bed and onto his back. Place top linen in place and make remainder of bed as described in Chart 6-1. Slip bath blanket out and fold in place on bed. Change pillow linen as described in Chart 6-1. Arrange pillows comfortably for patient. Put up bed siderails as necessary.		

Note: Some agency procedures recommend that both bottom and top linen be arranged before patient is assisted to that side of bed where bottom linen is clean. Follow agency procedure.

eating; using a toothpaste or powder containing stannous fluoride; and visiting the dentist regularly, at least once or twice a year.

The major cause of tooth loss in adults is gum disease. **Gingivitis** is an inflammation of the gums; a common cause is trench mouth. Severe inflammation of the gums, including bone tissue around the teeth, is called **periodontitis,** or **pyorrhea.** Regular dental care and good oral hygiene are the best ways to prevent periodontitis.

Toothbrushing and Flossing. The brush should be small enough to reach all teeth. The bristles should be firm enough to clean well but not so firm that they are likely to injure tissues. Many dentists recommend a soft-textured, multitufted toothbrush with a flat brushing surface. Others recommend brushes with widely spaced tufts. When tufts are widely spaced, the brush is easier to keep clean and dry.

Opinion differs concerning the best way to brush the teeth. Some dentists recommend that the brush be placed at a 45° angle at the area where the teeth and gums meet, with the tufts facing in the direction of the gums. This method is illustrated in Figure 10-11. Other dentists recommend that the brush be placed at the same angle but with the tufts facing away from the gum line. When assisting and teaching patients, the nurse will wish to follow the preference of the patient's dentist.

Automatic toothbrushes (electric or battery-operated) have been found to be as good as hand brushes. Water spray units are available to assist with oral hygiene. The unit is attached to the faucet and sprays water under pressure on areas to which it is directed. If too much pressure is used, damage to gum tissue may occur. It is helpful as an aid to brushing because it flushes material from around braces and dental bridges.

Many bacteria in the mouth become lodged between the teeth. The toothbrush cannot reach these areas well. Therefore, flossing several times a day is recommended by many dentists. The practice not only removes what the brush cannot, but helps to break up groups of bacteria. Figure 10-12 illustrates a recommended way to floss teeth. Table 10-1 further describes the process (see p. 181).

Mouth care is equally important for persons with false teeth, or **dentures.** Removable dentures are taken out and cleaned with a brush. There are brushes designed for dentures which are helpful for cleaning small areas. There are also preparations in which to soak dentures. Some dentists recommend that removable dentures remain in place except while they are being cleaned. If the patient has been instructed to remove his dentures while sleeping, a disposable, covered cup is convenient and easy to use. It is better not to place dentures in cups, glasses, or other dishes that are used for eating. Keeping the dentures out for long periods of time permits the gum lines to change, thus affecting the fit of the dentures.

Giving Oral Hygiene. The care of the mouth just described is used during illness. However, there are times when care must be modified because of the patient's condition. If the patient is able to assist with his mouth care, he should be provided with the necessary materials frequently. If he is helpless, the nurse will make certain that special attention is given as often as necessary to keep the mouth and teeth clean and moist.

Medicated mouthwashes may be used, especially if the patient likes

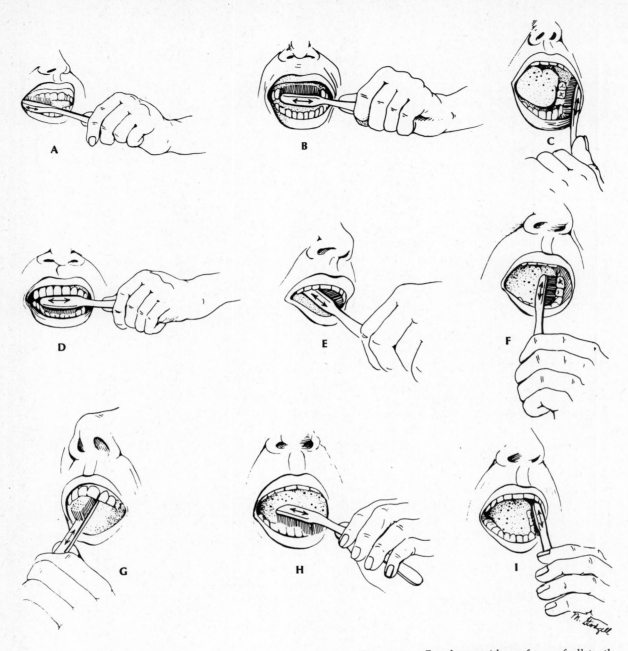

Fig. 10-11 For the outside surfaces of all teeth and the inside surfaces of the back teeth, position the brush with the bristles at the junction between the teeth and gums, as in A; note the exact position of the brush. Then move the brush back and forth with short strokes several times as in B through F. Study each figure carefully. For the inside surfaces of the upper and lower front teeth, hold the brush vertically, as in G and H, and make several gentle back and forth strokes over the gum tissue and teeth. To clean the biting surfaces brush back and forth as in I. (From Effective Oral Hygiene. Developed by USAF School of Aerospace Medicine, Brooks Air Force Base, Texas. Published by The Academy of Periodontology, Chicago.)

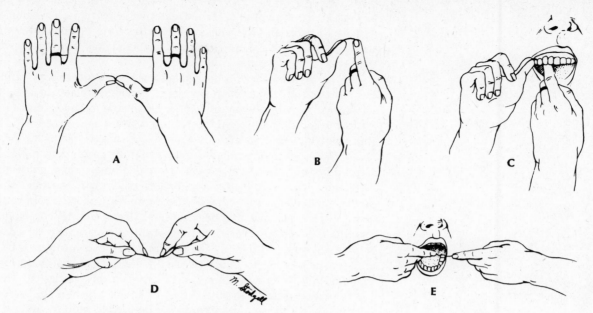

Fig. 10-12 Flossing technique, A. Wrap floss on middle fingers. B. Thumb to the outside for upper teeth. C. Flossing between upper back teeth. D. Holding floss for lower teeth. E. Flossing between lower back teeth. (From Effective Oral Hygiene. Developed by USAF School of Aerospace Medicine, Brooks Air Force Base, Texas. Published by The Academy of Periodontology, Chicago.)

Table 10-1 Suggestions for flossing and rinsing

1. The fingers controlling the floss should not be more than ½ inch apart.*
2. Do not force the floss between the teeth. Insert it gently by sawing back and forth at the point where the teeth contact each other. Let it slide gently into place.
3. With **both** fingers move the floss up and down six times on the side of one tooth, and then repeat on the side of the other tooth until the surfaces are "squeaky" clean.
4. Go to the gum tissue with the floss, but not into the gum so as to cause discomfort, soreness, or bleeding.
5. When the floss becomes frayed or soiled, a turn from one middle finger to the other brings up a fresh section.
6. At first flossing may be awkward and slow, but continued practice will increase skill and effectiveness.
7. Rinse vigorously with water after flossing to remove food particles and plaque that have been cut loose. Also rinse with water after eating when it is not possible to floss or brush. Rinsing alone will not remove bacterial plaque. Water spraying devices alone will not remove bacterial plaque because of the fatlike material in the plaque.

---

*Numbers 1 to 6 from Effective Oral Hygiene. Developed by USAF School of Aerospace Medicine, Brooks Air Force Base, Texas. Published by The Academy of Periodontology, Chicago.

the taste. However, plain or salted water will work equally well to loosen mucus particles and to cleanse the mouth. If the mucus and secretions are very sticky, a solution of half water and half hydrogen peroxide will help to remove them.

It may be necessary for the nurse to use some means for opening the patient's mouth if he is unconscious. A tongue blade usually works satisfactorily. After the mouth is opened, several methods can be used to clean the mouth and teeth. Prepackaged swabs moistened with lemon and glycerine are used in some agencies. A tongue blade wrapped with gauze that is secured with adhesive so that the gauze does not come off is good but may be too large to reach smaller areas. Small gauze squares held with a clamp are better for small areas, but care must be taken not to damage tissues and teeth with the clamp. Large cotton applicators are helpful. The cotton should be secured so that it will not come off in the mouth. The cotton is less irritating and the size can be varied easily, depending on the situation. The patient's toothbrush can be used if the nurse is careful not to injure tissues. If the tufts of the brush are stiff, running hot water over them helps to soften the bristles.

Whenever placing an object, such as a toothbrush or applicator, into a patient's mouth, a mouth gag should be used to hold the mouth open. The fingers should not be used. A human bite can be a dangerous wound because of the many organisms found in the mouth.

When introducing fluids into the mouth, the nurse keeps the patient's head in a position that will prevent choking. The patient can choke on even a small amount of fluid. When dipping applicators or gauze into a solution for cleaning the mouth, the nurse makes certain that it is moist, but not so wet that solution will gather in the mouth and choke the patient.

After cleaning all areas of the teeth, the nurse cleans the surface of the mouth and the tongue. Once the entire mouth has been cleaned, she moistens the mucous membrane with water. A cream may be applied to the lips to help prevent chapping. The skin on the lips is very thin and evaporation of moisture from the lips takes place rapidly, especially when the patient has a fever.

If the patient is able to take fluids by mouth, the nurse may moisten his lips and mouth frequently with water or chipped ice. This is an aid to oral hygiene.

If the patient has removable dentures, they should be cleaned as often as hygiene indicates. Care should be taken when cleaning dentures for the patient, because they are expensive and damage or loss can create problems. They should be cleaned over a basin of water or a soft towel so that they will not drop onto a hard surface, should they accidently slip from the nurse's hands. Warm water is used since hot water may warp the plastic material from which most dentures are made. When the patient's teeth are not in the mouth, they should be stored in a suitable container and in a safe place.

Caring for the mouth and teeth is an important nursing responsibility. A wide variety of solutions and moisturizers have been used, but studies show that the procedure of cleaning appears to be more important than the agent used. Many well persons would agree also that no mouthwash, breath freshener, ointment, or paste replaces a thorough cleaning of the mouth with a brush and with flossing.

Care of the eyes

The eyes often tell the nurse much about the patient's state of health. During illness, eyes may water or may appear glasslike.

Discharges should be removed carefully from the eyes as frequently as necessary. Dried and crusty secretions around the eyes and on the eyelashes are very uncomfortable. Cotton balls soaked in water or a mild salt solution (normal saline) may be used. The nurse wipes once with each cotton ball, from the corner of the eye toward the other side near the forehead.

Many patients wear glasses, and for some, they are essential for seeing. They represent a considerable financial investment. Therefore, the nurse should use every effort to prevent glasses from being broken or lost.

When cleaning glasses, the nurse allows warm water to flow over the lenses and frame. If there is material dried on the glasses, a little soap or detergent and water may be used. They are rinsed well, and dried carefully with a soft clean tissue. The lenses may be scratched if they are wiped with a tissue before washing them.

Plastic lenses have become popular because they are considerably lighter than glass lenses. Plastic lenses have one disadvantage, however; they are very easily scratched. The nurse will wish to remember this when handling them.

Contact lenses are small discs worn directly on the eyeball. Some eye defects can be corrected more easily with contact lenses than with regular eye glasses. In addition, they cannot be seen, which is why many people wear them for cosmetic purposes. Athletes often wear them during sports events because they are safer than regular glasses.

The nurse will wish to know if her patient wears contact lenses. Ordinarily, the patient will insert, remove, and take care of his own lenses. If his condition is such that he cannot remove them, it is best to seek assistance from someone familiar with the procedure. In emergency situations, the nurse should follow instructions as described in Figure 10-13. Contact lenses may cause damage to the eye if left in place too long or when removed improperly.

The patient wearing an artificial eye generally will wish to care for it himself. It is cleaned in warm water or a mild salt solution. If the patient is unable to remove the artificial eye, the nurse will wish to seek assistance from someone familiar with removing it.

Care of the ears and nose

The outer ear and the area in back of the ear are washed, rinsed, and dried when giving the patient a bath. No object should be placed into the canal of the ear. If the ear becomes plugged with wax, it may be necessary for a nurse experienced with the procedure, or a physician, to syringe the ear.

The best way to clean the nose is to blow it *gently*. Irrigating the nose is not often recommended because of the danger of forcing something up further into the nose. Small objects should not be placed in or near the nose because they may go up into the nose, become lodged, and then

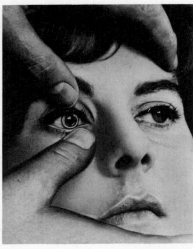

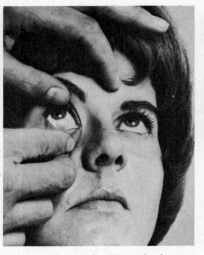

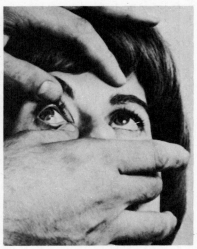

Directly over the cornea: This normal wearing position of the corneal contact lens is also the correct position for removing it. If the lens cannot be removed, however, slide it onto the sclera.

On the sclera only: Here the lens can remain with relative safety until experienced help is available; other white areas of the eye to the side or above the cornea might also be used. If the lens is to be removed, however, slide it to a position directly over the cornea.

On both the cornea and sclera: A lens in this position—or a similar one anywhere around the periphery of the cornea—should be moved as soon as possible. If the lens is to be removed, slide it to a position directly over the cornea; if the lens cannot be removed immediately, slide it onto the sclera.

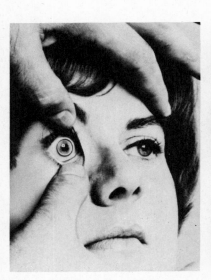

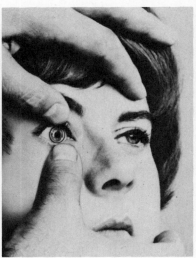

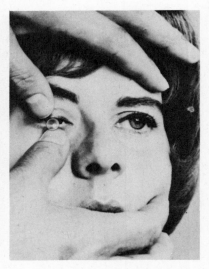

After the eyelids have been separated and the corneal contact lens has been correctly positioned over the cornea, widen the eyelid margins beyond the top and bottom edges of lens (as shown).

After the lower eyelid margin has been moved near the bottom lens edge and the upper eyelid margin has been moved near the top lens edge, (as shown) move under the bottom edge of the lens by pressing slightly harder on the lower eyelid while moving it upward.

After the lens has tipped slightly, move the eyelids toward one another, thus causing the lens to slide out between the eyelids (as shown).

Fig. 10-13 How to remove contact lenses. (From Contact Lens Emergency Care Information & Instruction Packet. Published by American Optometric Association Committee on Contact Lenses.)

become difficult to remove. Occasionally, secretions may dry around the outside of the nose. Mineral oil or a cream or lotion may be applied to the area to loosen and remove the secretions.

Care of the fingernails

The nails are a structure of the skin. The body of the nail is the exposed part. The root lies in a groove where the nail grows and is nourished by the bloodstream.

The fingernails are usually cared for at the time of the bath. They may be groomed by filing or cutting. The nails should not be trimmed too far down on the side because of the danger of injury to the cuticle and skin around the nail. Nail scissors should be used with great care to avoid injuring the skin.

Hangnails are dried and broken pieces of cuticle. Pushing the cuticle back gently after washing the hands helps prevent hangnails, as does using creams on the cuticles. Once they are present, they may be removed with cutting; this should be done with great care to prevent injury to the cuticle.

A blunt instrument, such as an orange stick or the large end of a flat toothpick, is used to clean under the nails. The nurse will wish to be careful to avoid injuring the area under the nail where it is attached to the skin.

Care is finished by lubricating the hands with a cream or lotion and massaging the hands from fingertips toward the wrists.

Care of the feet and toenails

Proper foot care is important at all times, especially when illness is present and for older patients.

Proper care starts with cleanliness. An important part of the bed bath is to soak the feet, rinse off soap well, and dry them thoroughly. Frequent bathing and using foot powder help when feet tend to perspire freely.

The toenails are trimmed. Cutting or digging deeply at the sides of the nails should be avoided. Patients with ingrown toenails may need medical attention. The area under the nail is cleaned in the same manner as that under the fingernails.

Toenails of the older patient are often brittle and thick. They should be soaked in water before being cut. If a basin of water is not convenient for soaking, the feet are wrapped in damp cloths and each foot is placed in a plastic bag for a period of time.

Foot care is completed by massaging the feet with a cream or lotion, beginning at the toes and moving toward the ankles. Or, plain powder is used if the skin is not dry or if the feet are perspiring. Special attention should be given to the heels and ankles. If there is redness present from pressure, the areas should be massaged well.

The nurse will wish to be aware of foot problems the patient may have, including infections, inflammations, ingrown nails, breaks in the skin, corns, calluses, and bunions. Such conditions should be reported since they may require a physician's attention. A patient with a diagnosis of diabetes needs special foot care also. This care is discussed in other nursing courses.

Care of the hair

Hair grows in follicles in the skin. A **follicle** is a small saclike structure. Hair receives its nourishment from the blood which circulates through each follicle.

Good general health is important for attractive hair. Cleanliness helps keep it attractive. Illness affects hair, especially when the body temperature is elevated, when the patient eats poorly, and when worry and tension are present.

Hair is exposed to the same dirt and oil as the skin. It should be washed as often as necessary to keep it clean. A weekly shampoo is sufficient for most persons but more or less frequent shampooing may be indicated for others. Brushing helps keep hair clean and also distributes oil along each hair shaft. In addition, it stimulates the circulation of blood in the scalp.

A comb is used for arranging the hair. Sharp and irregular teeth may scratch and injure the scalp and should be avoided. A large-toothed comb is recommended for very curly hair, for example, the hair of most black persons. The comb and brush should be washed each time the hair is shampooed and as frequently as necessary between shampoos.

If the hair is dry, an oil may be used. There are many preparations on the market, but pure castor oil, olive oil, and mineral oil are just as satisfactory. The hair of black people tends to be dry, and, therefore, the use of oil is usually necessary. If the hair is oily, more frequent shampooing is necessary.

When patients are ill, they may beg to have their hair left undisturbed. This can become a problem, especially if the hair is long. Hours of careful combing of small sections of hair may be necessary if the patient's hair is not combed even for one day. Tangling and matting can be prevented by braiding the hair if the patient does not object. The hair is parted in the middle at the back of the head and two braids are made, one on each side, so that the patient does not have to lie on one heavy braid. Bobby or hair pins or clips should be avoided because they may injure the scalp.

Most patients have a hair style they prefer. The nurse should observe this style when caring for the hair whenever possible.

Many health agencies have beauticians and barbers to assist with the care of the patient's hair, including shampooing. If these services are not available, the nurse shampoos the patient's hair.

When the patient is up and about, he may shampoo his hair when he showers or in a basin in the bathroom. If the patient is confined to bed but is able to be moved onto a stretcher, he can be taken to a convenient sink and have his hair shampooed as he lies on the stretcher.

If the patient is bedridden, his head and shoulders are moved to the edge of the bed, and a protective device is placed under the head. Many agencies use a plastic tray with a water trough, such as the one illustrated in Figure 10-14. The patient is placed so that water constantly drains from the tray, down the trough, and into a receptacle on the floor. This

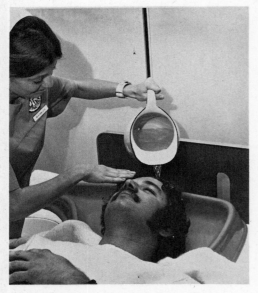

Fig. 10-14 The nurse is using a plastic tray with a trough that carries water from the shampoo to a receptacle on the floor. Note how the patient's neck is supported on the edge of the tray with a towel.

arrangement makes thorough washing and rinsing possible. Following the shampoo, the hair is dried quickly to prevent the patient from becoming chilled.

Pediculosis

Infestation with lice is called **pediculosis.** Lice live on the blood of the person they infest. There are three common types: one infests the hair and scalp; another infests the body; and the third infests the pubic and axillary hairs. Lice lay eggs, called **nits,** on hair shafts. Nits are white or light gray and look like dandruff. They cannot be brushed or shaken off the hair. Frequent scratching and scratch marks on the body and scalp suggest that the patient has pediculosis.

Pediculosis can be spread directly by contact with infested areas or indirectly through clothing, bed linen, brushes, and combs. The linen and personal care items of the patient with pediculosis require separate and careful handling to prevent spreading.

There are numerous preparations for the treatment of pediculosis. Some will destroy nits as well as the lice. Several treatments usually are necessary. Shaving off infested hair is done, especially when pubic and axillary hair are infested. Although shaving is a relatively simple way of handling pediculosis, shaving the scalp is rarely done.

Perineal care

An important part of personal hygiene is perineal care. There are times when care described with the bathing procedure in Chart 10-3 is not enough. Flushing and scrubbing the area then becomes necessary. The procedure is frequently referred to as an external douche. Chart 10-6 describes this type of perineal care.

The decubitus ulcer

A **decubitus ulcer** is an area where skin tissue has been destroyed and there is usually destruction of underlying tissue as well. The usual cause is insufficient blood supply to the area as a result of prolonged pressure. The terms, decubitus ulcer, **pressure sore,** and **bedsore** are used interchangeably.

Preventing Decubitus Ulcers. The earliest sign of a decubitus ulcer is pale skin on a part of the body. This is followed by reddened, irritated, and tender skin. The skin eventually breaks and a decubitus ulcer has formed. The nurse should watch for early signs of a decubitus ulcer, especially among patients most likely to develop pressure areas and on those parts of the body where they are most likely to develop.

A patient who is ill and possibly eating poorly is a likely candidate for a bedsore. Older patients whose skin is wrinkled and less resistant to irritation than younger persons are prone to develop decubitus ulcers, as are patients who have lost a great deal of weight and very thin patients. They occur in men more often than in women. If fever is present,

Chart 10-6 Perineal care
The purpose is to clean the external genitalia and perineal and crotch areas

Suggested Action	Reason for Action
Bring equipment and supplies to bedside, including solutions recommended by agency, usually one for cleaning and one for rinsing. Solutions should be warm, about 105°F.	Bringing everything to bedside conserves times and energy. A warm solution will be comfortable for patient.
Fan-fold top linen to foot of bed while replacing it with bath blanket. Or, pie-fold top bed linen to expose area. Place patient on bedpan, as described in Chart 10-2.	Proper draping prevents unnecessary exposure and chilling of patient.
While holding container about 6 inches above patient over genitalia, pour cleansing solution over area and follow with rinsing solution.	Cleansing solution will loosen dirt and organisms. Rinsing well will flush material into bedpan.
If flushing is not enough to clean area well, scrub, rinse, and then dry area. Use disposable material, as for example, cotton balls, for scrubbing. Material may be held with a forceps. Or, the nurse may don gloves and scrub and dry patient. Stroke from pubic area down toward anal area once and discard cotton ball. Repeat procedure as often as necessary for thorough cleaning. Rinse area well and dry area with cotton balls in same manner as described for scrubbing. In female, be sure to separate labia and carefully clean, rinse, and dry this area also.	Thorough washing and rinsing area removes dirt and organisms that cause skin irritation and unpleasant odors. Drying well helps prevent skin irritation and injury. Cleaning an area where there are fewer organisms before an area with many organisms helps prevent spreading organisms to cleaner areas.
Remove bedpan and turn patient on side. Clean and dry anal area well. Replace bed linen and help patient to comfortable position.	

Crotch, scrotum, penis, and anal area of male patient may be cleansed in same way as described above. Or, with towel under buttocks, area is thoroughly washed, rinsed, and dried but without flushing area with solution. If patient is not circumcised, the foreskin or prepuce is pulled back onto penis carefully; cleanse exposed area thoroughly and carefully. Be sure to pull prepuce back into place over glans penis after cleaning it to prevent injury to penis.

destruction of tissues may occur rapidly. Any area where there is pressure on the body may develop bedsores since blood cannot get to the part well enough to nourish skin cells.

Common areas where decubitus ulcers tend to develop are the area at the end of the spine (coccyx); the heels; the elbows; the ankles; the shoulder blades; the bony area at the top of the hips (iliac crests); and the back of the head.

The following are common nursing measures that help to prevent decubitus ulcers:

• Keep the skin dry and clean. This is especially important when patients have considerable drainage from wounds, when they are

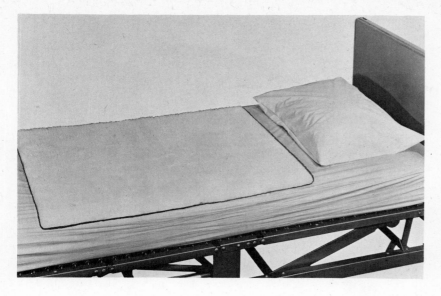

Fig. 10-15 This washable synthetic pad helps to protect a patient who is likely to develop decubitus ulcers, and also to promote healing for a patient with decubitus ulcers. (Photograph courtesy of the Posey Company)

unable to control voiding and defecating, and when they perspire a great deal.

- Change the patient's position often to prevent continuous pressure on one area of the body. The back-lying position should be used as infrequently as possible because it causes the greatest amount of pressure to many vulnerable areas.
- To help keep the skin dry, try to avoid using rubber and plastic on the patient's bed. If such protection is necessary, place the patient on sheepskin if possible. These are skins with wool cropped closely. The air spaces allow air circulation and help keep the area dry. Wool sheepskins can be washed by hand but they tend to become stiff and hard. They are usually used for one patient only because of the difficulty of cleaning them well. Synthetic sheepskins are also available. Figure 10-15 illustrates one. They can be washed and reused many times.
- Massage areas carefully and often where there is pressure on the body. This stimulates circulation and helps prevent the formation of a bedsore. Protect areas especially prone to pressure sores, as the coccyx, heels, and elbows. Figure 10-16 illustrates a type of protective heel device.
- A mattress that is too firm may cause too much pressure on parts of the body. A water mattress is useful to prevent pressure on areas of the body. Figure 10-17 illustrates how pressure is distributed on the water mattress. Alternating pressure pads placed over a regular mattress are helpful. These pads fill with air or fluid, part of the pad at a time, and then deflate; then another part inflates and deflates. In this way, no one part of the body has pressure on it for long continuous periods of time. Figure 10-18 illustrates another type of flotation pad. Be careful when using pins which can puncture and ruin these devices.
- Keep bed linens free of wrinkles, and dry and clean to prevent irritation of the skin.
- Do everything possible to help keep the patient in the best possible

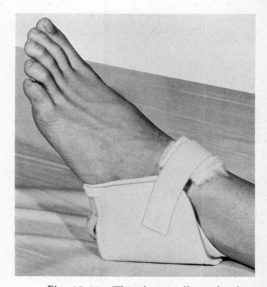

Fig. 10-16 This device allows for free movement as it protects the heel from pressure and contact with bed linens. (Photograph courtesy of the Posey Company)

The decubitus ulcer

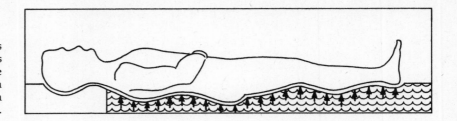

Fig. 10-17 The water mattress allows for even distribution of the patient's weight, thereby eliminating pressure areas. It can be used for the prevention of decubitus ulcers and as an aid in healing them.

physical condition. This includes seeing to it that he eats a nutritious diet, takes plenty of fluids, has sufficient rest, and gets exercise and activity to the extent possible.

Treating Decubitus Ulcers. A great variety of methods is used to treat decubitus ulcers. The nurse will wish to observe procedures of the agency where she gives care. No one method to date has proven very successful. By far the best treatment is to prevent the formation of decubitus ulcers with good nursing care.

Conclusion

Personal hygiene practices are an important part of health and grooming. These practices are also an important part of nursing care. In addition to helping patients meet personal care needs, the nurse as a health teacher uses opportunities as they arise to teach others good habits of personal hygiene.

References

Allen, Linda, ed., *The Look You Like*, American Medical Association, Chicago, Illinois, 1971, 182 p.

"Bedsores: Prevention and Care of Decubitus Ulcers," *Nursing Update*, 5:1, 3–14, December 1974.

Berecek, Kathleen H., "Etiology of Decubitus Ulcers," *The Nursing Clinics of North America*, 10:157–170, March 1975.

————, "Treatment of Decubitus Ulcers," *The Nursing Clinics of North America*, 10:171–210, March 1975.

Carbary, Lorraine Judson, "Bedsores, A Real Challenge," *Nursing Care*, 7:22–25, November 1974.

DeWalt, Evelyn M., "Effect of Timed Hygienic Measures on Oral Mucosa in a Group of Elderly Subjects," *Nursing Research*, 24:104–108, March-April 1975.

Griffin, Annie, "Doing It Better: Conquering Those Obstinate Decubiti: The Screen Box," *Nursing 75*, 5:25, March 1975.

Hardy, Jean, "Bathing Patients Without Soap and Water," *Nursing Care*, 7:25–27, February 1974.

Lang, Christine and McGrath, Anne, "Gelfoam for Decubitus Ulcers," *American Journal of Nursing*, 74:460–461, March 1974.

Miller, Marion E. and Sachs, Marvin L., *About Bedsores: What You Need To Know to Help Prevent and Treat Them*, J. B. Lippincott Company, Philadelphia, 1974, 45 p.

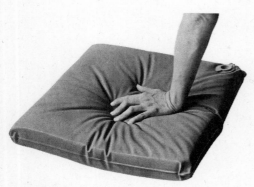

Fig. 10-18 This example of a flotation pad illustrates how weight can be distributed to relieve pressure areas. This type is especially handy for patients who are allowed to sit in a chair or a wheelchair. (Photograph courtesy of the Posey Company)

Pellegrino, Victoria Y., "Tips From the Experts: Unblemished Advice on Skin Care," *Today's Health*, 53:36–39, 53, 55, April 1975.

Reitz, Marie, and Pope, Wilma, "Mouth Care," *American Journal of Nursing*, 73:1728–1730, October 1973.

Taif, Betty, "Foods and Nutrition: Oral Health Counseling," *The Journal of Practical Nursing*, 25:14–15, 39, 40, March 1975.

Yentzer, Maryann, "Doing It Better: Conquering Those Obstinate Decubiti: Foam Leg Supports," *Nursing 75*, 5:24, March 1975.

Zucnick, Martha, "Care of an Artificial Eye," *American Journal of Nursing*, 75:835, May 1975.

11

measures to promote proper nutrition and to maintain fluid and electrolyte balance

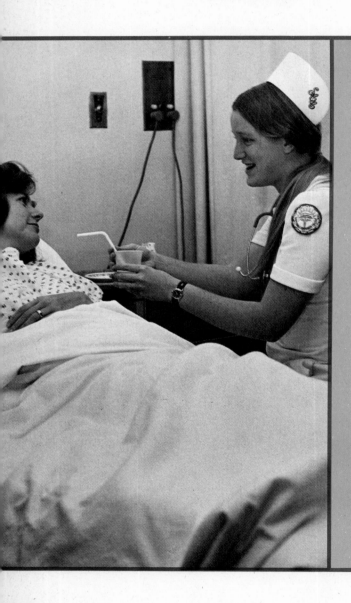

behavioral objectives

When mastery of content in this chapter is reached, the student will be able to

Define terms appearing in the glossary.

Describe briefly the basic nutritional needs of man.

List the four basic groups of food and give several examples of food in each group.

List several examples of cultural factors, other than those given in this chapter, that illustrate influence on eating habits.

List at least 15 ways in which the nurse can help when serving food to patients; list at least ten additional ways in which the nurse can help a patient to eat.

List at least six nursing measures that are often helpful when anorexia, nausea, and vomiting are present.

Describe briefly why it is important to help prevent patients from choking when they are eating or when they are vomiting, and list three or four measures the nurse can use that will help to prevent patients from choking.

Describe briefly why accurate and complete recording of intake and output are important.

List ways in which the nurse can assist the patient whose fluid intake should be considerably more than average normal amounts; whose fluid intake should be considerably less than average normal amounts.

Describe briefly special nursing care required by patients who are having gastric gavage or gastrostomy feedings and describe how these feedings are offered.

Discuss briefly how the body's acid-alkaline and fluid and electrolyte balance are normally maintained.

State five or six conditions that will suggest to the nurse that a patient is a likely candidate for fluid and electrolyte imbalance if preventive measures are not taken.

List eight or ten common signs that indicate fluid and electrolyte imbalances are occurring.

Discuss briefly how fluid and electrolyte disturbances are commonly corrected.

glossary

Acidosis A condition characterized by a proportionate excess of hydrogen ions in extracellular fluid.

Alkalosis A condition characterized by a proportionate lack of hydrogen ions in extracellular fluid.

Anorexia Loss of appetite or a lack of desire for food.

Belching The discharge of gas from the stomach through the mouth. Synonym for eructation.

Calorie The amount of heat necessary to raise the temperature of 1 kilogram of water 1°C.

Cellular Fluid The fluid within the cell. Synonym for intracellular fluid.

Electrolyte A substance capable of breaking into ions and developing an electrical charge when in solution.

Emesis Vomited content. Synonym for vomitus.

Eructation The discharge of gas from the stomach through the mouth. Synonym for belching.

Extracellular Fluid The fluid outside the cell; includes interstitial and intravascular fluid.

Gastric Gavage Introducing nourishment into the stomach with a tube inserted through the nose and esophagus.

Gastrostomy A surgical opening into the stomach through the abdominal wall.

Interstitial Fluid The fluid found between tissue cells.

Intracellular Fluid The fluid within the cell. Synonym for cellular fluid.

Intravascular Fluid The fluid found in the blood vessel (vascular) system. Synonym for plasma.

Ion An atom which carries electrical charge in solution.

Malnutrition The condition resulting from lack of proper food nutrients in diet.

Milliequivalent The unit of measure to describe electrolyte chemical activity. Abbreviated mEq.

Nausea The feeling of sickness with a desire to vomit.

Nutrition The process whereby the body uses foods and fluids to reach and maintain health.

pH The expression of hydrogen ion concentration and resulting acidity-alkalinity of a substance.

Plasma The fluid found in the blood vessel (vascular) system. Synonym for intravascular fluid.

Projectile Vomiting Vomiting with great force.

Regurgitation The act of bringing the stomach contents to the throat and mouth without vomiting effort.

Retching The act of vomiting without producing vomitus.

Vomitus Vomited content. Synonym for emesis.

introduction

You undoubtedly have or will have studied nutrition in a separate course. Therefore, only a brief review of some of the basic knowledge from the field of nutrition will be presented in this chapter. Much of the chapter deals with nursing care that will help patients maintain normal nutrition. The last part briefly discusses fluid and electrolyte balance and how the nurse can assist the patient in maintaining it.

Nutritional needs of man

Nutrition is defined as the process whereby the body uses foods and fluids to reach and maintain health. The science of nutrition has identified the normal needs of man. For example, we know that the body needs water, protein, carbohydrates, fats, vitamins, minerals, and calories in specific amounts for health.

Water. Approximately 75 to 80 per cent of our body tissue is water. Water content must be maintained at a fairly constant level in order to maintain health. Therefore, sufficient fluid intake is an essential part of wellness.

Protein. Protein is important to build and maintain body tissues. People who are poorly nourished are almost always on diets that are poor in protein content. Protein is usually considered the most important of all food substances. It is likely to be the most expensive nutrient in the diet except in sources such as peas and beans.

Carbohydrates. Carbohydrates are the main source of calories in most people's diets. They are important, however, for more than their caloric content. For example, the cellulose found in the stems and leaves of many vegetables gives the diet bulk that aids digestion and elimination. Carbohydrates also help to make the diet more tasty and attractive and are good sources of energy.

Minerals. In general, a well-balanced diet provides enough minerals for health. In some situations, the body may be short of certain minerals which must then be given to a patient in larger than usual quantities. An example is the pregnant woman. Her body will give up the mineral, calcium, to her developing baby. Therefore, she will need a larger intake of calcium to maintain her health. Similarly, iron is essential for the formation of hemoglobin in the blood. Lack of sufficient iron can become a serious problem unless steps are taken to increase the iron intake through foods and/or medications.

Vitamins. Vitamins are essential for normal tissue functioning. They are not manufactured by the body and some of them cannot be stored. Therefore, a daily intake of vitamins is important. Certain diseases are common when vitamin intake is poor. For example, vitamin D helps to prevent rickets, a disease in which bones are soft and will eventually become deformed.

Calories. The measurement for heat is called a calorie. A **calorie** is the amount of heat necessary to raise the temperature of 1 kilogram of water (about 2.2 pounds) 1°C. We speak of food as having caloric value. This means that food is able to furnish heat, or energy, to the body. Needs for calories vary and will depend on such factors as age, activity, and the sex of the person.

Nutritionists generally classify foods in four basic groups: meat, poultry, and fish; milk and milk products, including eggs and cheese; cereals and cereal products; and fruits and vegetables. Some foods from each group are recommended for daily intake.

When the diet is poor the person suffers from inadequate nutrition, and is said to be **malnourished.**

Culture and eating habits

Eating habits are generally learned early in life. They vary from culture to culture, as examples of eating habits in Chapter 3 illustrated. Factors related to food and eating habits include:

- Religious practices often influence eating habits. For instance, many Jews and Moslems avoid pork, and fasting is practiced in certain religions.
- Specific kinds of food are associated with certain nationalities. Hamburgers and hot dogs are associated with Americans; Italians favor pasta, such as spaghetti and macaroni; and the favorite dessert of Greeks is baklava.
- Some people favor eating their largest meal of the day at noon. Others prefer this meal in the evening.
- Family get-togethers are often centered around a holiday meal, as for example, Thanksgiving and Christmas dinners.
- Certain beverages and foods are associated with festive occasions. Champagne is the traditional wedding beverage; turkey is served for Thanksgiving; and candy is the gift of choice for St. Valentine's Day.
- Eating utensils differ. For example, Americans use knives, forks, and spoons; Far Easterners eat with chopsticks; and Arabs use bread to dip foods from common service containers.
- Food tends to relieve the tensions of worry for some people.

The nurse will wish to be aware of factors such as those just described, in order to help patients meet nutritional needs with as much pleasure and satisfaction as possible.

Eating habits are sometimes influenced by a fad. As a health teacher, the nurse has a responsibility to assist patients and their families to separate fads from facts. Chart 11-1 was prepared from material published by the Food and Drug Administration, U. S. Department of Health, Education, and Welfare, Public Health Service. It illustrates claims which often lead to fads that are not always consistent with the facts (see p. 198).

Serving food to patients

Nursing responsibilities in relation to food service will vary among health agencies. Most hospitals have a dietitian and centralized food services. However, nurses are still generally responsible for ordering and cancelling diets for patients, for assisting with the serving of meals, for helping patients eat, and for recording information concerning how well the patient is eating.

Most often, patients are served food at their bedsides. Some hospitals have cafeterias for patients who are up and about and some have areas where patients may eat together.

There are food services available now in many cities for the patient at home. For example, the U. S. Department of Agriculture has a program called "Drive to Serve Programs." There are community centers that provide food with "Meals-On-Wheels" service. Also, commercial vendors serve patients at home in some areas. In places where such services are not available, the nurse may be of help in teaching the patient and family members ways to meet nutritional needs for the patient at home.

The following are suggested ways nurses can assist in serving food to hospitalized patients:

- Avoid giving treatments immediately before and after meals whenever possible. Examples include enemas and dressing changes.
- Offer the patient a bedpan or urinal before meal hours. Offer mouth care as indicated.
- See that the patient is clean and in a comfortable position for eating. Change a soiled gown or bed linen, for example. Also, see that the room is tidy. Remove from sight supplies and equipment that may be annoying, such as a bedpan, urinal, dressing cart or tray, dead flowers, linen hampers, and other unattractive objects.
- Do whatever is needed to help the patient in pain. This will be discussed further in Chapter 13.
- When there are several patients in one room, it may be better in some cases to provide privacy for a critically ill patient while others are eating.
- A tired or excited patient is usually in no mood to eat. Try to provide a period of rest and quiet before meals. If the patient requires treatments that take considerable time, plan to allow sufficient time for him to rest before meal hours.
- Cooperate with the dietary department so that food is served promptly and the general appearance of the tray is orderly and tidy. Spilled liquids, out-of-place silverware, hot foods that have cooled, and cold foods that are wilted or melted do not increase appetite. Replace items missing from a tray, such as a napkin, silverware, or a glass or cup.
- Check carefully to see that the name on the tray corresponds with the name on the patient's identification bracelet. A tray served to the wrong patient can be a serious error.
- Place the tray so that it is easy for the patient to reach. Remove food covers.
- Open milk cartons and cereal boxes, butter toast, cut up meat, and otherwise assist as indicated. It is difficult for the patient to do these simple tasks when bedridden, even if he is not disabled.
- Serve trays last to those patients who need help with eating. It is unappetizing and often annoying for the patient to have food at his bedside while waiting for the nurse to finish other work.
- Note foods that the patient is not eating and report these findings. For example, if the patient is not eating his meat, a substitute may be offered. Or, if his dentures are not comfortable, he may eat ground meat more easily.
- Observe whether the patient feels satisfied with the amounts of food he is served. If he is hungry, servings may need to be increased. Or snacks may be offered between meals if the patient's condition permits. Also, note whether the servings seem too large. For patients who eat small portions, large servings may decrease their appetites.
- Some agencies allow family members to bring in certain foods when patients have eating problems. Observe agency policy concerning this practice. Some agencies may not allow it. When it is permitted, be sure food is refrigerated or stored properly, cover the food, and label it for

Chart 11-1 Common claims and facts concerning eating habits

Claim	Fact
You are what you eat.	In one sense, yes. You are also what heredity and environment have contributed.
Our soil has lost its vitamins and minerals; our food crops have little nutritional value.	In the commercial production of food crops fertilizers are applied in order to produce satisfactory yields. The nutrients which promote good plant growth are added to the soil in these fertilizers, and the food crops produced contain the expected nutritional value.
Chemical fertilizers are poisoning our soil.	Chemical fertilizers are not poisoning our soil. Modern fertilizers are needed to produce enough food for our population. Our increasing population further increases the need for these fertilizers.
Natural, organic fertilizers are not only safer than chemical fertilizers, but produce healthier crops.	Organic fertilizers cannot be absorbed, as such, by plants. They must be broken down by bacteria in the soil until they finally become the same chemical elements—potassium, phosphorus and nitrogen—that are supplied directly and more quickly by modern chemical fertilizers. Their use may also contribute to the spread of certain infectious diseases.
Pesticides are poisoning our nation.	When pesticides on food crops leave a residue, FDA and the Environmental Protection Agency (EPA) make sure the amount will be safe for consumers. The amount allowed, if any, is set at the lowest level that will accomplish the desired purpose, even though a larger amount might still be safe.
Modern processing removes most of the vitamins and minerals in foods.	This is not true. While any type of processing, including simple cooking, tends to reduce to some extent the nutrient content or quality of foods, modern processing methods are designed to keep such losses as low as possible. In many instances, nutrients are restored by enrichment after processing.
Aluminum cooking utensils are dangerous to health.	Aluminum is the second most abundant mineral element in the soil, and it, therefore, occurs naturally in many foods. Cooking in aluminum utensils is harmless.
Cooking with Teflon-coated utensils is dangerous.	Careful testing of this commercial product has proved that there is no danger from normal kitchen use, or the overheating which might occur in the kitchen.
If you have an ache or pain, or are just feeling tired, you are probably suffering from a subclinical deficiency.	Feeling poorly, lacking pep, or experiencing an ache or pain occurs in most persons at some time or another. These are symptoms which may be caused by overwork, emotional stress, disease, lack of sleep as well as by poor nutrition. If such symptoms persist, a person should see his physician. It is extremely difficult for the average person to accurately diagnose the cause of these symptoms.
You have to eat special foods if you want to correct overweight.	Your physician should prescribe any special diet you may need. Personal experimenting and fad diets can be highly dangerous to your health. Successful weight control depends primarily on self-control of one's total food intake while maintaining a reasonable level of physical activity.
Synthetic vitamins are dead and ineffective; vitamins from natural sources are much better.	Vitamins are specific chemical compounds, and the human body can use them equally well whether they are synthesized by a chemist or by nature.

Chart 11-1 continued

Claim	Fact
Everyone should take vitamins, just to be sure.	Very few of us eat exactly the same foods as our neighbors eat. There is some variation that makes our diet different from everyone else's. It is variety that helps to assure adequate nutrition for most of us. Most healthy individuals whose diet regularly includes even modest amounts of meat and eggs, milk products, fruits and vegetables, bread, and other cereal products need not resort to dietary supplements. Some persons under a doctor's care or in institutions need dietary supplements because of special conditions which greatly restrict their ability to eat a well-balanced diet. Modest supplementation with certain vitamins is generally recommended during infancy, pregnancy, and while breast feeding.

the patient. Also, care for leftover foods and dishes promptly and record extra foods the patient is eating.

- Be considerate of the patient on a special diet who may be denied food he likes because of a health problem. Explain that his diet is specially planned for him. It may help to visit him once or twice while he eats. Scolding patients who do not like their diets is not nursing. The patient needs the nurse's help and support.
- Remove trays as soon after eating as possible. If something has been spilled, see that it is cleaned up. Change linen as necessary. Leave the patient comfortable and clean.
- Offer the patient an opportunity to brush his teeth after eating. Assist him as necessary.
- Record the patient's intake according to agency policy.

Helping patients to eat

Some patients will need the nurse's help with eating. The suggestions offered in the previous section on serving food still apply. The following recommendations are also given:

- Assist the patient into a comfortable position. If permissible, raise the head of the bed. The sitting or semisitting position usually makes swallowing easier and choking less likely than the lying position.
- Protect the patient and top bed linen with a napkin.
- For patients who can eat without help but cannot handle food and utensils easily, open cooked eggs, butter the bread, cut meat into bite sizes, open milk containers, and so on.
- Provide a drinking tube for patients unable to use a cup.
- Sit in a comfortable position. Avoid appearing rushed or hurried. The nurse has an excellent opportunity while feeding the patient to develop good nurse-patient relationships, to learn to know her patient better, and to teach him as necessary.
- If the patient is allowed activity and can assist, encourage him to take part as he can. This helps him to develop independence to the greatest extent possible for him.
- Serve manageable amounts of food with each bite. Even patients sitting up can choke when the amounts of food are too large.

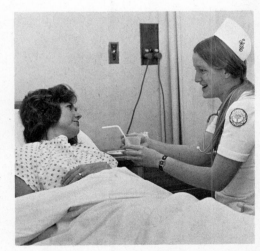

Fig. 11-1 The nurse illustrates various suggestions made in this chapter for assisting the patient to eat.

- Serve the food in the order of the patient's preference. Offer liquids and solids alternately. Give the patient sufficient time to chew and swallow his food thoroughly.
- Try not to leave a patient after starting to feed him until he has finished eating.
- Keep conversation friendly and discuss pleasant subjects. Avoid using mealtime as a question and answer period on the patient's condition.
- If the patient is blind, tell him what you are offering him. Use a system, such as hand touching, to indicate when he is ready for more food or when there is another bite ready for him.

Common problems that influence eating: anorexia, nausea, and vomiting

Anorexia is a loss of appetite or a lack of desire for food. There are many factors that may produce anorexia. Some are illness, general lack of interest in food, and feeling tense and worried. If the symptom continues and the patient is eating poorly, the physician may need to prescribe measures which will help the patient to receive adequate nourishment. An example is to provide the patient with nourishment intravenously, that is, to inject solutions directly into his veins. The intravenous injection of solutions is discussed further in Chapters 17 and 20.

Nausea is a feeling of sickness with a desire to vomit. It may be associated with feeling faint or weak. Often, dizziness, perspiration, skin pallor, a rapid pulse rate, and a headache are present. **Retching,** which is the act of vomiting without producing vomitus, may also be present.

Vomiting results when the contents of the stomach are forced out through the mouth. It is also called **emesis.** The vomited content is called **vomitus.** Nausea is usually present before vomiting occurs.

Projectile vomiting refers to vomiting with great force. Nausea may be present. Projectile vomiting is often noted in certain disease conditions, such as increased pressure on brain tissues or when gastrointestinal bleeding is present.

Bringing stomach content to the throat and mouth without the effort of vomiting is called **regurgitation.** It occurs quite commonly among infants after eating.

Eructation or **belching** is a discharge of gas from the stomach through the mouth.

The following measures are often helpful when anorexia, nausea, and vomiting are present:

- Check to see that suggestions offered in the last two sections of this chapter are being observed. Something as simple as an annoying odor or sight may produce anorexia, nausea, and even vomiting. Having to use a bedpan or urinal, an uncomfortable position in bed, and being served foods that the patient finds distasteful are other causes for these symptoms.
- Avoiding abrupt movements and limiting the patient's activities may help prevent nausea and vomiting, especially if motion seems to bring on the symptoms.
- Taking deep breaths is often helpful during periods of nausea.
- Limiting the patient's food and fluid intake temporarily until the symptoms subside is advised. Then offer fluids in small sips. Chipped ice may be helpful.

- Bland foods are usually better than spicy foods or foods high in fat content. Carbonated beverages are often tolerated when others are not.
- When a patient is vomiting, it becomes important to prevent choking and having vomitus go to the lungs. Should this happen, the patient is likely to develop an infection in lung tissue, or he may choke to death by suffocating. Turn the patient's head to one side while he is vomiting and is in the lying position. Elevate his head on a pillow or raise the head of the bed slightly. This position will help vomitus leave the mouth. Usually the patient is more comfortable if he can lie down, rather than remain in a sitting position. If the head is lower than the stomach, vomiting may increase. In some cases when the patient is very weak or unconscious, it may be necessary to use a suction machine to remove vomitus from the mouth and throat in order to prevent choking.
- If the patient has a wound in his abdomen, offer firm support when he is vomiting or retching. The nurse may hold her hands over the affected area or place a firm pillow against the abdomen; an abdominal binder will also offer support.
- After he vomits, help the patient with oral hygiene as soon as possible. Wash his hands and face and change linen as indicated. The sight, taste, and odor of vomitus are often enough to cause more vomiting.
- Help reduce tension as much as possible. Give the patient a backrub and see to it that his room is quiet and that it is comfortable in relation to temperature, ventilation, and light.
- Measure, or estimate if necessary, the amount of vomitus and note its appearance and odor. Vomitus is recorded as output on the patient's record. Send a specimen to the laboratory if ordered. Report and record the findings according to agency policy. Have your supervising nurse check the vomitus if you have any questions, especially if you notice an unusual odor, such as the odor of fecal material or alcohol.
- When anorexia, nausea, and vomiting continue, the physician may find it necessary to prescribe drugs to help relieve the symptoms.

Recording the patient's fluid intake

Chapter 10, included a discussion on measuring the patient's output. As stated there, most patients whose output is measured and recorded need to have intake measured and recorded as well. Intake and output are often abbreviated I and O.

Health agencies generally have tables readily available to tell the nurse the amount of fluid that common serving dishes, glasses, and cups contain. The unit of measure usually is a cc. or ml. Also, if water containers are left at the patient's bedside, the nurse learns the amount of water they contain. She follows agency procedures concerning measurement of the fluid a patient takes from the container and the times of day when the amount is measured and recorded.

Recording intake includes all liquids the patient takes—those he takes with meals, as milk, soup, coffee, and tea; the water he drinks during the course of each 24-hour period; the liquid nourishment he may have, as a malted milk or a soft drink; and intravenous solutions he has had. Ice cream, sherbet, and thin cereals are recorded as liquids in most hospitals.

The nurse will use the form supplied by the agency for recording intake. Most forms will contain spaces where she records fluid taken with each meal and where entries can be made between meals. At the end of the 24-hour period, the nurse (or some other person charged with this duty) totals the amount, records it according to agency procedure on the patient's record, and begins a new form for the next day.

For home care, the nurse may need to teach the patient or family members how to measure and record fluid intake. Using a common household measuring cup, the fluid content of the patient's cup, glass, soup dish, or whatever, can be determined. Then it becomes an easy matter to measure and record the intake. Home measurement is usually stated in ounces. The patient should be made to understand why his intake is to be recorded and why it is important to do so accurately.

Recording a patient's intake and output sometimes seems a humdrum affair. Carelessness becomes all too frequent. Yet measuring and recording intake and output are very important nursing duties. Much of the patient's care may be planned around his intake and output. If the patient appears not to be taking enough fluids, for example, the physician may order a solution to be given intravenously. Decisions in relation to prescribing certain drugs and determining proper dosages may be based on the patient's intake and output. Other examples could be cited but the importance of complete and accurate records of intake and output is obvious, and carelessness in this nursing responsibility represents poor-quality care.

Figure 11-2 illustrates a form used to record the patient's intake.

Forcing or limiting fluid intake

There are times when the patient's fluid intake should be either more or less than he normally would take. The first is referred to as **forcing fluids;** the latter is usually called **restricting fluids.** Most often, the amount the patient should take is indicated. For example, if the patient is to have fluids forced, the amount may be stated as 3000 cc. or ml. each day. Or, if fluids are restricted, the amount will be 800 or 1000 cc. or ml. It often takes a great deal of ingenuity on the nurse's part to assist the patient when fluids are forced or restricted. The nurse will wish to offer understanding and support and encourage the patient's efforts.

When fluid intake is to be high, fluids should be handy at the bedside at all times, and kept in containers the patient can manage. It is of little value to leave a pitcher of water at the bedside that he cannot handle. A variety of fluids should be offered often during the day. Goals are set for the amount that should be taken, for example, every two hours, or by noon or dinner time. Food high in water content, such as fresh fruits, should be offered. Fluids should be served at the proper temperature. Normally, during the night the patient takes little or no fluids. Therefore, he is usually able to take a proportionately greater amount during early hours of the day.

When fluids are restricted, they are kept out of sight as much as possible. Small containers are used. Fluids or foods that are likely to make the patient feel more thirsty should be avoided, such as dry, salty,

	INTAKE					OUTPUT					
	ORAL	I.V.	I.V.	BLOOD	COMMENTS	GASTRIC TUBE	URINE	STOOL	VOMITUS	OTHER	COMMENTS
7-8	370cc										
8-9											
9-10											
10-11	100cc										
11-12											
12-1	350cc										
1-2	75cc										
2-3	200cc										
8 HR. TOT.	1095cc										
3-4											
4-5	50cc										
5-6											
6-7	400cc										
7-8	200cc										
8-9	125cc										
9-10	100cc										
10-11											
8 HR. TOT.	875cc										
11-12											
12-1											
1-2	50cc										
2-3											
3-4											
4-5											
5-6	75cc										
6-7	75cc										
8 HR. TOT.	250cc										
24 HR. TOT.	2220cc										
	TOTAL INTAKE					TOTAL OUTPUT					

INTAKE AND OUTPUT CHART

Fig. 11-2 An example of a form used to record the patient's oral intake. Note that there are three 8-hour totals as well as the 24-hour total on this form. Recording output was discussed and a form was illustrated in Chapter 10.

and sweet foods. The spacing of fluids he is allowed is planned with the patient. Oral hygiene is maintained as necessary and the lips are kept lubricated to prevent drying and chapping. Rinsing the mouth with water often helps reduce thirst. Chipped ice is generally helpful. The resulting liquid amounts to about one-half the volume of the ice.

When fluids are forced or restricted, a careful record of the patient's intake should be kept. To neglect to do so gives an inaccurate picture of the results of the patient's plan of care.

Gastric gavage and gastrostomy feedings

When patients are unable to take fluid or food by mouth, other methods are used to maintain nutrition. Giving solutions intravenously has already been mentioned. Another method is gastric gavage. **Gastric gavage** means introducing nourishment into the stomach with a tube that is inserted through the nose. It is used when the patient has no disturbances of the stomach and small intestines. An example is the patient

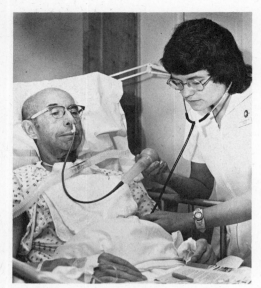

Fig. 11-3 The nurse checks to be sure that the gavage tube is in the patient's stomach before offering nourishment. In this case she introduces air with the bulb syringe, while simultaneously using a stethoscope to listen for the sound of air entering the patient's stomach.

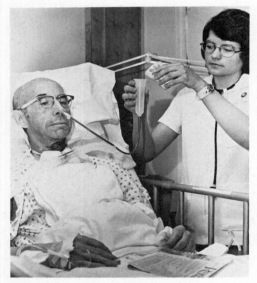

Fig. 11-4 Once the tube is in the patient's stomach, the nurse removes the bulb from the syringe and pours nourishment. The rate at which nourishment flows into the stomach is determined by the height of the syringe: the higher the nurse holds the syringe, the faster the flow of nourishment and vice versa.

who has had mouth or throat surgery. Occasionally, an unconscious patient is fed by gavage. It is also used for patients too weak to eat or drink. Infants born prematurely are often fed by gavage in order to save their strength.

An experienced nurse or physician introduces a tube through the nose and into the stomach. Proper nourishment in liquid form is prepared, generally by the dietary department of a hospital. It consists of basic food requirements. Drugs ordinarily taken by mouth may be added to the liquid nourishment, as ordered by the physician.

Before giving nourishment, it is a good precautionary measure to check the position of the tube so that nourishment will not accidentally be introduced into the lungs. One of these three methods may be used: (1) Placing the end of the tube in a container of water. If air bubbles appear, the tube is not in the stomach but most likely in a bronchus leading to the lung. (2) Attaching a syringe onto the end of the tube. If stomach contents can be aspirated, the tube is then in the stomach. (3) Attaching a syringe onto the end of the tube. While listening with a stethoscope over the upper abdomen, the nurse will hear air entering the stomach as she injects air with the syringe.

Either of two methods is used to introduce nourishment. When the patient is to receive a rather large amount several times a day, an asepto syringe (a syringe without a barrel) or a funnel is attached to the tube. The nourishment is poured into the syringe or funnel *slowly* and allowed to flow steadily into the stomach by gravity. The flow can be regulated simply by raising or lowering the syringe or funnel. Raising it will increase the flow; lowering it will decrease the rate of flow.

It is best to warm the nourishment to about 105°F. before introducing it into the stomach. This helps prevent the patient from feeling chilly. While pouring the nourishment, the nurse does not let the syringe or funnel empty. If this happens, air will be forced into the stomach when she fills the funnel or syringe. After the nourishment has been introduced, a small amount of water, an ounce or two, is given. The water washes the remaining nourishment in the tube into the stomach. Between feedings, the tube is clamped in order to prevent stomach contents from escaping.

Another method uses a special receptacle that will hold a pint to a quart of nourishment. It is attached to the tube and hung on a standard at the patient's bedside. An adjustable clamp on the tube regulates the rate of flow into the stomach. The patient receives nourishment very slowly and continuously with this method. Pre-warming the nourishment is not recommended. The liquid will warm sufficiently before it reaches the stomach as it passes through the tube. Also, most nourishments contain milk or cream which will sour quickly if warm too long before reaching the stomach.

In most instances, the tube is left in place. However, it is generally removed and a clean one inserted every two or three days for sanitary purposes.

There is another way to introduce nourishment directly into the stomach. A **gastrostomy** is a surgical opening into the stomach through the abdomen. A tube is placed into the stomach through the surgical opening in the abdominal wall. Nourishment is then given through the tube. Methods for giving gastrostomy feedings and the care and preparation of nourishment are the same as for a gastric gavage.

Patients who are fed in either of the two ways just described are in need of special mouth care frequently. The mucous membrane and lips should be kept lubricated also. When the tube is placed through an opening in the abdominal wall, the skin around the wound will require care and attention. Wound care is discussed in Chapter 18.

The amount of nourishment the patient receives is measured and recorded according to agency procedures.

Fluid and electrolyte balance: definition of terms

During the last three decades or so, remarkable progress has been made in our knowledge of body fluids and the elements they contain. We know that our lives depend on maintaining the proper amount of body fluids and their chemical elements, their proper place in the body and their proper relationship to each other.

Normally, physiological processes in the body maintain fluid and electrolyte balance. However, many illnesses and even certain circumstances in the healthy person threaten that balance. For example, participating in extensive outdoor physical activity on a hot day, going for a long period of time with a poor fluid intake, or eating a poorly balanced diet for an extended period can cause disturbances in fluid and electrolyte balance. Disorders resulting in vomiting, diarrhea, and high fever may cause imbalances. Certain conditions such as diabetes, burns, surgical procedures, and infectious diseases frequently create disturbances. Some drugs, such as those that promote the excretion of urine, may also result in imbalances.

Fluids are present in two body spaces. There is fluid within each of the body's cells. This is referred to as **cellular** or **intracellular fluid.** All fluid outside of the cells is **extracellular fluid.** It consists of intravascular and interstitial fluid. Fluid within the blood vessel (vascular) system is called **intravascular fluid** or **plasma;** fluid in which tissue cells are bathed is called **interstitial fluid.**

All body fluids contain electrolytes. An **electrolyte** (sometimes called a salt or a mineral) is a substance capable of breaking into ions and developing an electrical charge when dissolved in solution. An **ion** is an atom which carries an electrical charge in solution. The unit to describe electrolyte chemical activity is a **millequivalent,** abbreviated mEq.

The element, hydrogen, is the basis for pH calculations. The term **pH** is an expression of hydrogen ion concentration. The pH calculation describes the acidity-alkalinity of a substance. The pH of pure water is 7.0, which is neutral. As the hydrogen ion increases, a solution becomes more acid and the pH becomes less than 7.0. When the concentration of hydrogen decreases, the solution is alkaline and the pH is greater than 7.0. The strongly acidic gastric secretions have a pH of about 1.0 to 1.3. Strongly alkaline secretions from the pancreas have a pH of about 10. Normal blood plasma is slightly alkaline with a pH of about 7.35 to 7.45. **Acidosis** is the condition in which there is an excess of hydrogen ions in

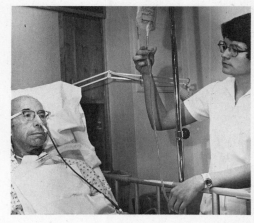

Fig. 11-5 An illustration of how nourishment is introduced into the stomach continuously and slowly via the gastric gavage tube. The nourishment has been placed in a container that is suspended on a standard. The nurse regulates the rate at which nourishment is given, drop by drop, with a clamp and drip meter.

the body's extracellular fluid and the pH falls below 7.3. **Alkalosis** is the condition in which the extracellular fluid has a pH exceeding 7.45. Normal acid-alkaline balance is maintained by the body's ability to take up or discharge hydrogen ions, by carbon dioxide excretion from the lungs, and by the ability of the kidneys to select or reject ions.

Maintaining fluid and electrolyte balance

Healthy persons maintain fluid and electrolyte balance automatically. They take in a wide variety of materials in various quantities and dispose of wastes and excesses as a result of complicated chemical mechanisms in the body. Water and electrolytes for the body arrive from the ingestion of fluids and food and from metabolic processes. Water and electrolytes are normally lost from the body through the kidneys, intestinal tract, skin, and lungs. Fluid and electrolyte intake and their losses from the body vary with the individual and circumstances but are kept in careful balance in the healthy person. Tables 11-1 through 11-3 illustrate

Table 11-1 Average daily adult fluid sources

Amount of fluid	Sources of fluid
ml.	
1200–1500	Ingested water
700–1000	Ingested food
200–400	Metabolic oxidation
2100–2900	

Table 11-2 Average daily adult fluid losses

Amount of fluid	Exit route
ml.	
1200–1700	Urine
100–250	Feces
100–150	Perspiration, insensible losses
350–400	Skin
350–400	Lungs
2100–2900	

Table 11-3 Average daily water losses of healthy adults under varying circumstances*

Exit route	When body temperature is normal	When pyrexia is present	Following prolonged exercise
	ml.	*ml.*	*ml.*
Urine	1400	1200	500
Feces	200	200	200
Perspiration, Insensible losses	100	1400	5000
Skin	350	350	350
Lungs	350	250	650
	2400	3400	6700

*Adapted from Shepard, R. S.: Human Physiology. p. 390. Philadelphia, J. B. Lippincott, 1971.

average daily adult fluid sources and losses and average daily water losses of adults under varying conditions.

The major electrolytes required by the body are sodium, potassium, chloride, calcium, and bicarbonate. They are normally present when persons are eating and taking fluids properly.

Many measures are ordinarily taken to aid in maintaining the patient's fluid and electrolyte balance. For example, helping the patient maintain proper nutrient and fluid intake is very important. Drugs are often ordered to handle an infectious process that predisposes to imbalance. Every effort is made to help patients take adequate nourishment and fluid when anorexia, nausea, and vomiting are problems. Fluid intake is encouraged or guarded, depending on the circumstances. Efforts are made to avoid the development of decubitus ulcers which, if allowed to occur, can result in drainage that may upset balance. The inactivity of bed rest often accompanying illness may result in such disturbances as an increased excretion of nitrogen. Hence, high protein diets are often ordered for patients requiring long periods of bed rest. Calcium is taken from bone tissues during long periods of inactivity. Hence, nursing measures, to be discussed in Chapter 12, are used to promote activity to the greatest extent possible.

Successful prevention of fluid and electrolyte imbalances must often actively involve the patient. The nurse may find that an extensive teaching program for the patient and his family could result in the prevention of serious illness for the patient who is not maintaining fluid and electrolyte balance.

The nurse's observations are particularly important in order to detect early signs of imbalance. The frequency of observing patients likely to develop imbalances should be increased. Once imbalances occur, the nurse should observe common symptoms and report them promptly so that preventive measures can be started immediately.

Signs of fluid and electrolyte disturbances

Fluid and electrolyte imbalances usually occur in combination. While observations of the patient are important, laboratory studies are usually used to help determine the exact nature and type of imbalance. Advanced nursing texts discuss characteristic symptoms of the numerous imbalances that can develop during illness. A brief summary is presented here.

The nurse will want to be familiar with the patient's health state, the history of his present illness, and the medical plan for therapy. Any one, or any combination of factors may predispose to fluid and electrolyte imbalance. Because balance is maintained normally when the intake of fluid and electrolytes are in proper proportion to their output, anything that upsets the scale on either side acts as a warning to the nurse. These are a few typical questions for which the nurse will wish to seek answers: Has the patient's normal food and fluid intake changed? If so, for how long has it differed from the usual? Have there been restrictions on what the patient could eat or drink? Has there been any abnormal loss of body fluids? What particular body fluids were involved? What is the patient's intake and output of fluids?

Any situation in which the patient has lost excessive fluids and electrolytes warns of imbalance problems. Examples include extreme perspiration, vomiting or diarrhea, wound or body drainage, or blood loss. With fever, patients lose more fluids than when their body temperature is normal, as Table 11-3 illustrates. Inadequate fluid and electrolyte intake can result from nausea, a poorly balanced diet, or the unavailability of food or fluids. Excessive intake of fluids or electrolytes can also be a problem. Patients who are on gastric or duodenal suction, which will be discussed in Chapter 20, are especially susceptible to fluid and electrolyte disturbances unless preventive measures are taken. Because the young and the elderly have less effective physiological processes than normal adults, they will tend to be higher risks for imbalances.

No single symptom in itself necessarily indicates fluid and electrolyte imbalance. All must be reviewed in relation to the patient's state of health. Probably more important than any particular sign is how the symptom compares with the person's usual characteristics. These are some signs that often indicate imbalances are occurring:

- When fluid intake is below normal, the skin and mucous membranes become dry. The lips may be chapped and a whitish coating may be present. The eyes appear sunken. When the skin is pinched between the fingers, it remains in folds or returns slowly to its normal position.
- An excess of fluid in tissues produces swelling, or edema. This can often be seen around the eyes, in the fingers, at the ankles, and in the lower part of the back.
- Electrolyte imbalances may cause the muscles to appear limp, or to be tense and twitch or cramp involuntarily.
- The patient may be sleepy and disoriented. He may go into a state of unconsciousness. Or, in other imbalances, he may be very apprehensive, active, and tense. Convulsions may occur.
- Personality changes may occur. For example, the active, outgoing person may become withdrawn and quiet, or vice versa.
- Any changes in the vital signs are important to note. For example, the pulse and respiratory rate and volume may change from normal. Body temperature may be elevated.. Blood pressure may be increased or decreased from normal.
- Fluid intake in relation to output may be out of balance. This can be determined most accurately by careful measurement of the patient's intake and output.
- The patient may be gaining or losing weight out of proportion to his intake.
- Anorexia, nausea, and vomiting commonly accompany certain electrolyte imbalances.
- Laboratory analyses of the urine and blood will indicate changes in their composition, specific gravity, and pH.

Fluid and electrolyte imbalances are likely to occur in conjunction with many different types of illnesses. Some examples include uncontrolled diabetes, perforated peptic or duodenal ulcers, pneumonia, infections, injuries, chronic alcoholism, asthma, emphysema, various kidney and heart diseases, and burns. Imbalances also often result from the indiscriminate use of diuretics (drugs that increase the production of urine), morphine or meperidine (Demerol), vitamin D, salt, sodium bicarbonate, and plain water enemas. In fact, it is the rare illness or indiscretion that offers no threat to eventual fluid or electrolyte disturbances.

Correcting fluid and electrolyte disturbances

Certain guides help in planning action when measures to correct fluid and electrolyte disturbances become a necessary part of the patient's care. Any deficits the patient has need to be corrected. After deficits are met, the normal fluid and electrolyte requirements of the body must be maintained. Any abnormal losses of water and electrolytes, such as, for example, losses due to wound drainage, vomiting, or diarrhea, must be replaced on a continuing basis as required.

The degree and type of fluid and electrolyte imbalances and the body's ability to cope with them determine the type and intensity of the therapy needed. The physician prescribes the therapy in accordance with each patient's needs. Nursing measures also depend on each patient's individual situation. Whenever possible, it is highly desirable to have the patient help plan his own care and participate in it to whatever extent he can.

There are several measures commonly used to help correct fluid and electrolyte imbalances. Fluid intake may be encouraged or restricted; nursing measures to assist the patient were discussed earlier in this chapter. Encouraging or restricting certain foods is another way to correct disturbances. Intravenous infusions are often used to increase fluids and whatever specific electrolytes the patient needs. Blood transfusion may be used. Infusions and transfusions are discussed further in Chapters 17 and 20.

Conclusion

The nurse is assuming an important duty when she takes steps to help patients meet nutritional needs. Finicky eating often goes along with illness and possibly not every problem can be solved. But a poorly nourished patient faces still one more problem in addition to the others he already has. Therefore, anything the nurse can do to encourage proper eating and drinking is to the patient's benefit.

Maintaining fluid and electrolyte balance often depends on how well the patient's nutritional and fluid needs are being met. Observing the patient carefully is especially important. At the first sign of imbalance, proper remedial steps can be taken, thereby preventing the patient from experiencing the serious problems that can accompany fluid and electrolyte disturbances.

Science has explained many exceedingly complex processes that at best, had been left largely to guesswork in the past. In health, the body has remarkable abilities to maintain normal fluid and electrolyte balance. But in illness states, when the body needs assistance to maintain fluid and electrolyte balances, the demands for high-quality and exacting care can be seen.

References

Beaumont, Estelle and Wiley, Loy, eds., "Innovations in Nursing: Nourishing Recipes for the Patient on Liquid Feedings," *Nursing '74*, 50, August 1974.

del Bueno, Dorothy J., "Electrolyte Imbalance: How to Recognize and Respond to It. Part 1." *RN*, 38:52–54, 56, February 1975.

———, "Electrolyte Imbalance: How to Recognize and Respond to It. Part 2." *RN*, 38:54–55, March 1975.

Feigenberg, Myrtle and Sotman, Judith W., "A Toddler With a Malabsorption Syndrome," *American Journal of Nursing*, 75:978–979, June 1975.

Feingold, Ben F., "Hyperkinesis and Learning Disabilities Linked to Artificial Food Flavors and Colors," *American Journal of Nursing*, 75:797–803, May 1975.

Gaffney, Terry Weiler and Campbell, Rosemary Peterson, "Feeding Techniques for Dysphagic Patients," *American Journal of Nursing*, 74:2194–2195, December 1974.

Grotta-Kurska, Daniel, "Before You Say 'Baloney' . . . Here's What You Should Know About Vegetarianism," *Today's Health*, 52:18–21, 73, 74, October 1974.

Kee, Joyce L., "Fluid Imbalance in Elderly Patients," *Nursing '73*, 3:40–43, April 1973.

Kroog, Emily, "Helping People Stretch Their Grocery Dollars," *American Journal of Nursing*, 75:646–648, April 1975.

Lawler, Marilyn R., "Consultation: Meals for Toothless Patients," *Nursing '74*, 4:70, February 1974.

Lee, Joyce L. and Gregory, Ann P., "The ABC's (and mEq's) of Fluid Balance in Children," *Nursing '74*, 4:28–36, June 1974.

McCarter, Donna, "Nourishing the Solute-Sensitive Patient," *American Journal of Nursing*, 73:1935–1936, November 1973.

Sharer, Jo Ellen, "Reviewing Acid-Base Balance," *American Journal of Nursing*, 75:980–983, June 1975.

Taif, Betty, "Foods and Nutrition: Dietary Assessment: A Blueprint for Change," *The Journal of Practical Nursing*, 24:14–17, August 1974.

———, "Foods and Nutrition: Health Foods and Food Fads," *The Journal of Practical Nursing,* 23:14–17, 33, July 1973.

Tudor, Lea Layton, "Feeding the Helpless Patient Requires A Special Technique," *Nursing Care,* 7:22–24, October 1974.

"When Vomiting Signals a Geriatric Emergency," *Nursing Update,* 6:12–15, June 1975.

12 measures to promote exercise and activity

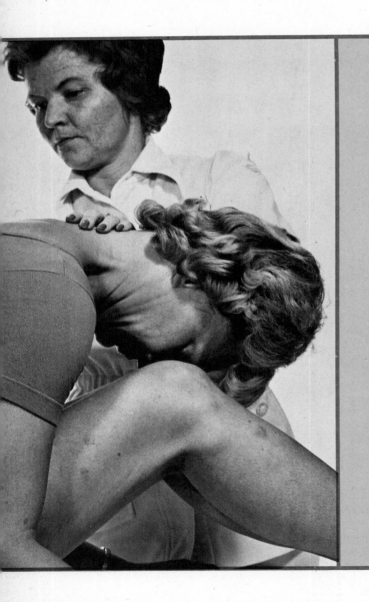

behavioral objectives

When mastery of content in this chapter is reached, the student will be able to

Define terms appearing in the glossary.

List eight dangers to patients resulting from inactivity.

Explain how the 12 devices described in this chapter help to provide safety and comfort for the patient confined to bed and give one common problem each device helps to prevent.

Describe how patients are positioned to provide comfort and proper body alignment in the back-lying, side-lying, face-lying, and semisitting (Fowler's) positions.

Demonstrate how each joint is placed through its range of motion and explain what each exercise accomplishes.

Describe a way in which the nurse properly lifts a patient up in bed and two ways in which two nurses properly lift a patient up in bed.

Describe how a patient can be carried from a bed to a stretcher, using the three-carrier lift.

Describe how one nurse can move a patient from a bed to a chair; from a chair to a bed.

Describe four exercises that can be carried out by the bedridden patient which help prepare him for getting out of bed and walking.

Explain what dangling is and why it is used.

Describe how to help a patient out of bed and to his feet.

Describe four ways in which a patient can be assisted to walk.

State two ways in which a patient is measured for crutches.

List several exercises that help a patient prepare for crutch walking.

Describe three types of crutches.

Discuss how a patient can be helped to handle crutches before he starts to use them for walking.

Explain how the patient supports his weight when using axillary crutches.

Explain four crutch-walking gaits.

List several leisure-time activities that help the patient to exercise and to become active.

glossary

Abduct To move a body part away from the middle of the body.

Active Exercise An exercise performed by a person without assistance from others.

Adduct To move a body part toward the middle of the body.

Axillary Crutches Crutches that fit under the upper arms into the axillae.

Canadian Crutches Crutches that fit the forearms by means of frames or metal cuffs. Synonym for Lofstrand crutches.

Cervical Referring to the neck.

Contracture The abnormal shortening of muscles that makes normal movement at the joint difficult or impossible.

Dangling The position in which the person is sitting on the edge of the bed with his legs and feet hanging freely over the side of the bed.

Extension Action that increases or straightens an angle between two adjoining parts.

Flexion Action that reduces an angle between two adjoining parts; bending.

Footdrop A condition in which the foot falls forward; the toes often point outward.

Fowler's Position The semisitting position.

Hyperextension Action that increases an angle between two adjoining parts further than its average normal range.

Lofstrand Crutches Crutches that fit the forearms by means of frames or metal cuffs. Synonym for Canadian crutches.

Passive Exercise An exercise in which one person moves the body parts of another person.

Platform Crutches Crutches on which the patient bears his weight on his forearms.

Pronation The position of the forearm in which the palm of the hand faces downward, or of the body when one is lying on one's abdomen.

Quadriceps Drills Contracting and relaxing the muscles on the front of the thigh (quadriceps femoris).

Range of Motion The normal extent of movement in a joint.

Rotation The process of turning.

Supination The position of the forearm in which the palm of the hand faces upward, or of the body when one is lying on one's back.

introduction

Research has shown that activity is important for health. Therefore, patients confined to bed or those with physical limitations require care that includes activity and exercise.

Chapter 5 discussed principles of body mechanics and how the nurse uses them in her work. The discussion continues in this chapter. In addition, this chapter describes how to protect the patient from problems that could develop when he is inactive due to illness or disability. This type of care is often referred to as rehabilitation nursing care.

Terms commonly used when discussing exercise and activity

Abduct means to move a body part away from the middle of the body. **Adduct** is the opposite—the body part is moved toward the midline or middle of the body. **Extension** refers to the action that increases or straightens an angle, while **flexion,** or bending, is the action that reduces an angle between two adjoining parts. The trunk of the body is in a state of extension when one is lying flat on one's back, and in flexion when one is sitting. **Hyperextension** means that the angle at a joint is made larger than its average or ordinary range. The neck is hyperextended when one is looking at the ceiling overhead.

Muscles contract, that is, become shorter, to produce flexion or bending at a joint. The shortening of muscles over a period of time results in a **contracture,** a condition that makes normal movement at a joint difficult, or impossible in severe cases. Patients often refer to a contracture as a "locked" or "frozen" joint. For example, if a patient has his knees flexed for a long time, the muscles will become shorter and the patient will have difficulty straightening his knees. Contractures can develop relatively quickly—in a matter of a few weeks—and can be painful and difficult to correct. Therefore, helping a bedridden patient assume a proper posture in bed and having him exercise are important measures to help prevent contractures.

In the standing position, the foot is at a right angle to the leg, with the toes pointing straight forward. When the patient is in bed on his back, the foot tends to drop and the toes usually point outward. If this position is maintained for a period of time, a condition known as **footdrop** occurs. The muscles at the back of the ankle and leg shorten. This condition makes walking difficult, or impossible in severe cases. Footdrop is a contracture of the heel cord (Achilles tendon). Footboards and foot blocks, discussed later in this chapter, can be used to help prevent footdrop. Also, using pleats in the top bed linen keeps the linen from forcing the foot into a footdrop position.

Rotation is the process of turning. For example, the neck is rotated when the head is turned from side to side. The leg rotates outward when the toes point outward. **Pronation** refers to the position of the forearm in which the palm of the hand faces downward. It also refers to the position of the body when one is lying on one's abdomen. **Supination** is the position of the forearm when the palm of the hand is facing upward, or the position of the body when one is lying on one's back. Most of the terms just described are illustrated in Figure 12-1. Supination and pronation of the body are illustrated in Figure 12-2 on page 217.

There are two ways in which patients receive exercise. **Active exercise** means the patient performs the movements for himself without assistance from others. **Passive exercise** means that movement of parts of the patient's body is done by another person, such as the nurse. When possible, active exercise is encouraged. But when the patient cannot move a part of his body, the nurse may be required to move it for him.

Dangers of inactivity

Bed rest and limited activity go along with most illnesses. The dangers of inactivity illustrate the importance of nursing care that includes activity and exercise in the patient's plan of care.

The patient generally suffers psychologically from inactivity. It is normal to be up and about, to work, to exercise, and to enjoy leisure-time activities. When the patient is denied these normal functions because of illness or physical handicaps, his mental attitude and spirit

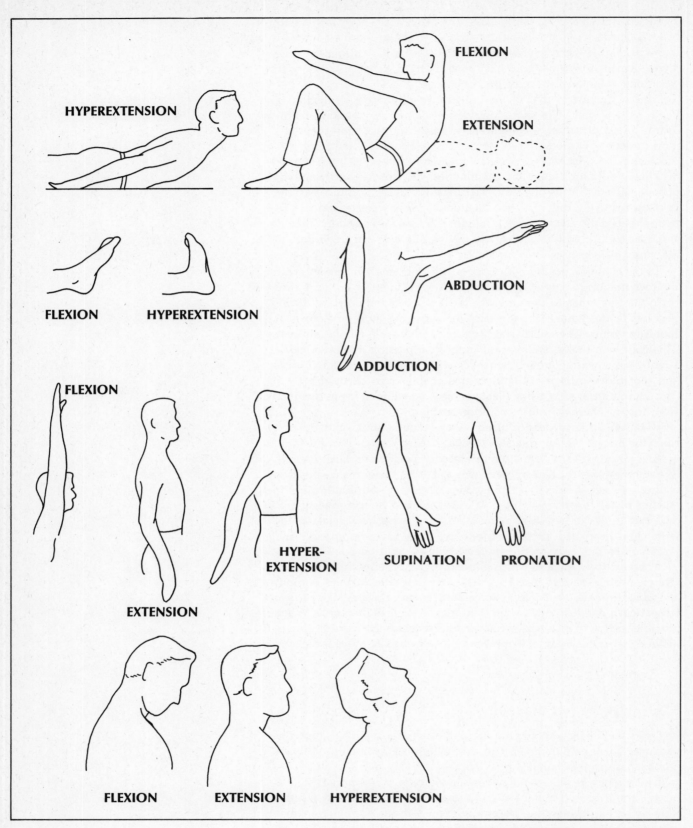

Fig. 12-1 These sketches illustrate some of the terms commonly used when describing movement of body parts.

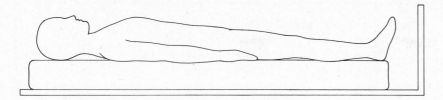

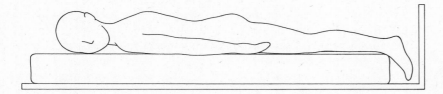

Fig. 12-2 (Top) The body in the supine position. (Bottom) The body in the prone position.

generally suffer. Therefore, helping him to reach or to maintain psychological well-being includes encouraging activity to whatever extent is possible. It includes helping the patient regain his independence as a normal human being. These concepts were discussed in Chapter 1 when rehabilitation was described as an important part of nursing care.

The patient also suffers physiologically from inactivity. Damage to the musculoskeletal system will occur. Muscular weakness develops quickly with inactivity. Recall a time when you were ill with the flu or some other acute infection. Just a few days in bed no doubt left you feeling weak and unsure of foot due to muscle weakness. When inactivity is prolonged, muscular weakness may become so severe that the effects are more damaging than the original illness. In addition to muscular weakness, lack of activity may lead to these problems: the joints of the body become "frozen"; endurance to perform an activity diminishes; and deformities and lack of coordination may develop.

The patient's circulatory system suffers when he is inactive. Blood clots may form that can become a threat to the patient's life. When muscles contract, they squeeze veins, an action which helps to move blood back to the heart. Lack of activity reduces this circulatory assistance. Poor posture, whether one is active or inactive, also tends to slow down circulation. In addition lack of activity hinders good circulation within the lymphatic system, as is the case when the feet swell after standing for a long period of time.

The exchange of oxygen and carbon dioxide in the lungs is influenced by body activity, as well as by posture. Inactivity and poor posture decrease the ability of the lungs to function at their best.

The movement of food in the gastrointestinal tract, intestinal elimination, and the production and excretion of urine are functions influenced by activity. Inactivity places extra work on these functions.

As discussed in Chapter 10, when patients are inactive and remain in one position for long periods of time, decubitus ulcers may develop. Keeping the patient as active as possible and changing his position frequently help to prevent bedsores.

Dangers of inactivity 217

The balance of certain chemicals in the body is often upset when patients remain inactive. This may result in brittleness of bones, as for example, when the calcium balance is upset.

Usually patients feel satisfaction and enjoy whatever activity their plan of care allows. This makes it easier for nurses to help prevent complications due to inactivity. Occasionally, however, a patient may resist the nurse's efforts to promote activity and exercise. He may prefer remaining inactive and receiving care to meet his needs. Sometimes, this desire to remain inactive is due to fear. For instance, a patient recovering from surgery may be afraid to move, fearing his wound may open. An arthritic patient may say he is too stiff and achy to get out of bed. A patient who has had a leg amputation may feel that the effort to relearn to walk on crutches and then on an artificial leg is just too much for him. Helping such patients means that the nurse must show understanding, kindness, and patience. She will wish to build on the patient's abilities and encourage any efforts that he makes. The patient will need to be taught the importance of activity. Explanations are also necessary so that he understands that activity and exercise are part of his medically prescribed care. The nurse promotes a feeling of security by helping the patient know that someone cares as she helps him to stay as active as his condition permits.

It can be seen from this discussion that patients should be encouraged to carry out activities of daily living to the greatest extent possible. By so doing, they feel more independent and are helping to prevent complications that result from inactivity.

Orders for and the recording of exercise and activity

Policies concerning orders for and the recording of exercise and activity vary. A physician's order may be necessary in some situations. In others, the nursing team leader takes responsibility for writing nursing orders for the patient's exercise and activity. It is recommended that the nurse follow orders on the nursing care plan and consult with her supervising nurse if she has any doubts about exercise and activity for the patient.

Recording is also a matter of agency policy. While the types of activity and exercise may not be recorded every time they are used, the progress of and effects on the patient nearly always are. The nurse should observe agency policies concerning recording.

Devices for the safety and comfort of the patient confined to bed

It is just as important for the body to be in good alignment and posture when a person is lying down as it is when he is standing or sitting. There are many devices that help to maintain good body alignment in bed and to prevent discomfort or pressure on various parts of the body.

Pillows. The primary purposes of pillows are to provide support for and elevation of a body part. A pillow under the arm of a patient in the semisitting (Fowler's) position helps prevent pulling the shoulders downward and into a poor posture, as illustrated in Figure 12-19. Small pillows are ideal for support or elevation of the head, extremities, shoulders, or incisional wounds. Specially designed, heavy pillows are useful to elevate the upper part of the body when an adjustable bed is not available, as for example, in the home.

Mattress. For a mattress to be comfortable and supportive, it must be firm but have sufficient "give" to permit good body alignment. Figure 6-1 on page 75 shows the effect of a supportive and nonsupportive mattress on body alignment. Note the unnatural curvature of the spine in the lower drawing.

Bed Board. If the mattress does not provide sufficient support, a bed board may help to keep the patient in better alignment. Bed boards usually are made of plywood or some other firm material. The size varies with the needs of the situation. If sections of the bed can be raised, such as the head and the foot, it may be necessary to have the board divided and held together with hinges. For home use, full bed boards can be purchased, or, they can be made at home from materials on hand.

Adjustable Bed. The adjustable bed was described in Chapter 6. When in the high position, this bed is helpful for the nurse when giving care. When in the low position, it enables the patient to get in and out of bed with greater ease. Raising the head of the bed helps the bedridden patient to see and to look about without twisting and bending his neck. Also, he is in a nearly vertical position without the effort of standing, which helps to prepare him for the day when standing and walking will begin. The foot of the bed may be raised to prevent the patient from sliding down in bed when he is in the semisitting position.

Rocking Bed. The rocking bed is mounted on a frame rather than on the usual bedstead, and by means of an electric motor, it can be made to rock rhythmically up and down in seesaw fashion. It has a footrest to help keep the patient from sliding and also to help keep the feet in good alignment. The bed ordinarily is adjusted to rock at the same rate as the patient's respirations. By shifting the abdominal organs, the rocking bed aids respirations for the patient having difficulty with breathing. This helps move the diaphragm upward and downward, thus helping the patient to breathe. In addition, the constant change in position aids the flow of blood.

Chair Bed. Another type of bed used in the care of patients requiring bed rest is one that can be placed into a chairlike position. These beds are designed primarily for patients who have certain heart conditions. They are also called cardiac beds.

Circular Bed. The circular bed operates with an electric motor. It has a 6 or 7 foot metal frame with a diameter support for the patient. This type of bed is used most often for the patient who will be completely helpless for a long time. As illustrated in Figure 12-3, the patient can be placed in any number of positions which helps prevent the dangers of inactivity described earlier.

Stryker and Foster Frames. A Stryker frame, illustrated in Figures 12-4 through 12-7 has two canvas-covered frames. The patient is secured well between them with safety belts and then turned to his back for the supine position or to his abdomen for the prone position. Once the patient is in position, the upper frame is removed (see pp. 221-222).

The frame on which the patient lies when on his back has an opening

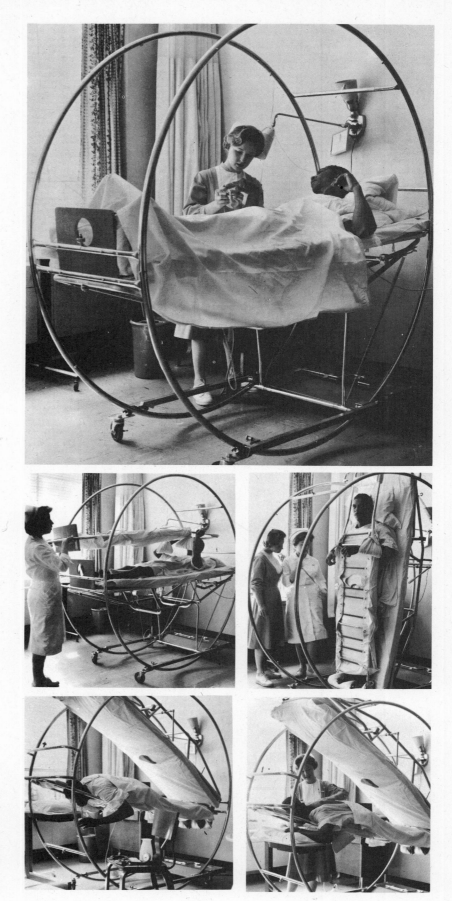

Fig. 12-3 The CircOlectric bed permits the patient to be placed in any number of positions. An electrically powered motor turns the large circular frame. The patient is secured to the part on which he lies with another similar part in a manner like that used with the Stryker frame.

220

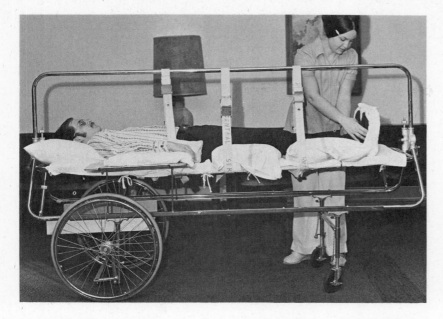

Fig. 12-4 The patient model is positioned on his back on the Stryker frame. Note the support for the feet to prevent footdrop. The knees are kept free of pillows to prevent pressure on blood vessels and nerves in the posterior areas of the knees. The arms and hands are positioned in good alignment.

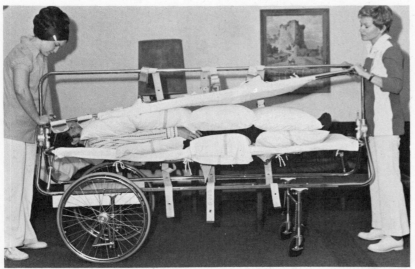

Fig. 12-5 The nurses have protected the patient with pillows and are positioning and securing the top frame in preparation for turning him onto his abdomen.

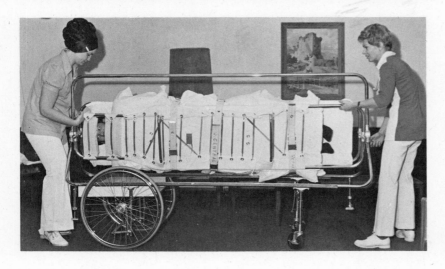

Fig. 12-6 The patient is being turned on the Stryker frame.

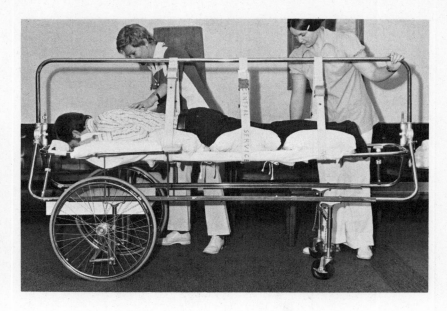

Fig. 12-7 After the turn, the frame on which the patient has been lying is removed, and he is checked for proper alignment and comfort. Note that the feet extend over the edge of the pillow support to prevent poor alignment of the legs and feet. The face is exposed where the forehead and chest supports separate. This frame has large front wheels. The patient able to do so can move himself about by propelling the bed in the same manner as a wheelchair.

for a bedpan and a support to prevent footdrop. The frame on which he lies when on his abdomen has an opening between the forehead and shoulders so that his face is exposed. He can then see objects placed under this area, such as reading materials, food, fluids, and so on. The canvas ends at the ankles so that the patient's feet can rest in the normal position over the bottom edge when he lies on his abdomen. The canvas pieces above and below the openings are covered with bed linen that is pinned under the frame. A Foster frame is similar to a Stryker frame except that it is larger and sturdier.

Patients are placed on Stryker or Foster frames when they are to be immobilized so that healing may occur, for example the patient whose spine has been fractured. They also are used by patients who are paralyzed, for example, patients who have paraplegia (paralysis of both lower extremities) or quadriplegia (paralysis of all four extremities).

Footboard and Foot Block. Footboards and foot blocks are used primarily to keep the foot in the normal walking position, that is, the feet at right angles to the legs and the toes pointed straight forward. This position prevents footdrop. The board is placed between the foot of the bedstead and the mattress. If the patient is short and cannot reach the board, a foot block can be used. The block can be a sturdy box, carton, or wooden block covered with appropriate linen. Another type fastens to the sides of the mattress with a clamp. It can then be placed on the mattress at an appropriate place for the patient. Footboards are illustrated in Figures 12-8 and 12-9.

If a block or footboard is not readily available, an improvised foot support can be made with a pillow and a large sheet. The pillow is rolled in the sheet, and the ends of the sheet are twisted before being tucked under the mattress. The ends should be tucked under the mattress at an angle toward the head of the bed to help keep the pillow in place. A pillow support does not provide the firmness of a board or block and therefore, is better used on a temporary basis only.

Cradle. If the top bed linen must be kept off the patient's feet or legs, a cradle may be used. A cradle is a frame, usually made of metal and constructed so that it can be secured well under the mattress. It is often used over patients with burns and with fractures of the leg. A high footboard may also be used to help keep the bed linen off the patient's feet and legs, as can be seen in Figures 12-8 and 12-9.

Sandbags. Sandbags are used when an extremity needs firm support. For example, the patient may tend to turn his leg outward. To prevent his lying in this position for long periods of time, the leg can be held in good alignment by placing sandbags alongside the outer surface of the leg from the hip to the knee or ankle. When sandbags are properly filled, they are not hard or firmly packed but pliable enough to be shaped to fit body contours. They should not be placed so that they create pressure on bony prominences, such as the bony area at the hip. This precaution helps to prevent the development of a ducubitus ulcer.

Sandbags of various sizes can be purchased. Figure 12-10 illustrates several commonly used sizes.

Trochanter Rolls. The femur is the long, large bone in the thigh. The trochanter is a bony process at the head of the femur near the hip. If sandbags are not available to prevent the legs from turning outward, trochanter rolls, as illustrated in Figure 12-11, can be made.

To make a trochanter roll, fold a sheet lengthwise in half and place it under the patient. Avoid a large piece of linen because of the bulkiness under the patient's back. Place a rolled bath blanket or two bath towels under each end of the sheet that extends on either side of the patient. Roll the sheet around the blanket so that the roll is under. In this way, it cannot unroll itself, and the weight of the patient helps to hold it securely. When the trochanter rolls are properly in place, the patient will be lying on a piece of linen which has a large roll on either side of him. Fix these rolls close to the patient and firmly against the hip and thigh. The leg then does not turn outward. If the roll is not sufficiently long, very little support along the leg can be expected. Pillows properly placed in the same manner can also serve as trochanter rolls, but pillows tend to slip out of place easily.

Hand Rolls. In the resting position, the thumb is held away from the hand slightly and at a moderate angle to the fingers. A rolled washcloth or a ball secured into the hand can be used to maintain this position. There are several hand supports available which are especially helpful if the patient needs hand and thumb support for extended periods of time. Figure 12-12 on page 225 illustrates a type of hand support.

Bed Siderails. Bed siderails are often used for the patient's safety, as described in Chapter 6. They also are valuable to help patients in need of activity in bed. For example, with siderails in place, the patient can safely roll himself from side to side and sit up in bed. These activities help patients regain muscle strength after periods of time when they had to lie quietly in bed.

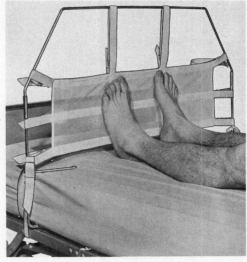
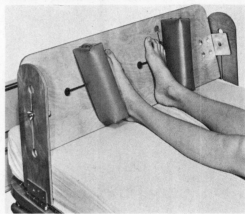

Fig. 12-8 Two types of supports to prevent footdrop. (Top) This support can be secured with clamps at any level along the side of the mattress, depending on the patient's height. The frame of the support is high enough to prevent linen from touching the patient's feet and legs. (Bottom) This support can also be fastened at any level along the side of the mattress. Special supports help to prevent the feet and legs from rotating outward. (Photograph courtesy of the Posey Company)

Positioning the patient confined to bed

Changing the position of patients in bed helps add to their comfort and offers the exercise of movement. The patient's position should be changed frequently if he does not move about by himself. For the very weak, helpless, or unconscious patient, changing position every one to three hours may be necessary to help prevent complications of inactivity. Unless the patient is in good posture, however, complications and discomfort are likely to occur.

The Back-Lying (Supine) Position. In the back-lying position, the feet and neck are in need of particular attention. The greatest danger to the feet occurs when they are not held perpendicular to the legs and footdrop develops. The greatest danger to the neck occurs when the patient uses pillows to tilt the head forward in order to improve his field of vision. This produces flexion of the cervical spine. The word, **cervical,**

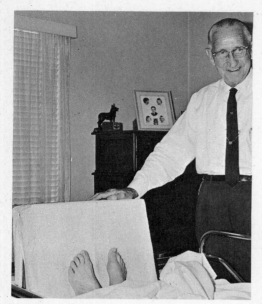

Fig. 12-9   This man prepared a good foot support for his wife who is cared for at home. It is sufficiently high to keep linens off the feet and legs.

Fig. 12-10   These sand-filled positioning weights can be purchased in a variety of sizes, and can be used effectively to support the patient's legs and ankles in proper alignment. (Photograph courtesy of the Posey Company)

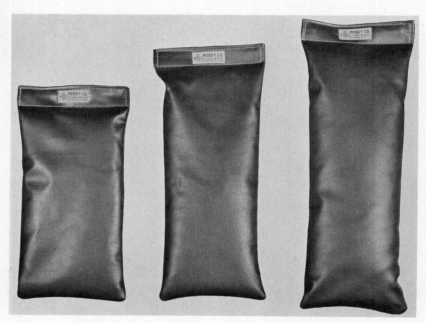

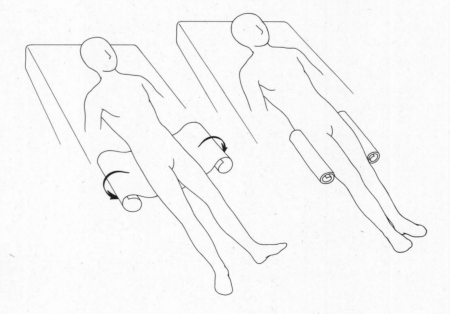

Fig. 12-11   These two sketches illustrate how trochanter rolls are made and used to support the patient's legs so that they do not rotate outwardly.

refs to the neck. Chart 12-1 describes the proper back-lying position and the complications proper positioning can help to prevent.

Side-Lying Position. Lying on the side is a welcomed relief after periods of lying on the back. The toes are not being pulled downward by gravity and footdrop is less likely to develop. The neck is also held in a more erect position. The primary concerns for the patient are the positions of the thigh and arm on the upper side of the body. The pull created by both of these extremities as they fall to the bed causes fatigue. Also, the arm pulls the shoulder forward, thus making breathing more difficult.

Chart 12-2 describes the proper side-lying position and the complications proper positioning can help to prevent. Figures 12-13 through 12-15 illustrate the side-lying position.

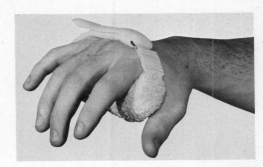

Fig. 12-12 An example of a palm grip that helps prevent contractures of the fingers and thumb. (Photograph courtesy of the Posey Company)

Chart 12-1 Back-lying position

Complication to be Prevented	Suggested Preventive Measure
Exaggerated curvature of spine and flexion of hips	Provide firm supportive mattress. Use bed board if necessary.
Contracture of neck	Place pillows under upper shoulders, neck, and head so that head and neck are held in correct position.
Internal rotation of shoulders and extension of elbows (hunched shoulders)	Place pillows or arm support under forearms so that upper arms are alongside body and forearms are pronated slightly.
Extension of fingers and abduction of thumbs (clawhand deformities)	Make hand rolls or use small towels for hands to grasp. If patient is paralyzed, use thumb guides to hold thumbs in adducted position.
External rotation of femurs	Place sandbags or trochanter rolls alongside hips and upper half of thighs.
Hyperextension of knees	Place small roll under knees, sufficient to fill space behind knees but not to create pressure and not to exceed a 5 to 10° flexion.
Footdrop	Use footboard or block to hold feet in proper position, at right angles to lower legs.

Chart 12-2 Side-lying position

Complication to be Prevented	Suggested Preventive Measure
Lateral flexion of neck	Place pillow under head and neck so that neck is in position of extension.
Inward rotation of arm and interference with respirations	Place pillow under upper arm.
Internal rotation and adduction of femur	Use one or two pillows as necessary to support leg from groin to foot so that leg does not fall onto bed.

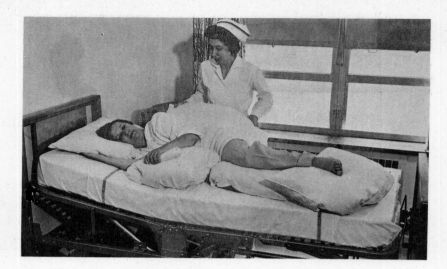

Fig. 12-13 The nurse places pillows properly to keep the patient in good body alignment while in the side-lying position. A pillow at the patient's back prevents her from rolling into the supine position.

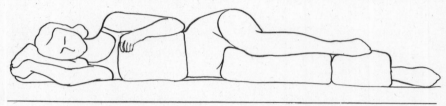

Fig. 12-14 Proper positioning and support of the patient in the side-lying position.

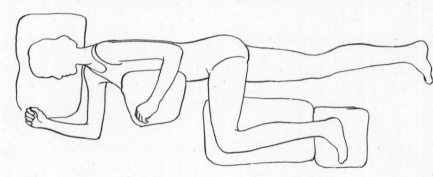

Fig. 12-15 A further illustration of proper positioning in the side-lying position.

Face-Lying (Prone) Position. Lying on the abdomen can be a comfortable and relaxing position. It is especially helpful for the patient with bedsores or one who is likely to develop them from pressure when lying on his back or side. The feet need special support or they should be allowed to go over the end of the mattress. Otherwise, they are forced into footdrop and the legs will turn inward or outward.

Chart 12-3 describes the proper face-lying position and the complications proper positioning can prevent. Figures 12-16 through 12-18 illustrate the face-lying position.

Semisitting or Fowler's Position. The semisitting position is often called **Fowler's position.** This position helps the heart and respiratory system to function, and aids elimination. It also makes eating, conversing, and seeing easier than a lying position. If it is adjustable, the head of the bed is raised to the desired angle. Wedge-type supports and pillows may be used to place the patient in a semisitting position when

Chart 12-3 Face-lying position

Complication to be Prevented	Suggested Preventive Measure
Footdrop	Move patient down in bed so that his feet are over edge of mattress. Or, support lower legs on pillow just high enough to keep toes from touching bed.
Flexion of cervical spine	Place small pillow under head.
Hyperextension of spine and impaired respirations	Place some suitable support under patient between end of ribs and upper abdomen if there is space there and this facilitates breathing.

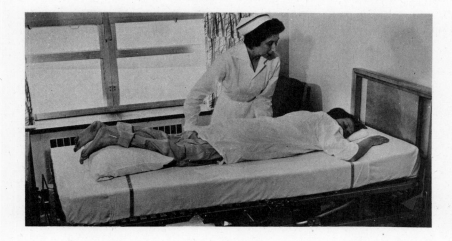

Fig. 12-16 The nurse places pillows properly to keep the patient in good alignment in the face-lying position.

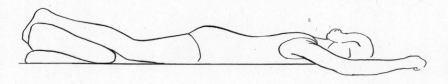

Fig. 12-17 Proper positioning and support of the patient in the face-lying position.

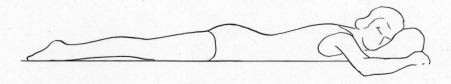

Fig. 12-18 A further illustration of proper positioning and support of the patient in the face-lying position.

the bed is not adjustable. The chair bed, mentioned earlier, is designed to keep patients in the Fowler's position.

Chart 12-4 describes the semisitting position and the complications proper positioning can help to prevent. Figure 12-19 illustrates the position.

Chart 12-4 Semisitting or Fowler's position

Complication to be Prevented	Suggested Preventive Measure
Contracture of neck	Allow head to rest against mattress or be supported by small pillow only.
Exaggerated curvature of spine	Use firm support for back. Position patient so angle of elevation starts at his hips.
Dislocation of shoulder	Support forearms on pillows so they are elevated sufficiently to prevent pull on shoulders.
Contracture of wrists	Support hands on pillows so they are in natural alignment with forearms.
Edema of hands	Support hand so it is slightly elevated in relationship to elbow.
Impaired lower extremity circulation and knee contracture.	Elevate knees for brief periods only. Avoid pressure on vessels on back side of knee.
Footdrop	Support feet in position at right angles to lower legs.

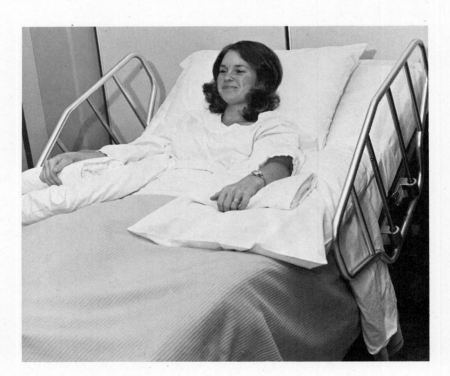

Fig. 12-19 Proper positioning and support for the semisitting, or Fowler's position. Note that good support of the arms and hands prevents pulling the shoulders into poor alignment.

Range of motion exercises

Changing positions and keeping patients in good alignment while in bed may be the only activities possible for some patients. When the patient is permitted some exercise, additional measures should be considered to help him stay in good physical condition and prevent the dangers of inactivity.

The framework of the body is the skeleton. The bones of the skeleton are of various sizes and shapes and are held together by ligaments and tendons. The points where bones join are the joints of the body. It is by means of the muscles and the joints that body motion is possible. The type of movement differs at various joints and depends on the shape and the number of bones forming the joint. Each joint has a **range of motion,** that is, each joint is allowed certain movement that is determined by its structure. For example, the joint at the shoulder allows one to move the arm in a complete circle; it is a ball-and-socket type joint. The joint at the elbow moves like a hinge.

A good exercise for the patient, especially one confined to bed, is to move each joint through its full range of motion. Routine tasks, such as bathing, eating, dressing, and writing, help to put certain joints through full range of motion. When the patient is not carrying out such activities, the joints should be put through full range of motion by purposeful exercising to the extent the illness allows.

Range of joint exercises may be carried out by the patient as active exercises, or by the nurse as passive exercises. Or, the patient may do some of them on his own while the nurse assists or carries out others for him. Before starting exercises, the nurse must be sure the patient understands what is being done, why, and how to do it. A patient at ease and relaxed can more actively take part in the exercises.

The patient should not be forced to exercise to the point of fatigue. The joint should be moved until there is resistance but not pain. Certain exercises may need to be delayed until the patient's condition allows, as for example those that require a standing position. The nurse starts gradually and in such a manner that the patient does not experience discomfort while he works toward improving his range of motion. All movements should be smooth and steady. Irregular and jerky movements are usually uncomfortable.

When she moves body parts, the nurse must be sure to support the part well. For example, she picks up the leg by placing the patient's heel into her cupped hand and rests the upper leg, just below the knee, in her other hand. She holds the arm by the wrist and the elbow or just above the elbow.

Some hospitals use powder boards to assist the patient in exercising his legs. The board is made of smooth material, such as plywood or fiberboard, and sprinkled with powder to reduce friction.

Range of motion exercises can be performed at least once a day. Each joint, or those listed on the nursing care plan, should be exercized daily. Many of the exercises can be carried out when the patient is being bathed and thereby become a part of that procedure. Those joints needing special care should be placed through range of motion exercises two to five times, twice a day if possible. Chart 12-5 offers suggested exercises for range of joint motion.

Chart 12-5 Providing exercises for range of joint motion

The purpose is to help keep the patient's musculoskeletal system in the best possible condition in order to carry out normal activities

Body Part	Exercise	Figure to Illustrate
Neck and Head	Move head backward, chin up.	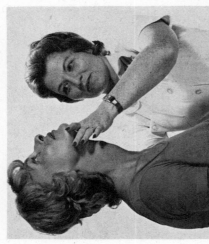 Fig. 12-20 The head is moved backward, chin up, for hyperextension of the cervical spine.
	Move head forward, chin on chest.	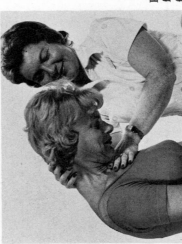 Fig. 12-21 The head is moved forward, chin toward chest, for flexion of the cervical spine.

Turn head from side to side.

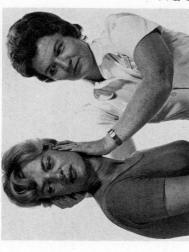

Fig. 12-22   The head is turned from side to side for rotation of the cervical spine.

Shoulders and Arms

Move arms over and alongside head. Return them to side of body.

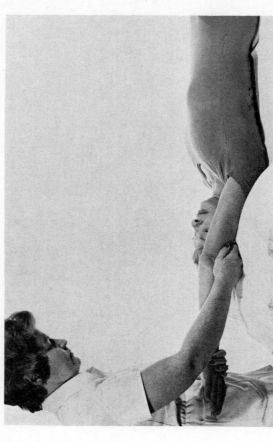

Fig. 12-23   The arm is moved over the head for extension of the shoulder.

Chart 12-5 continued

Body Part	Exercise	Figure to Illustrate
Shoulders and Arms	Move arm across chest toward opposite shoulder and then back straight out to patient's side.	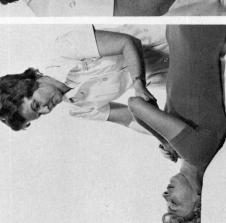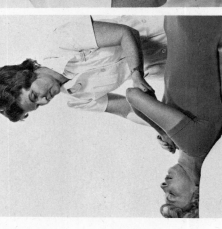

Fig. 12-24 (Left) The arm is moved across the chest for rotation of the shoulder and adduction of the arm. (Right) Bringing the arm out to the side rotates the shoulder and abducts the arm. |
| | With patient on abdomen, lift arms off bed toward ceiling. Or, with patient in standing position, bring patient's arm straight backward from body. |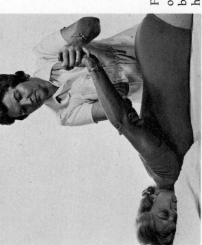

Fig. 12-25 While the model lies on her abdomen, the arm is lifted back and toward the ceiling for hyperextension. |

With patient in standing or sitting position, arm extended at side, move arm in circles.

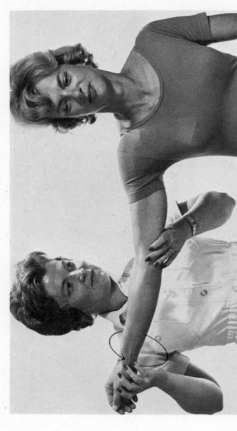

Fig. 12-26 The arm is extended to the side and moved in a circle for rotation of the shoulder.

Elbows

Bend elbow and then straighten it.

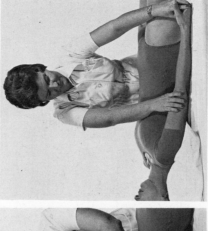

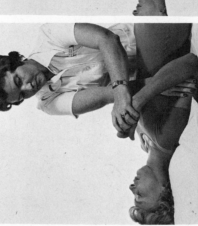

Fig. 12-27 (Left) The elbow is flexed and then (right) straightened for flexion and extension.

Chart 12-5   continued

Body Part	Exercise	Figure to Illustrate
Forearms, Wrists, and Fingers	With arm placed alongside of body, turn hand so that palm is facing upward and then turn so that palm is facing downward.	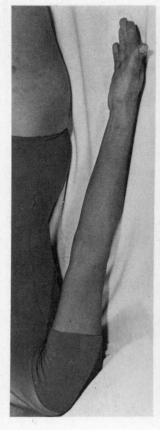 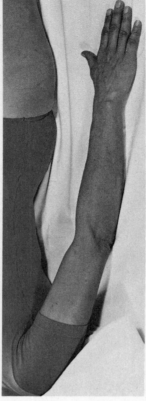 Fig. 12-28 (Top) The hand and forearm are placed in the supine position and (bottom) then in the prone position.
	Bend hand backward and then forward.	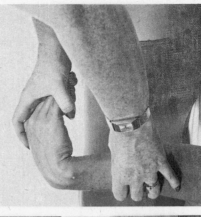 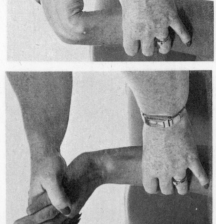 Fig. 12-29 (Left) The hand is bent backward and then (right) forward for hyperextension, extension, and flexion of the wrist.

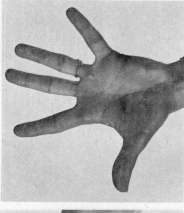

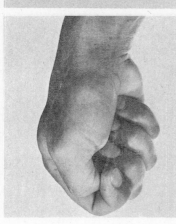

Make a fist with fingers and thumb and then open fist.

Fig. 12-30 (Left) A fist is made and then (right) opened for flexion and extension of the fingers and thumb.

Move fingers and thumb apart and then bring together.

Move thumb in circular motion.

Bend and straighten thumb joint.

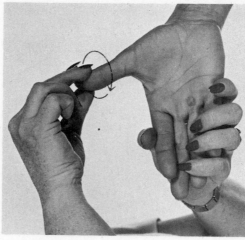

Fig. 12-31 The thumb is moved in a circle for rotation, and the thumb joint bent and straightened for extension and flexion.

Chart 12-5 continued

Body Part	Exercise	Figure to Illustrate

Knees, Legs, and Hips

Bend and straighten knee.

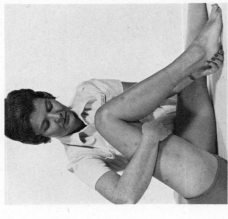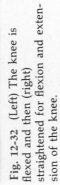

Fig. 12-32 (Left) The knee is flexed and then (right) straightened for flexion and extension of the knee.

Bring flexed knee up toward chest. Then straighten knee and bring leg back down on bed.

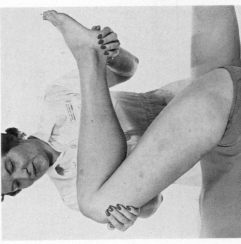

Fig. 12-33 The knee is flexed and then brought up toward the chest for flexion of the knee and hip. The knee and leg are then brought down onto the bed, and the knee is straightened for extension of the knee and hip.

Move leg out to side of body and then bring back to body.

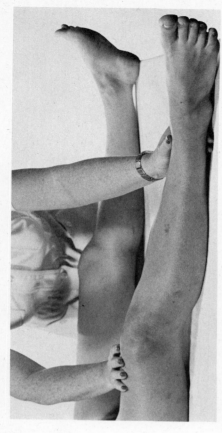

Fig. 12-34 The leg is moved away from the body for abduction of the leg. Adduction occurs when the leg is moved back to the opposite leg.

With knee bent, move leg away from body and then back toward other leg.

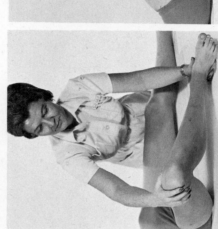

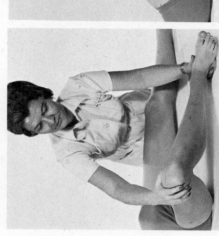

Fig. 12-35 (Left) With the knee bent, the leg is moved away from the body and then (right) toward and over the opposite leg for rotation of the hip.

Chart 12-5 continued

Body Part	Exercise	Figure to Illustrate
Knees, Legs, and Hips	Turn leg inward with toes pointing in, and then outward with toes pointing out. With patient on abdomen, lift leg off bed toward ceiling.	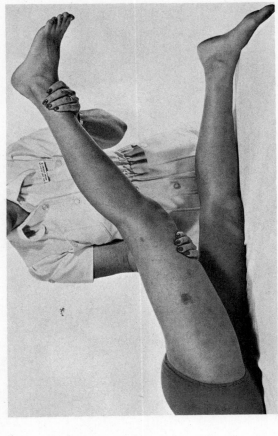 Fig. 12-36 While the model lies on her abdomen, the leg is moved up and toward the ceiling for hyperextension of the leg.

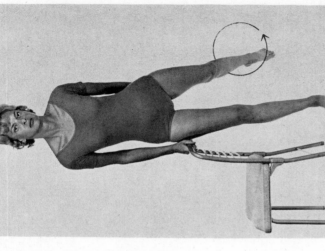

With patient in standing position and holding onto chair, swing leg in full circle.

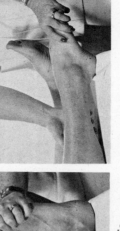

Fig. 12-37   While the model stands and supports herself on a chair, the leg is moved in a circle for rotation of the hip.

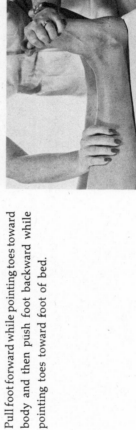

Fig. 12-38   (Left) The foot is moved forward, toes toward body, and then (right) backward, toes toward the foot of the bed, for flexion, extension, and hyperextension of the ankle.

Pull foot forward while pointing toes toward body and then push foot backward while pointing toes toward foot of bed.

Ankles and Toes

Chart 12-5 continued

Body Part	Exercise	Figure to Illustrate

Body Part

Ankles and Toes

Exercise

While keeping leg straight, turn foot in full circles.

Move toes toward under side and then toward upper side of foot.

Figure to Illustrate

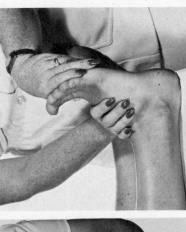

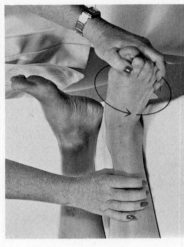

Fig. 12-39 The leg is held as the foot is moved in a circle for rotation of the ankle.

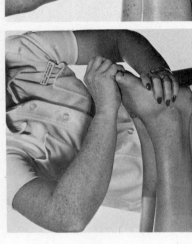

Fig. 12-40 (Left) The toes are moved toward the under side of the foot and then (right) toward the upper side of the foot for flexion, extension, and hyperextension of the toes.

Ankles and Toes

With patient in standing position, raise body on toes. Then lower body back onto floor until feet are flat on floor.

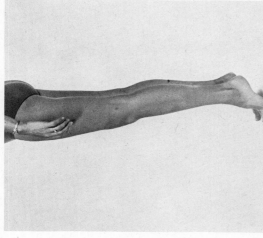

Fig. 12-41 While standing, the model raises herself onto her toes to flex the toes. The toes are then extended as she lowers herself and places her feet flat on the floor.

Spine

With patient on his abdomen, lift head and chest off bed.

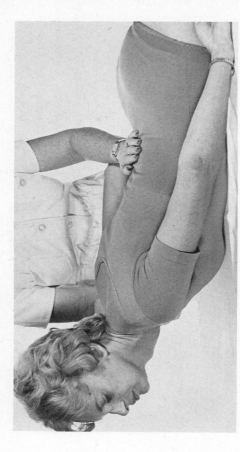

Fig. 12-42 The head and chest are lifted off the bed while the model lies on her abdomen for hyperextension of the spine.

Chart 12-5   continued

Body Part	Exercise	Figure to Illustrate
Spine	Curl spine forward by bringing head down toward waist while patient is in sitting position.	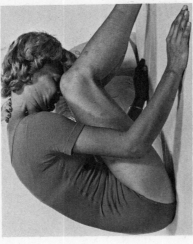 Fig. 12-43 The spine is curled by bringing the head down for flexion of the spine.

Any uncomfortable reaction should be reported promptly and exercises halted until further instructions are obtained.

Turning, moving, lifting, and carrying the patient

Frequently a patient needs to be turned, moved, lifted, or carried while he is being given care. He should be kept in good alignment during these procedures and protected from injury. Also, the nurse will avoid strain and injury to her muscles when she turns, moves, lifts, and carries the patient properly. She will wish to observe principles of body mechanics, as discussed in Chapter 5.

Friction burns can occur when pulling a patient across the bed or by pulling his bed linens or a bedpan from underneath him. Reducing friction by using powder or cornstarch sprinkled on the patient's skin and/or linen can be helpful. Rather than pulling the patient, rolling and turning him when possible help to avoid skin injury. Elderly patients in particular require careful handling since their skins tend to be tender and injure easily.

Protection also means supporting muscles and joints properly. The nurse should avoid grabbing and holding an extremity by its muscles. This can injure muscles as well as joints. Rather, she should support the extremity well, especially at the joints.

Nurses need to be realistic about what they can safely do without injuring themselves. For example, two small-statured women cannot safely lift and carry a patient weighing 250 pounds, even though they observe good body mechanics. Pushing, pulling, or sliding the patient requires less energy than lifting him. Whatever method is used to help a patient move from one place to another, the nurse should seek adequate assistance, as the situation indicates.

Mechanical devices are often available in health agencies for moving very heavy patients. Some persons also have such devices in their homes. Care should be taken to make certain that the operator understands how to use the device, that the patient is properly secured, and that he is informed of what will occur. Patients who do not understand or are afraid may not be able to cooperate and possibly, may suffer injury as a result.

Turning the Patient on His Side. The nurse will often wish to turn the patient on his side, either to give care or to place him in the side-lying position. To turn a patient toward her, the nurse places her hands on the patient's shoulder and hip on the far side, as illustrated in Figure 12-44, and gently rolls him toward her. While doing so, she provides herself with a wide base of support with one foot well behind the other. As she rolls the patient, she rocks backward, using her body weight to assist her arms in the rolling process. After the patient is on his side, she raises the bed siderail so that there is no danger of the patient falling from the bed. Then, she moves to the far side of the bed and puts her feet in position to rock. She places her hands under the patient's hip and shoulder, rocks back, and as she does so, pulls him toward the middle of the bed.

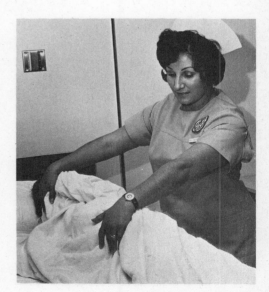

Fig. 12-44 The nurse turns the patient toward her by supporting him in the shoulder and hip areas. She rocks back as the patient turns.

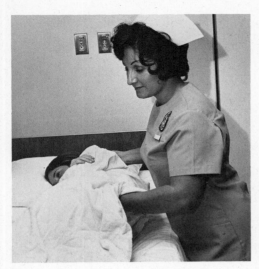

Fig. 12-45 The nurse turns the patient away from her by supporting her in the shoulder and hip areas and rocks toward the patient. The patient's arms are crossed at her chest and the upper knee is flexed. Bed siderails are in place opposite the nurse for the safety of the patient.

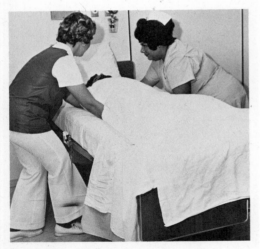

Fig. 12-46 These two nurses support and join hands under the heaviest part of the patient's body. A pillow at the head of the bed serves as a precaution to prevent the patient from injuring his head on the headboard. With a wide base of support, the nurses are ready to slide the patient up in bed.

To turn a patient away from her, the nurse puts the bed siderail up on the side opposite her. This is especially important so that there is no danger of the patient rolling off the bed. She has the patient flex his knees if possible with the leg nearest her on top of the leg resting on the bed, and crosses the patient's arms on his chest. She gives herself a wide base of support and flexes her knees. She places her hands under the patient's shoulders and hips and gently rolls him over. Figure 12-45 illustrates this procedure. With the patient on his side, she moves him to the center of the bed as described above.

Moving the Patient up in Bed. Before moving the patient up in bed, the nurse locks the wheels on the bed and places the adjustable bed in the flat position. She removes the pillows from under the patient's head and places one at the head of the bed so that the patient's head does not accidently hit the bedstead as she moves him up.

Children and lightweight adults are relatively easy for one nurse to slide toward the head of the bed. She places one hand under the patient's shoulders and the other under his hips, and assumes a position of "hugging" the patient as she flexes her knees. Then she places her feet so that she rocks toward the head of the bed as she slides the patient up in bed.

Moving a heavy helpless patient requires two persons. If the patient is able to assist by pushing with his feet, he is asked to flex his knees. One nurse stands on one side of the bed and the other nurse on the other side, near the patient's chest and head. Both nurses face the head of the bed. Each nurse places the arm nearest the patient under the patient's axillary area. One nurse assumes responsibility for supporting the patient's head. Both nurses flex their knees, place one foot forward, and come down close to the patient. Upon a signal given by one of the nurses, the patient pushes with his feet, and the nurses rock forward, thus moving the patient up in bed.

If the patient is unable to assist by pushing with his feet, the nurses stand at either side of the bed and face each other at a point between the patient's waist and hips. Both nurses give themselves a wide base of support, flex their knees, and lean close to the patient. They join hands under the widest part of the patient's hips and under his shoulders. At a given signal, both rock toward the head of the bed and slide the patient on the bed. The procedure may need to be repeated if the patient is heavy and far down in bed. Care should be taken to avoid injury to the patient's neck and head. Figure 12-46 illustrates this procedure.

Using a Drawsheet to Move the Patient up in Bed. While the method described previously may be necessary or convenient, the amount of effort expended by the nurses can be reduced. A drawsheet or a large sheet may be placed under the patient so that it extends from the head to below the buttocks. The sides of the sheet are rolled close to the patient so that they may be grasped easily. The patient's knees are flexed. The nurses stand at opposite sides of the bed at a point near the patient's shoulders and chest and face the foot of the bed. They have a wide base of support with the leg nearest the bed behind them and the other leg in front. Holding the sheet securely at a point near the patient's neck and middle to lower back, they first lean forward and then rock backward. As they rock backward, the weight of their bodies helps to slide the drawsheet and the patient. At the completion of the rocking

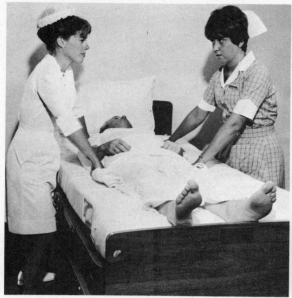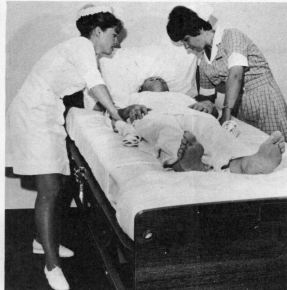

Fig. 12-47 (Left) Nurses in position to rock back and slide patient up in bed. Each one has a hand grasping the rolled drawsheet under the patient near his neck in order to support it. When they have a grasp of the sheet close to the patient's body in the hip area, one will give the signal and they will rock back. (Right) Nurses in position following completion of the draw sheet pull.

motion, each nurse usually has the elbow nearest the patient on the mattress. Figure 12-47 illustrates. The procedure can be done with the nurses facing the head of the bed. However, it seems easier when the backward rock is used.

Moving the Patient from the Bed to a Stretcher. Considerable care must be taken when moving a patient from the bed to a stretcher, or vice versa, to prevent him from being injured. If he is unconscious or helpless, the extremities and the head must be well supported. The most convenient way to move the patient is to place a sheet underneath him and then to pull carefully on the sheet to slide the patient from one surface (the bed) to the other (the stretcher). However, there are instances when patients must be lifted and carried. This can be done by means of a three-carrier lift. If done properly, the patient will feel secure, and those lifting will not suffer strain. The three-carrier lift is described in Chart 12-6 and illustrated in Figures 12-48 through 12-50.

When lifting the patient to the bed from the stretcher, the same principles are observed. However, the carriers should first place the patient onto the bed, leaving him at the edge. Then, one member of the team supports the patient on the edge of the bed to prevent his falling while the other two members go around to the opposite side of the bed and place their arms underneath the patient in preparation for sliding him to the center of the bed. Once the two persons on the opposite side of the bed have a good grip on the patient, the third person is able to join

Chart 12-6 The three-carrier lift

The purpose is to move a patient with safety from a bed to a stretcher with minimum effort for those who are carrying the patient

Suggested Action	Body Mechanics for the Nurse	Figure to Illustrate
Place stretcher at right angle to foot of bed so that it will be in position for carriers after they pivot away from bed. Lock wheels of bed and of stretcher.	Having stretcher and bed close to each other decreases distance to carry patient. Locked wheels help prevent accident, should bed or stretcher tend to move while patient is being lifted.	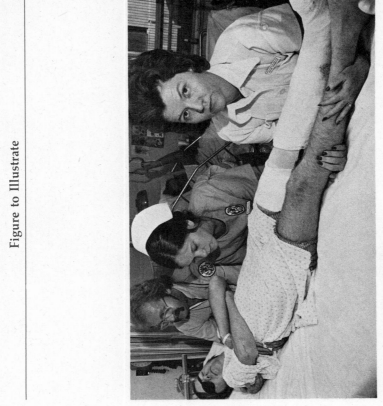
Arrange carriers according to height, with tallest person at patient's head.	Tallest carrier usually has longest arm grasp, making it easier for him to support patient's head and shoulders.	Fig. 12-48 The three carriers have come down close to the patient in preparation for lifting him. Because of this patient's cast, one nurse uses both of her arms to support the legs. Since the patient is not heavy, the middle and upper carriers can safely lift his body.

Stand facing patient and prepare to slide arms under him. Carrier in middle position places his arms directly under patient's buttocks. Carrier at head has one arm under patient's head, neck, and shoulder area and other arm directly against middle carrier's arm. Carrier at patient's feet has one arm also against middle person's arm and other arm under patient's legs and ankles. Figure 12-48 illustrates.

Slide arms under patient as far as possible and get in a position to slide patient to edge of bed.

Lean over patient and on signal simultaneously rock back and slide patient to edge of bed next to carriers.

Place arms further underneath patient. Prepare to "logroll" patient onto chests of all three carriers at same time patient is being lifted from bed.

Greatest weight is in area of buttocks. Having middle carrier's arms spread smaller than that of other two carriers helps prevent strain on this person. Having arms of first and third carriers touch arms of middle carrier provides additional support to heaviest area of patient's body.

Place one leg forward, thigh resting against bed and knees flexed, and put on internal girdle.

Movement is accomplished by rocking backward and attempting to "sit down." Weight of carriers and power of their arms, hips, and knees move patient.

Place one leg forward, flex knees, and put on internal girdle. "Logrolling" patient onto carriers brings center of gravity more directly over base of support, thus increasing stability of group and reducing strain on carriers.

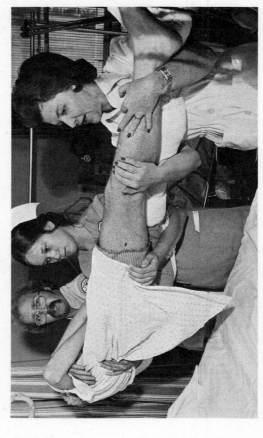

Fig. 12-49 The nurse carrying the patient's legs signals directions as the patient is lifted and then logrolled onto the carriers' bodies.

Chart 12-6 continued

Suggested Action	Body Mechanics for the Nurse	Figure to Illustrate
Pivot to stretcher and, on signal, lower patient onto stretcher.	Flex knees, have one foot forward, and bring body down with patient, thus letting large leg and arm muscles do work of lowering patient.	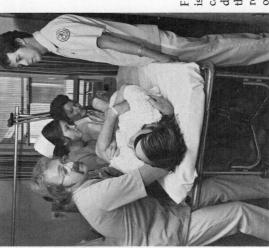 Fig. 12-50 On signal, the patient is placed on the stretcher as the carriers flex their knees and come down with the patient. Because of the heavy cast, a fourth nurse is ready to assist as necessary and offer support to the stretcher.

them and assist in sliding the patient to the center of the bed. Sliding the patient requires much less effort than attempting to place him directly onto the center of the bed. Also, the patient is less likely to be dropped onto the bed.

The three-carrier lift is used in various other situations, such as lifting a patient who has fallen to the floor, or lifting a patient out of a chair and onto the bed. Once the principles of such a lift are mastered, it becomes relatively easy to analyze situations in which it may be used advantageously.

For patients who present special problems because of their weight or a cast, the three-carrier lift may not be sufficient. It may be necessary to have an additional person to support the heaviest or most cumbersome part of the patient. The persons distribute their arms while carrying so that the heaviest part is well supported.

Moving the Patient from the Bed to a Chair. There are occasions when a patient is permitted to be out of bed but loss of various body functions makes it impossible for him to assist in getting out of bed. If the patient is able to help by using his arms for support, the problem is reduced considerably. However, some patients cannot use their arms. In a health agency, several persons usually are available to lift the patient from the bed to a chair. Whenever possible, lifting is preferred to sliding or pulling the patient because it prevents skin injury from friction. To a great extent the technique is dependent on the size and the weight of the patient and the style of chair that he is to use. Chairs often complicate the procedure because the backrest and the arms get in the way of the persons lowering the patient.

It is possible for only one person to get a helpless patient into a chair. The single-person technique is a valuable procedure for nurses to know for the home care of invalids and for emergency use. Often, only one family member is available to assist the patient out of bed and to return him to bed. The technique is described in Chart 12-7 and illustrated in Figures 12-51 and 12-52.

Preparing the patient for walking

Preparing patients confined to bed for short periods of time for increased activity may be simply a matter of assisting them out of bed and helping them to walk. However, there are some patients who may require preparation, especially those who have been in bed for long periods of time. In addition to range of motion exercises, certain other exercises and activities can be done in bed that will help prepare the musculoskeletal system for walking.

The muscles on the front of the thigh, the quadriceps femoris, are important for walking and climbing stairs. To help reduce weakness in these muscles, the patient should be encouraged to exercise them frequently. The patient contracts these muscles by pulling the kneecap toward the hips. He will feel that he is pushing his knee down into the mattress and pulling his foot upward. The exercise, frequently referred to as **quadriceps drills,** can be done two or three times hourly but should not be done to the point of fatigue. Counting slowly to four helps establish a rhythm as the muscles are exercised.

Chart 12-7 One person moving a patient from bed to chair and from chair to bed

The purpose is to move a patient out of and into bed when his weight makes it possible for only available person to lift him

Suggested Action	Body Mechanics for the Nurse	Figure to Illustrate
Place chair facing and against bed at a point near patient's buttocks to receive patient and to use a brace.	Having chair as close as possible to patient decreases distance to move patient.	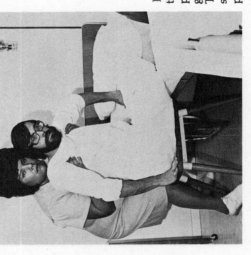
Slide upper portion of patient's body to edge of bed. This makes patient lie diagonally on bed.	Place arms under patient's head and shoulders, one foot forward, and rock backward.	
Place arms well under patient's axillary areas from rear, as illustrated in Figure 12-51. Patient's head and shoulders may be resting on nurse.	Support upper portion of patient's body on self to reduce weight to be moved.	
Move around to back of chair, pulling patient into chair while so doing, as illustrated in Figure 12-51.	Lean against back of chair to keep it from moving and to brace self. Rock back while pulling patient into chair.	Fig. 12-51 With the chair near the bed and while supporting the patient from the back, the nurse gently moves him onto the chair. The nurse has a wide base of support and will rock back as the patient slides to the chair.
Pull chair away from bed until patient's feet are on edge of bed, being careful not to pull chair out from under patient.	Flex knees, grasp chair near seat, and rock back, pulling chair with patient away from bed.	
Support patient's legs while lowering his feet to floor.	Flex knees while lowering patient's feet to floor to decrease strain on back.	

To move patient into bed from chair, bring chair directly alongside bed with patient facing foot of bed. Place pillow on arm of chair if chair has an armrest.

Life patient's legs onto edge of bed, as illustrated in Figure 12-52.

Go behind chair, grasp patient in axillary areas from rear, and roll him onto bed, as illustrated in Figure 12-52. Have wide base of support and rock to move patient onto bed.

Move chair and help patient into desired position. Slide chair away with foot and brace self against bed to prevent patient from falling.

Sliding chair with patient requires less energy than lifting. If floor has polished surface, slide chair on small rug or cloths.

Flex knees, lower body, and support both patient's legs when coming to erect position.

Rolling rather than lifting patient, having a wide base of support, and rocking reduces strain on muscles.

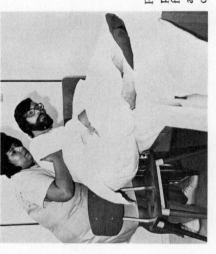

Fig. 12-52 The nurse places the patient's feet and legs on the bed first. Then she rocks toward him as she rolls him off the chair and onto the bed.

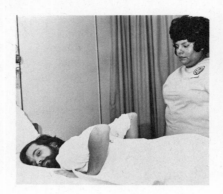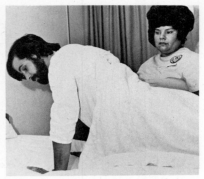

Fig. 12-53 (Left) The patient is in position to begin push-ups. (Right) He lifts himself off the bed as he straightens his elbows, then lowers himself by flexing his elbows to return to his original position.

Exercises referred to as push-ups strengthen muscles of the shoulders and arms. These muscles are important for holding onto a chair as the patient begins to walk again. Also, they are needed for patients who must learn to walk on crutches or with a cane.

The patient sits up in bed without support to begin one type of push-up exercise. He then lifts his hips off the bed by pushing with his hands down on the mattress. If the mattress is soft, a block or books are placed on the bed under the patient's hands.

Another method of doing push-ups is to have the patient lie on his abdomen. The hands are placed near the body at approximately shoulder level, palms down on the mattress with elbows bent sharply. The patient straightens his elbows while lifting his head and shoulders off the bed, as illustrated in Figure 12-53. This same exercise can be done when the patient sits in an armchair. He places his hands on the arms of the chair and then raises his body out of the seat. Push-ups usually are done three or four times a day.

Many other activities help patients prepare for being out of bed, for example, placing the signal device on the bed so that the patient can exercise his arm and shoulder muscles as he reaches for it. However, it should not be placed where it could cause the patient to fall from the bed as he reaches for it. Bed siderails should be in position to prevent falling. The patient is encouraged to wash his back and feet, comb his hair, and put on his socks in bed. These as well as other activities that require the patient to use various muscles will help prepare him for walking and moving about.

Another exercise that helps prepare the patient for being out of bed is referred to as **dangling.** The patient is helped to sit on the edge of the bed with his feet and legs hanging freely over the side of the bed, as illustrated in Figure 12-54. The nurse should be sure to stay with him when he is in this position until she is certain he is not weak or likely to faint or fall from the bed.

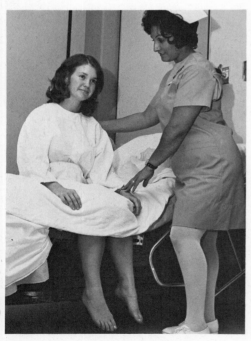
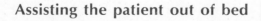

Fig. 12-54 The patient dangles in preparation for getting out of bed. The nurse remains in readiness should the patient feel weak or faint.

Assisting the patient out of bed

Before assisting the patient out of bed, the nurse has the chair, preferably one that is not upholstered or a wheelchair in readiness. She places the chair or wheelchair parallel to the bed in a convenient place and locks the wheels of the bed and the wheelchair.

The nurse brings the patient to the side of the bed and helps him to a sitting position. She may elevate the head of the bed to give the patient extra support if necessary. She pivots the patient while supporting his shoulders and legs so that his legs are off the side of the bed, and dresses him appropriately as he sits at the edge of the bed. If he is going to walk, the nurse helps him as necessary to put on shoes and stockings. Hard-soled and well-fitting shoes will give him more support than loose, floppy slippers. An adjustable bed is lowered so that the patient's feet are on the floor. Or, if the bed is not adjustable, a sturdy footstool is placed under his feet.

While facing the patient, the nurse will give herself a wide base of support by putting one foot forward and bending her knees. The patient puts his hands on the nurse's shoulders while she places her hands in the patient's axillary area. Grasping the patient on his chest wall as she helps him is uncomfortable for him and restricts his breathing. The patient now lifts himself to a standing position as the nurse assists by lifting the upper part of his body. Figure 12-55 illustrates this. If a footstool has been used, the nurse assists the patient off it while continuing to hold him.

The nurse allows the patient to stand a few seconds until she is sure he is not feeling faint. Then, she pivots him, and herself, while she faces him, giving herself a wide base of support. She lowers the patient into the chair or wheelchair. As she lowers the patient, she lowers herself by bending her knees. If there are armrests on the chair, the patient can assist by holding onto them as he is being lowered into the chair.

Assisting the patient to walk

The nurse should walk alongside the patient, keeping her arm under his in an arm-in-arm manner. If the patient begins to feel faint, the nurse can quickly slide her arm up and into his axillary area. She then places one foot out to her side to form a wide base of support for herself. The patient rests on the nurse's hip until additional help arrives to assist.

A walking belt is helpful for some patients. An example of one is illustrated in Figure 12-56. The patient has the security of support until he feels ready to walk on his own.

Canes can be used to help the patient walk. One type is a straight walking stick with a rubber cup on the end to help prevent the cane from sliding along the floor. Another type, the "quad" cane, has four legs which gives extra support for the patient. Figure 12-57 illustrates the "quad" cane. A patient may use one cane, or two, depending on the amount of support he needs.

A walker offers considerable support and is often used by patients who are learning to walk again after prolonged periods in bed. A patient using a walker is shown in Figure 12-58 (see p. 255).

Some health agencies have parallel bars that help patients begin to walk. The patient grasps a bar on either side of him and starts to walk as he supports himself on the bars. When parallel bars are not available, almost any two *stable* pieces of furniture can be used. Examples include the backs of two heavy chairs, the footboards of two beds, or a hall rail and a chair. Figure 12-59 illustrates this technique using two sturdy chairs and a chair and doorknob (see p. 255).

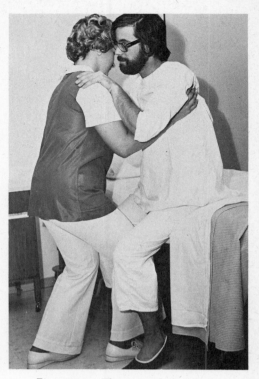

Fig. 12-55 The nurse helps the patient out of bed and into the standing position. Note the nurse's wide base of support and flexed knees. She supports the patient in his axillary area while he places his hands on the nurse's shoulders.

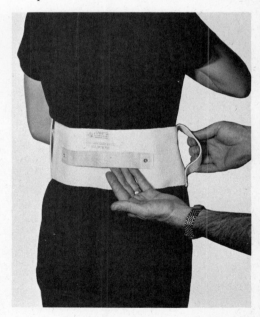

Fig. 12-56 This is an example of a walking belt. Handles on the sides and in the back give firm grips for the person assisting the patient. (Photograph courtesy of the Posey Company)

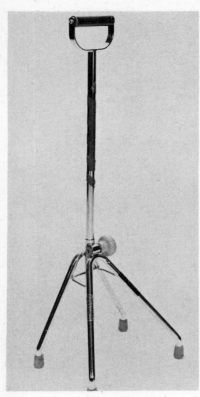

Fig. 12-57 A cane with four legs, usually referred to as a "quad" cane. The knob near the legs is used to adjust the overall length of the cane.

Crutch walking

In some health agencies, a physical therapist teaches the patient how to use crutches. However, it is important for the nurse to understand how the patient uses his crutches so that she can assist him after the initial teaching has been done. Also, in some agencies and in the home, the nurse may be responsible for teaching patients how to use crutches.

Several exercises will help a patient prepare for crutch walking. Push-ups, as described earlier, help strengthen the arm and shoulder muscles. The muscles of the hand also need exercising. Squeezing a ball 50 times or so a day will help to strengthen hand muscles. Hand grips can be purchased that are also used for this purpose.

There are two common methods of measuring a patient for **axillary crutches,** that is, crutches that fit under the arm into the axillary area. With the patient in bed on his back and wearing shoes, the nurse measures the distance from the fold at the axillary area to the feet and adds 2 inches. Or, she measures the distance from the fold at the axillary area to a point 6 to 8 inches away from the patient's heel. The measurement of crutch length includes the axillary pads and crutch tips. The handgrips are adjusted so that with the patient standing, the elbows are slightly bent, about 30°, and the wrists are bent backwards (hyperextended) slightly. Safety rubber suction tips on the ends of crutches prevent slipping. It is important to be sure they are clean and not worn.

When the patient is ready to get out of bed, the nurse assists him into a chair which is close to a wall. Then he can be helped to stand against the wall and the crutches placed in his hands. Next, while the patient stands slightly away from the wall, he should sway from side to side on the crutches. This helps the hands and arms to become used to weight bearing.

After this practice, the patient should be asked to lean against the wall and pick up one crutch about 6 inches from the floor and then place it back down on the floor. He should do the same thing with the other crutch and repeat this exercise several times. Then, while still leaning against the wall, he should pick up both crutches from the floor and place them down again and repeat this exercise several times. It helps the patient learn how to manage his crutches. He is ready to start to walk after he has shown that he can handle his crutches with ease and comfort.

The patient's posture with the crutches should allow the line of gravity to go through the base of his support. The base of support should be wide. The crutches should be placed about 4 to 8 inches in front and about 4 to 8 inches to the side of the feet for good balance.

The patient should be taught that he is to support himself on the crutches with his arms and hands. If he supports himself by placing his weight on the axillary area, he may irritate the skin of that area. Also, the weight tends to cut off circulation and places pressure on nerves to the arms and hands, which may result in crutch paralysis.

There are crutches with no axillary support. Rather, a frame or metal cuff extends beyond the handgrip for the lower arm to help guide the crutch. This type of crutch generally is used by well-experienced patients and by those who need permanent assistance with walking. These crutches are called **Lofstrand,** or **Canadian crutches.** They are illustrated in Figure 12-60.

Another type of crutch is called the **platform crutch.** It is especially useful for patients unable to bear weight on their hands and wrists. Many patients with arthritis use them. As Figure 12-61 illustrates, the patient's weight is distributed over the entire forearm.

There are four basic gaits for crutch walking. The two-point gait requires that the patient be permitted to bear weight on both feet. The pattern is as follows: right crutch and left foot forward; left crutch and right foot forward. It resembles a normal walking pattern.

The four-point gait requires that the patient be permitted to bear weight on both feet also. The pattern is as follows: right crutch forward; left foot forward; left crutch forward; right foot forward. This pattern also resembles the normal walking pattern but uses four bases of support. It is illustrated in Figure 12-62.

The three-point gait is used when weight bearing is permitted on one foot. The other foot cannot bear weight or can bear only limited weight. The pattern is as follows: both crutches and the leg that cannot bear weight move forward and then the foot permitted to bear weight comes through. The crutches are brought forward immediately and the pattern is repeated. The three-point gait is illustrated in Figure 12-63.

The swing-through gait can be used when the feet (or foot) can bear weight. Both crutches are brought forward and the leg(s) are brought through quickly and placed in front of the crutches, and then the crutches are brought forward. This gait is illustrated in Figure 12-64. It is used by the patient accustomed to crutches who wishes to move about quickly, and is often used by the patient with a leg amputation.

Leisure-time activities

The concept of rehabilitation includes active involvement of the patient. Patients often are or can be encouraged to become involved, and to exercise and move about while enjoying leisure-time activities. When helping patients select such activities, remember that most people enjoy some variety. Few care to do one thing all day long. Children and young adults are especially likely to become bored without variety.

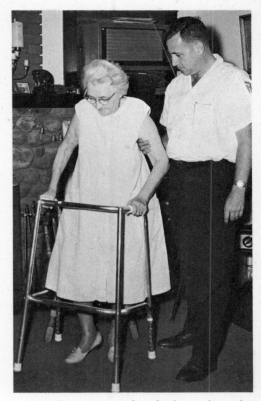

Fig. 12-58 After discharge from the hospital many patients require supervision by other health workers in addition to a visiting nurse. In this instance, the physical therapist is helping the patient in her struggle for more mobility. The nurse will be aware of this as she visits the home, and she too can supervise the patient in her efforts. (Courtesy Good Samaritan Hospital, Phoenix, Arizona)

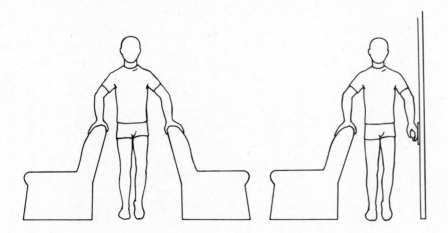

Fig. 12-59 This sketch illustrates how a patient using two sturdy chairs, or a chair and a doorknob, helps support himself as he prepares to walk.

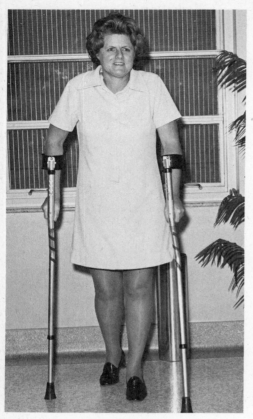

Fig. 12-60 Lofstrand or Canadian crutches have bands to fit around the forearm to help keep the crutches in place.

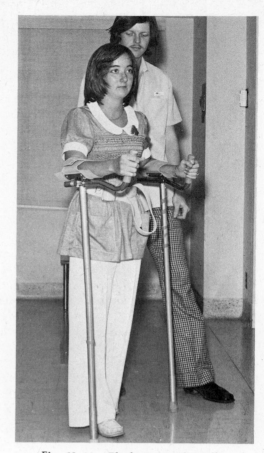

Fig. 12-61. Platform crutches allow the patient to distribute weight bearing on the forearm. The belt the patient is wearing is a type of walking belt. The person assisting the patient holds onto the belt in the back to offer support and security until the patient has mastered the skill of walking with crutches.

Fig. 12-62 This patient is using the four-point gait for crutch walking with axillary crutches. (Left) The left crutch is placed forward first, and the patient moves her right foot forward in position to receive weight. (Right) The right crutch is then placed forward, and her left foot is brought forward in position to receive weight.

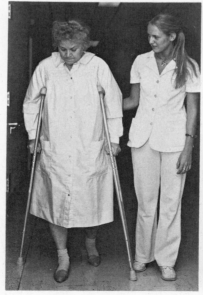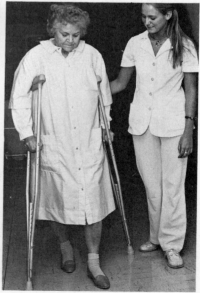

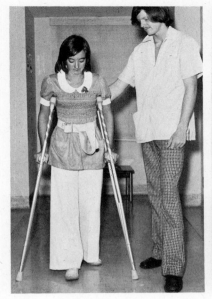 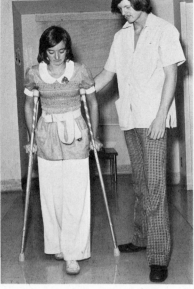

Fig. 12-63 (Left) When using the three-point gait, one foot is permitted to bear weight, in this case, the patient's left foot. She is placing both crutches and her right foot, which can bear only limited weight, forward. (Right) After shifting her weight from her left foot to her crutches and her foot with limited weight-bearing ability, she then brings her left foot through and in front of her to receive her weight.

Many persons enjoy at least some reading during their leisure time. Books, magazines, and newspapers are usually available in most health agencies. For those unable to visit the library, volunteers in many agencies bring reading materials to the patients. The nurse can inform patients of available reading materials in the agency where she gives care.

Some persons also enjoy writing while hospitalized. Chronically ill patients may have pen pals. New mothers usually plan to write birth announcements while hospitalized.

While reading and writing do not involve much exercise and activity, writing and handling books, magazines, and newspapers help to exercise

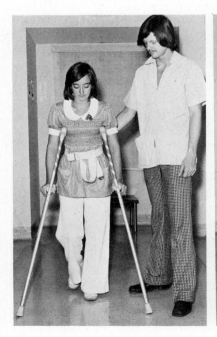 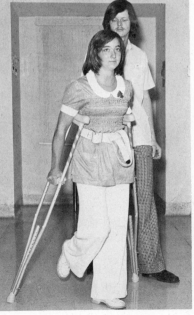

Fig. 12-64 This patient is starting the swing-through gait. She cannot bear weight on her right foot. (Left) The patient shifts her weight from her left foot onto her two crutches which she has placed in front of her. She then lifts her left foot, swings it through her crutches and then (right) places her weight on her left foot. At no time has there been weight on her right foot.

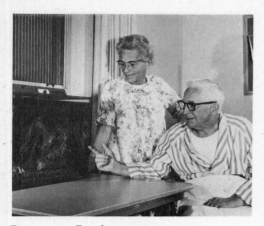

Fig. 12-65 For these patients in a chronic disease unit, a visit to the aquarium in the patient's lounge offers an opportunity to socialize, pleasant diversion, and the exercise of moving about.

arm, fingers, and thumbs. Also, the sitting or semisitting position helps patients prepare for being out of bed.

Most health agencies and homes have provisions for patients to use television and radio sets. For patients who are up and about, sets often are available in patient lounges and recreation rooms. Many people enjoy watching television or listening to a radio for at least part of each day. Except for the very ill and the very young, this is usually appropriate. It should be remembered that television and radio programs may be a source of annoyance for other persons in a health agency. Therefore, the volume should be kept at a moderate to low level.

Arts and crafts can often be rewarding leisure-time activities. They are especially helpful when they benefit the patient by providing exercise also.

Toys can be the source of much pleasure for the bedridden child, but they should be carefully selected with safety in mind. Toys with small, removable parts should be avoided because of the danger of being swallowed. Also, toys with sharp edges or points should be avoided. Interesting and inexpensive toys can be made from common objects found in the home.

Almost no one likes to eat alone. Efforts to bring the patient to the family table or into a dining area with other patients usually are rewarding. Many of the hospitals for the chronically ill have patient dining rooms, and often patients may go to the dining room or cafeteria for meals.

Patient lounges are available in most health agencies. Here, patients can enjoy games together, chat, watch television, and find company. For persons who do not socialize readily, a patient lounge with opportunities to meet or be near others can make the difference between loneliness and the satisfaction of being active and one of a group.

Usually, patients enjoy visits with family members and friends. At one time most health agencies observed very limited visiting privileges, the reason being that visitors often were thought to upset patients as well as hospital routines. However, most hospitals have become increasingly lenient with visiting privileges as health personnel have observed the value visitors have for patients.

Some agencies permit visitors to assist with the patient's care. For instance, they may assist him with eating, walking, and exercises, and help with the care of nails and hair. However, the nurse is still responsible for the care of her patients; assistance from visitors does not free her of this duty.

At one time patients were expected to help each other and to assist with work in health agencies when such work did not interfere with their recovery. However, using patients as helpers is uncommon today. In those agencies where this system has been used carefully, the results have been impressive. For some patients, being able to help is gratifying. It gives them a feeling of personal accomplishment, relieves their boredom, and offers exercise and activity. A few examples of things patients can do to help include acting as interpreters when language barriers occur, reading to other patients, making telephone calls, writing letters for others, making beds, and assisting with landscaping or gardening.

Some agencies have facilities for swimming, movies, canteens, and so on. In general, it seems that as facilities and opportunities for diversion increase, patients' attitudes toward health agencies often improve. Places of long-term confinement need not be as dreary, lacking in things to do, and impersonal as they may have been in the past.

Community recreational facilities promote exercise and activities such as singing, dancing, group exercises, craft work, and game playing for all ages. Special activities for the handicapped and chronically ill in their homes or in community centers are sometimes available.

The nurse will wish to be familiar with leisure-time facilities and activities in the agency and in the community where she gives care. Assisting the patient to use these facilities can very well help him to reach high-level wellness.

Conclusion

Helping to keep the patient in the best psychological and physical condition is an important part of nursing care. To neglect this aspect of care may result in complications that are more serious than the patient's original illness. The nurse will wish to see to it that her patient is active and exercising to the extent his condition permits. At the same time, she observes principles of body mechanics in order to prevent strain and injury to herself.

References

Beaumont, Estelle, "Product Survey: Wheelchairs," Nursing '73, 3:48-57, November 1973.

Brower, Phyllis and Hicks, Dorothy, "Maintaining Muscle Function in Patients on Bed Rest," American Journal of Nursing, 72:1250–1253, July 1972.

Downs, Florence S., "Bed Rest and Sensory Disturbances," American Journal of Nursing, 74:434–438, March 1974.

Foss, Georgia, "Breaking the Architectural Barrier with Crutches, Wheelchairs, & Walkers," Nursing '73, 3:16–31, October 1973.

"How to Negotiate the Ups and Downs, Ins and Outs of Body Alignment," Nursing '74, 4:46–51, October 1974.

Jordan, Helen S. and Kavchack, Mary Anne, "Transfer Techniques," Nursing '73, 3:19–22, March 1973.

Lavin, Mary Ann, "Bed Exercises for Acute Cardiac Cases," American Journal of Nursing, 73:1226–1227, July 1973.

May, Christine M., "Wheelchair Patient for a Day," American Journal of Nursing, 73:650–651, April 1973.

Young, Sr. Charlotte, "Exercise: How To Use It To Decrease Complications in Immobilized Patients," Nursing '75, 5:81–82, March 1975.

13 measures to promote comfort, rest, and sleep

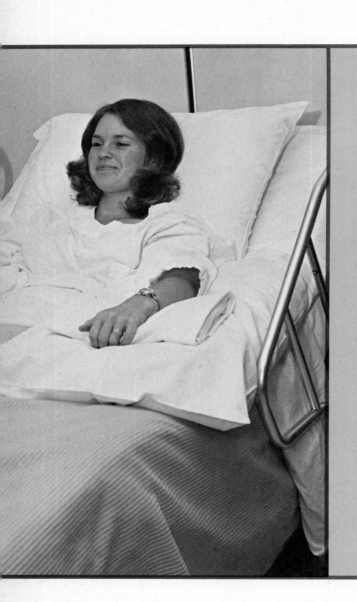

chapter outline

behavioral objectives

When mastery of content in this chapter is reached, the student will be able to

Define terms appearing in the glossary.

Describe various characteristics of pain.

List typical questions, the answers to which will help the nurse plan care for a patient in pain.

State four typical signs of pain, other than what the patient tells the nurse, that indicate that he is in pain.

Describe six or eight nursing measures that often help to relieve pain.

List the average number of hours of sleep persons at various ages generally need to feel refreshed.

List eight or ten typical symptoms of fatigue.

Explain why some patients feel that hospitals are poor places to rest.

List four common disorders of sleep and describe nursing measures that may be used for each.

List three principles that guide the nurse in promoting rest and sleep for her patients.

List ten or twelve nursing measures that often help patients to relax, rest, and sleep.

State three items of interest to nursing and health team members that the nurse caring for a patient in pain will record.

State three items of interest to nursing and health team members that the nurse caring for a wakeful and restless patient will record.

List two or three subjects in a teaching plan that the nurse will wish to discuss with patients suffering with pain and with those who are wakeful and restless.

Explain why inability to sleep can be described as a painful experience, using the definition of pain and symptoms of fatigue given in this chapter as guides.

glossary

Diffuse Pain Discomfort covering a large area.

Dull Pain Discomfort of a gnawing type; not as intense or acute as sharp pain.

Enuresis Involuntary urination, usually occurring during sleeping hours.

Insomnia Difficulty in falling asleep, intermittent sleep, and early awakening from sleep.

Intermittent Pain Discomfort that comes and goes.

Pain The sensation of physical and/or mental suffering or hurt that usually causes distress or agony to the one experiencing it.

Phantom Pain Pain that does not have physiological or pathological substance.

Referred Pain Pain in an area removed from that part of the body which is diseased or injured.

Relax To become less rigid and to decrease effort and tension.

Rest To decrease the state of activity, resulting in a feeling of being refreshed.

Sharp Pain Quick, sticking, and intense discomfort.

Shifting Pain Discomfort that moves from one area to another.

Sleep A state of relative unconsciousness.

Somnambulism Sleepwalking.

introduction

Chapter 12 discussed the importance of activity and exercise. Seeing that patients are receiving adequate rest and sleep and are comfortable is equally important. This chapter discusses common measures that help to promote comfort, rest, and sleep.

Description of pain

Pain is a subjective symptom, that is, it can be described only by the person having it. It has been defined in many ways. This text describes **pain** as a sensation of physical and/or mental suffering and hurting that usually causes misery or agony for the one experiencing it.

Pain has various characteristics. For example, there may or may not be damage to body tissue when pain occurs. The pain of grief when a loved one dies causes mental suffering that does not involve tissue damage. On the other hand, the hurt of a fracture or of a heart attack is associated with damage to body tissue.

The amount of pain experienced is not necessarily in proportion to the amount of damage occurring in the body. For example, a patient may not complain of pain until a cancerous growth is beyond hope of cure. Similarly, a soldier may be severely wounded and not be aware of pain until he is removed from combat. On the other hand, a patient who has had surgery for hemorrhoids (piles) may describe severe pain even though the condition is unlikely to be life-threatening.

Some people experience the pain of anticipation. For example, a person may suffer misery as he anticipates the pain he is likely to feel when the dentist will drill and repair a cavity. The misery of anticipation may be so great that people have been known to postpone necessary medical and dental care.

People view pain differently. The person who wishes to be thought of as sturdy and brave may describe pain casually, as though it hardly existed, even when it is considerable. Another person may show great concern and anxiety about his pain.

Consciousness and attention are necessary to experience pain. The unconscious patient does not experience pain. However, even the conscious person, it appears, needs to pay attention in order to experience pain. For example, an athlete hurt while playing football may not be aware of pain until after the game when he directs his attention to his injury. Also a child's attention can often be distracted from a procedure that causes pain. He may become so interested in a favorite toy that he is unaware of the pain of an injection.

Observation is important for the nurse to determine the nature of the patient's pain. She will wish to determine the amount and location of the pain, and to know what tends to produce the pain and what tends to relieve it. How did it start? How long has the patient had pain? What is his diagnosis and his physician's plan of care? How did the patient handle pain in the past? Can the family help the nurse to understand the patient's reaction to pain? Answers to such questions will help the nurse to understand the patient in pain and to plan nursing care to meet his needs.

Listed below are some commonly used terms to describe different kinds of pain.

Sharp Quick, sticking, and intense.

Dull Not as intense or acute as sharp pain, possibly more annoying than painful.

Diffuse Covering a large area. Usually, the patient is unable to point to a specific area without moving his hand over a large surface, such as the entire abdomen.

Shifting Moving from one area to another, such as from the lower abdomen to the upper abdomen.

Intermittent Coming and going. It may or may not be regular.

In some instances, the patient may complain of pain in an area removed from the diseased or injured area of the body. This is called **referred pain.** For example, people with gallbladder disease often complain of pain in the upper back or shoulder area.

Patients often complain of pain in an amputated extremity. This is called **phantom pain.** It shows that pain can be felt without having tissue damage present and without nerve routes from the painful area to the brain.

When a patient has pain, he usually has signs that will tell the nurse something about it. Most people will have a characteristic expression on their faces or carry out certain actions that show they are in pain. For instance, the patient may frown, grimace, or cry. He may pace the floor, grip onto a bed or chair, or clench his jaws or fists. Another sign of pain is tense, firm muscles in the affected area. For example, the muscles of the abdomen may become tense and feel firm when a patient has appendicitis. The patient in pain often shows signs of anger, fear, or worry.

There are signs of pain which the patient cannot control. For example, he will often perspire freely. His pulse and respiratory rates will increase. His blood pressure may be elevated or he may faint.

The patient in pain needs careful observation. He needs the nurse's support and concern. Listening to what the patient says and looking for signs of pain will help the nurse plan her care to meet the patient's needs.

Nursing measures to promote comfort

From the previous discussion, the nurse learns that she needs to understand the patient and the nature of his pain before starting care. Nursing measures will depend to a large extent on this type of information.

The nurse will want to try to decrease or remove the cause of the pain whenever possible. The following examples will illustrate: loosening a tight binder; seeing that the patient's urinary bladder is emptied; taking steps to relieve constipation or flatus; changing the patient's position in bed; giving the patient a backrub when his muscles are tense and sore; and changing soiled linens.

The following nursing measures also will often help. If the patient is tired, he may need rest. The nurse may need to explain the situation to visitors who may be tiring the patient. Usually, a darkened, well-ventilated room is restful and comfortable. The hungry or thirsty patient may feel better when he has a snack or fresh fluids. A soaked dressing may need changing. An extremity in a cast often feels more comfortable when it is elevated on a pillow.

Experience has shown that the patient who has confidence in his health practitioners, in general, needs less treatment for the relief of pain than the patient who has little confidence in those caring for him. Without confidence, nothing seems to help. Staying with a patient in pain and using touch, for example, holding his hand firmly, have been found helpful for some patients. Nurses have also found that discussing pain with the patient and having him help select a method to relieve it have been effective measures in some instances. In addition they have found these measures to be helpful for some patients: explaining why the patient has pain; helping him understand that pain is common; and assuring him that it is normal and acceptable to express his pain. These nursing experiences show that the patient in pain is easier to help when he feels he has support, interest, and concern from those caring for him.

There are times when the patient will need medication prescribed by the physician to relieve pain. When necessary and used with good judgment, medication is a desirable measure. However, using drugs as a substitute for good care is not considered a part of high-quality nursing practice.

Description of rest and sleep

To **relax** means to become less rigid and to decrease effort and tension. One can relax without sleeping. However, sleep rarely occurs until one relaxes.

Rest means a condition in which the body is in a decreased state of activity. It results in a feeling of being refreshed. For some, rest occurs while leisurely enjoying a break in the day's activities. For others, it may not come until sleep.

Sleep is a state of unconsciousness. The depth of unconsciousness varies. During certain periods of sleep, the person can be wakened easily. During others, it is difficult to do so. The depth of unconsciousness for the sensory organs also varies. For example, the depth is greatest for the sense of smell, which may explain why home fires gain headway since sleeping occupants do not smell the smoke. The depth is least for pain and hearing. This explains why ill persons often are wakeful when pain is present and when only a small but strange noise disturbs them.

For no known reason, eight hours of sleep is generally recommended for well adults. Yet, some people need more to feel refreshed and some require less. Such factors as metabolism rate, age, physical condition, type of work, and amount and kind of exercise influence the amount of sleep people need. Despite such differences, in general, infants sleep from 18 to 20 hours a day; growing children require from 12 to 14 hours; adults average seven to nine hours. The sleep pattern of older persons varies, but they tend to need less sleep than younger persons.

Most people work during the day and sleep during the night. However, many nighttime workers learn to sleep well during the day. Some people tend to work best during early morning hours while others prefer working later. There is no indication that any one of these patterns is better than the other.

Lack of sleep and rest produces rather typical symptoms. As weariness begins, normal performance fades with lapses in attention and concentration. Unpleasant sensations such as blurred vision, itching eyes, nausea, and headache are common signs of tiredness. Imagining unusual sights and thoughts and mental confusion finally may occur. There may be a lack of memory and an attitude of not caring what happens.

Shortchanging one's sleep occasionally does not produce dramatic changes in personality. However, a tired person often is irritable and depressed, and he usually is not able to perform as well in his work.

Hospitals are frequently thought of as poor places to rest. It may well be. Many patients, already fearful because of illness, suffer with added problems such as being surrounded by complicated and noisy equipment in a monotonous environment; being interrupted frequently with nursing and medical measures; and being bombarded with the noise of loudspeaker systems, talking and housekeeping chores. Patients often complain that they are awakened to take sleeping pills and are aroused at early morning hours to prepare for breakfast long before it is served.

The importance of sleep for well-being is well known. Lack of sleep can result in errors and tragedy as judgment fails. Today's living, requiring many split-second decisions, depends to a great extent on a rested person. Therefore, it is important for the nurse to use measures to promote rest and sleep for her patients. Also, she will wish to observe sensible sleep habits herself so that she can function effectively and safely.

Common disorders of sleep

Insomnia. Difficulty in falling asleep, waking during sleeping hours, and early awakening from sleep describe **insomnia.** The condition can lead to such distress that further wakefulness occurs. There are some physical conditions that cause wakefulness but insomnia is usually the result of worry and stress. When the patient complains of being wakeful, the nurse should investigate and take all steps possible to aid in promoting relaxation and sleep.

Somnambulism. Somnambulism is sleepwalking. It is seen more commonly in children than in adults. Most children outgrow sleep-walking. The danger of this disorder is that the patient may suffer injury. Measures to provide safety include having secure locks on doors. If a patient with a history of sleepwalking is admitted to a hospital, a record should be made of this and proper precautions taken to prevent injury.

Enuresis. Enuresis is involuntary urination and is often called bed-wetting. Since it usually occurs at night, it is commonly considered a disorder of sleep. The cause is unknown. Most texts dealing with the care of children describe common measures to assist in preventing bed-wetting, such as limiting fluid intake for several hours before bedtime and being sure that the bladder is empty prior to bedtime. It is an uncommon disorder among adults.

Sleep Talking. From observations, it appears that almost everyone talks in his sleep at some time. It rarely presents a problem unless the talking interfers with the rest of persons sharing the same room.

Nursing measures to promote rest and sleep

Research has taught us several important things about sleep.

- The body requires periods of rest and sleep to refresh itself.
- Rest and sleep generally occur best when the person is relaxed and tension and worry are reduced.
- The amount and kind of sleep and rest necessary for well-being vary among people.
- The quality of sleep influences well-being.

These observations serve as principles to guide the nurse in promoting rest and sleep for her patients, as the following nursing measures will illustrate.

The nurse is not casual or forgetful about the sleepless or restless patient. She knows rest and sleep are important for health and well-being. Therefore, she uses every effort to assist patients to obtain sufficient rest.

Relaxing is an individual matter. Promoting relaxation requires knowing the patient and learning how he can be helped to relax. Relieving monotony is often relaxing. This is especially important for patients who are bedridden for long periods of time. Some of the leisure-time activities discussed in Chapter 12 will help to relieve monotony. Exciting activities, such as watching a tension-filled television mystery drama, do little to promote relaxation.

Some people find relaxing exercises helpful. For example, while the patient is in a comfortable position, have him take several deep breaths. On the last breath after exhaling, encourage him to try to feel as limp as possible, as though he were about to sink deeply into the mattress. Instruct him to contract the muscles of his legs and then purposely allow them to go limp. Do the same for the gluteal muscles (those in the buttocks), the arms, the shoulders, and the face. Stress the importance of purposefully contracting each group of muscles and then allowing them to go as limp as possible.

Most people have certain habits that help prepare them for rest and sleep. For example, some like a snack before bedtime. Others may wish a glass of milk, hot chocolate, or tea. A cup of coffee may relax some people although most seem to feel that the caffeine in the coffee keeps them awake. Reading, listening to the radio, or watching television can be relaxing activities. Children often want a favorite stuffed animal or blanket. For many, preparation for sleep includes brushing the teeth, washing the hands and face, and going to the bathroom. A bath or shower may be relaxing for some patients. Most people have a regular bedtime hour. Being aware of such habits and helping the patient to follow them are helpful measures to promote rest and sleep.

In addition the nurse will wish to consider the following measures as she prepares patients for rest and sleep: placing the patient in a comfortable position; being sure the bed linen is clean and in order; giving a backrub; seeing to it that the room is quiet and darkened; providing privacy; providing for comfortable ventilation and temperature in the room; and observing measures that will help relieve pain, tension, and worry. Once a patient is asleep, every effort should be made not to waken him unnecessarily.

The physician may prescribe medications for helping the patient rest and sleep. Certainly there are times when patients need these drugs. They should be given after all other preparations for sleep have been completed so that the patient will obtain full benefit from them. However, the nurse will wish to use good judgment when administering them. As was true for relieving pain, drugs are not an acceptable substitute for good nursing care.

The sleeping person is just as much an individual with a unique personality as is the awake person. Therefore, to be of most help, care must be individualized. Something relaxing and restful for one patient may not be so for another.

Recording observations in relation to pain and sleeplessness

Members of the nursing and the health team will wish to be made aware of the patient's pain and of his sleeping patterns. Therefore, the nurse caring for the patient will record her findings. Usually, she will record this information in the nurses' notes. If not, she records according to agency policy.

The patient's record should indicate the nature of the pain. The section on Description of Pain early in this chapter will serve as a guide. In addition, the nurse will wish to record measures she used to promote comfort and the results of these measures.

The nurse will record the nature of the patient's resting and sleeping, as well as measures she used to promote rest and sleep and the results of these measures.

Teaching in relation to comfort, rest, and sleep

A great variety of medications for relieving pain and sleeplessness are available. Many can be bought without prescription. Some have been shown to be of very little value. Others have been proven to be dangerous. Using them may cause the patient to delay medical attention he needs. The nature of these drugs and dangers associated with their use are discussed in other courses in nursing. While giving care, the nurse has an excellent opportunity for teaching patients about these drugs. She will wish to share appropriate information with her patients. Also, she can use opportunities to teach patients how to relieve pain and sleeplessness with measures described in this chapter before turning to drugs.

Drug abuse is a serious problem in this country. It is not limited to narcotics. High-quality nursing care includes teaching patients and members of their families about the danger of careless use of all drugs, including those for relieving pain and sleeplessness.

Conclusion

Pain and sleeplessness are commonly associated with illness. Often, the nurse needs to use considerable ingenuity and skill to help patients plagued with these problems. Certain drugs may be used effectively in some situations. However, their use does not eliminate the need for high-quality nursing care that includes measures to promote comfort and rest. An important part of her care is demonstrating a sincere interest and concern for the patient as an individual.

Many over-the-counter medications are available for relieving pain and sleeplessness. The nurse will wish to help patients through teaching programs when they are observed to be using these medications indiscriminately.

References

Albert, Ira B. and Albert, Sharon E., "Penetrating the Mysteries of Sleep and Sleep Disorders," *RN*, 37:36–39, August 1974.

Beaumont, Estelle and Wiley, Loy, eds., "Bad Dreams, Bad Moods, and Bedrest," *Nursing '74*, 4:16, March 1974.

Branson, Helen Kitchen, "Insomnia," *Nursing Care*, 8:28–29, 35, January 1975.

Fagerhaugh, Shizuko Y., "Pain Expression and Control on a Burn Care Unit," *Nursing Outlook*, 22:645–650, October 1974.

Grant, Donna Allen and Klell, Cynthia, "For Goodness Sake—Let Your Patients Sleep!" *Nursing '74*, 4:54–57, November 1974.

Isler, Charlotte, "New Approach to Intractable Pain," *RN*, 38:17–21, January 1975.

McCaffery, Margo, *Nursing Management of the Patient with Pain*, J. B. Lippincott Company, Philadelphia, 1972, 248 p.

Norris, Catherine M., "Restlessness: A Nursing Phenomenon in Search of Meaning," *Nursing Outlook*, 23:103–107, February 1975.

"Nurses' Notebook: Sleep Discovery," *Nursing 75*, 5:64, June 1975.

"Pain and Suffering," A Special Supplement, *American Journal of Nursing*, 74:489–520, March 1974.

Strauss, Anselm, et al, "Pain: An Organizational-Work-Interactional Perspective," *Nursing Outlook*, 22:560–566, September 1974.

Wiley, Loy, ed., "Nursing Grand Rounds: Intractable Pain: How Nursing Care Can Help," *Nursing '74*, 4:54–59, September 1974.

14 measures to promote elimination from the large intestine

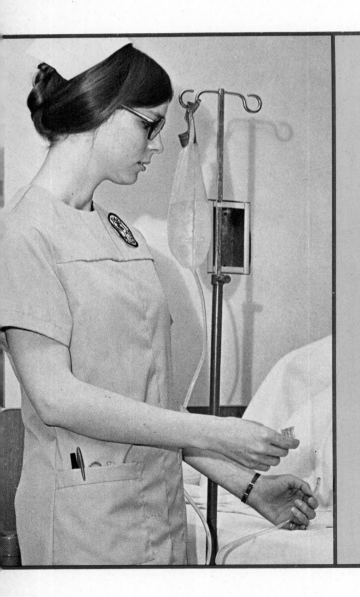

chapter outline

behavioral objectives

When mastery of content in this chapter is reached, the student will be able to

Define terms appearing in the glossary.

Explain how contents are normally propelled along the gastrointestinal tract.

Explain how defecation normally occurs.

Describe the normal stool.

Design a teaching program that will aid to establish and promote normal elimination from the large intestine. Include in this program plans to teach the dangers of the habitual use of laxatives, cathartics, and enemas.

List common problems of elimination and their common symptoms; state nursing measures that are helpful when caring for patients with these problems.

Describe briefly how each of these procedures is carried out: removing a fecal impaction; using a rectal tube for distention; inserting a suppository; giving a cleansing enema when using up to 1000 ml. of solution and when using 120 ml. of hypertonic solution; giving an oil retention enema; irrigating a colostomy; and obtaining a stool specimen.

List the primary purpose of each of these procedures: Harris flush; colonic irrigation; carminative enema; anthelmintic enema; emollient enema; nutritive enema.

glossary

Anal Incontinence The inability to control the discharge of feces and flatus.

Anthelmintic Enema An enema to help destroy intestinal parasites.

Carminative Enema An enema to help in the expulsion of flatus.

Cathartic A substance to induce defecation.

glossary cont.

Cleansing Enema An enema to help in the expulsion of feces.

Colonic Irrigation A washing out or flushing of the large intestine.

Colostomy A surgical opening into the large intestine.

Constipation The passage of dry, hard stools.

Defecation The process of evacuating waste products from the large intestine.

Diarrhea The passage of watery, unformed stools.

Emollient Enema An enema to help protect and soothe the intestinal mucous membrane.

Enema The introduction of a solution into the lower intestinal tract.

Fecal Impaction A hardened mass of feces in the rectum.

Flatulence An excessive amount of gas, or flatus, in the gastrointestinal tract.

Harris Flush The alternate filling and draining of the large intestine with a solution to help relieve distention.

Hemorrhoids Distended rectal veins.

Hypertonic Having a greater osmotic pressure than blood plasma.

Ileostomy A surgical opening into the small intestine.

Intestinal Distention Abdominal swelling due to an accumulation of flatus in the gastrointestinal tract. Synonym for tympanites.

Laxative A substance to induce defecation.

Nutritive Enema An enema to help supply the body with nutrients and/or fluids.

Ostomate A person with an ostomy.

Ostomy The creation of a surgical opening into the body. Used as a suffix or a noun.

Peristalsis Contractions of the gastrointestinal tract muscles which propel contents.

Retention Enema An enema to be retained; not intended to be expelled.

Stoma A surgical opening into the body.

Suppository A solid substance which melts at body temperature; intended for insertion into a body cavity.

Tympanites Abdominal swelling due to an accumulation of flatus in the gastrointestinal tract. Synonym for intestinal distention.

introduction

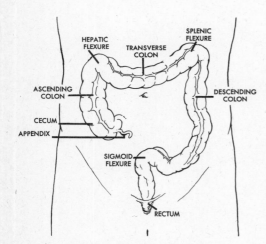

Fig. 14-1   Diagram of the large intestine.

Food is digested and absorbed in the gastrointestinal tract. Much of the waste of digestion is excreted from the intestinal tract. Excretion of waste is important for life and must continue during illness as in health. This chapter reviews briefly the process of intestinal elimination and discusses measures that help to promote it.

Elimination from the large intestine

Anatomy and Physiology of the Intestines. You will recall from science courses that the intestinal tract consists of the small and large intestines. Stomach contents empty into the small intestine. Wastes are received by the large intestine from the small intestine, and are eventually excreted via the rectum and anal canal. The various parts of the large intestine are shown in Figure 14-1.

The contents entering the large intestine are normally semiliquid or watery in nature. Water is absorbed as the contents pass through

272

the large intestine. As much as 800 to 1000 ml. are absorbed daily. This absorption of water accounts for the formed, semisolid nature of the normal stool. When absorption does not occur properly, the stool is soft and watery. If too much water is absorbed, the stool is dry and hard.

The tissues of the large intestine contain arteries and veins. Distended or swollen veins in the lower part of the large intestine (rectum) are called **hemorrhoids.** The nurse must be especially careful when introducing a tube into the rectum when hemorrhoids are present. The tissues are easily injured and therefore, the tube should be well lubricated and inserted gently, slowly, and without force. The same precautions are used when inserting a thermometer into the rectum.

Peristalsis is the process of moving contents along the gastrointestinal tract by muscular contraction. There are times when nervous tension brings on peristalsis. However, more commonly, mechanical and chemical means bring on contractions. The bulk of the contents in the tract mechanically stimulates nerve receptors which then cause muscles to contract. The action of bacteria normally found in the gastrointestinal tract produces substances (e.g., organic acid) that chemically stimulate nerve receptors and muscle contraction. The action of bacteria also produces flatus in the tract which normally helps to stimulate muscle contraction.

There are two sphincters in the anal canal. The sphincters are ring-shaped bands of muscles that control the discharge of feces and flatus from the large intestine. The internal sphincter cannot be controlled voluntarily. The external sphincter, located at the anus, is normally under voluntary control.

Defecation is the process of evacuating waste products from the large intestine. When the urge to have a bowel movement is noted, the sphincters relax; the intestinal, abdominal, and pelvic floor muscles contract; and feces are expelled from the anus. The urge to defecate can be voluntarily delayed in which case the external sphincter is not allowed to relax.

Normally, the act of defecation is painless. When pain is present, the symptom should be noted and reported promptly.

Frequency of having a bowel movement varies among healthy persons. For example, some people have a daily movement. Others normally defecate three or four times a week. The frequency of the patient's bowel movements should be noted. However, judgments in relation to frequency should be made only after the nurse knows the patient's usual habits of elimination.

The Normal Stool. The stool normally contains wastes of digestion, organisms of various kinds, secretions from intestinal glands, bile pigments, and water. The nurse should note and report any unusual contents, such as worms, their eggs, pus, blood, foreign objects (e.g., a swallowed button, ring, or coin), and so on.

Feces are normally brown in color and have a characteristic odor. The odor is caused by bacterial action on foods that are eaten. An unusual color or odor should be reported since either may be a symptom of disease. For example, tarry-black stools with a strong offensive odor are often due to bleeding high in the gastrointestinal tract. Clay-colored stools often are a sign of gallbladder or liver disease.

The stool is a formed, semisolid mass that assumes the shape of the rectum. An unusually dry or a watery stool is not normal and should be reported. A change in the shape of the stool is significant if it persists. For example, a growth in the intestine that is partially closing off the passage may cause the stool to be pencil-like in shape. The size of the stool varies, depending on the type and amount of food the person has eaten.

Normally, flatus moves along the gastrointestinal tract and is excreted in much the same manner as feces. Passing unusually large amounts or no flatus should be noted and reported. Certain foods may cause excessive flatus. The offending foods vary and, therefore, eliminating or limiting their intake becomes an individual matter.

Observing the stool and the frequency of defecation is an important nursing responsibility. Changes from normal may be significant symptoms of disease and should be reported. Sometimes changes are temporary and unimportant, such as the result of a change in the diet. Asparagus, for example, adds to the odor of excreted matter. Certain fresh vegetables may cause the stool to be darker than normal in color. Beans and cabbage also influence the appearance of the stool and frequency of defecation. In certain instances, the physician may need to change drugs or their dosage because of symptoms the patient has, diarrhea or constipation being examples.

Factors Normally Influencing Elimination. In general, factors influencing elimination fall into these categories: diet; fluid intake; exercise and activity; habits of elimination; and emotional factors. The nurse will wish to be familiar with these factors and how they influence elimination. She can then make sounder judgments and can offer the patient more helpful information in relation to promoting normal elimination.

As mentioned earlier, the stool acts to stimulate muscular contractions and evacuation. Therefore, a diet with sufficient residue or bulk is important to produce feces and movement in the intestinal tract. If the patient is having bowel movements too frequently, possibly a diet with less roughage and bulk will help. High-residue foods, such as fresh fruits and vegetables, tend to promote elimination. Low-residue foods, such as lean meats, rice, and eggs, tend to decrease peristalsis.

Fluid intake influences stool consistency. When the stool tends to be dry and hard, increased fluid intake often is helpful. Therefore, the nurse will wish to be sure the patient takes enough liquids to prevent constipation. Some persons find that drinking hot liquids on arising, or fruit juices, such as prune or orange, helps to stimulate defecation.

Exercise and activity help elimination by promoting muscle tone and by stimulating the appetite and peristalsis. The person who has little activity, as the hospitalized and ill person, generally finds that his elimination patterns become irregular. Encouraging daily activity and exercise to the extent possible often becomes an important part in helping patients to establish and maintain good elimination habits.

Bowel habits begin in early childhood. They generally have psychological aspects and often grow out of cultural considerations, such as privacy, cleanliness, and frequency.

Usually having a bowel movement is easier when a person is relaxed. Stress and worry or being away from home and unusual routines may disrupt bowel habits. This often happens to the hospitalized patient.

Most people have an urge for a bowel movement at a particular time of the day. Ignoring the urge may cause the feces to become hard and dry as increased water absorption occurs in the intestine. In addition, the intestinal tract eventually becomes insensitive to the normal stimulation to defecate. Repeatedly ignoring the normal desire to defecate is possibly the most common cause of constipation. Individual patterns of living influence the selection of a convenient time. The urge to defecate often occurs following a meal, especially after breakfast. Responding to the urge to defecate is an important factor in establishing and maintaining good elimination habits.

Positioning during a bowel movement usually influences ease of emptying the rectum. The semisquatting or sitting position permits the best use of muscles for defecation. A short person may need a footstool as he sits on the toilet. Having the bedridden patient sit on a bedpan with his feet over the edge of the bed and resting on a chair is helpful. A patient who cannot be in this position will usually find it easier to use the bedpan when the head of the bed and his knees are elevated. Or, if allowed, the patient may be assisted to a commode at the side of the bed.

This section has offered the nurse information for helping and teaching patients how to promote good habits of elimination. Irregularity and constipation are among the commonest and oldest of all complaints. Yet, they are very often preventable. Teaching plans and a program to assist patients with elimination should become a part of the patient's nursing care plan.

Common problems of intestinal elimination and suggested nursing care

Constipation. Constipation is defined as the passage of dry, hard stools. This definition makes no mention of frequency. Some persons may be constipated and yet have a daily bowel movement. Others who defecate no more than three times a week are not necessarily constipated. The consistency of the stool rather than the frequency determines whether constipation is present.

Certain diseases cause constipation. However, when no changes due to disease are involved, constipation is usually the result of poor elimination habits, low-residue diets, inadequate fluid intake, and/or lack of activity and exercise. Through teaching programs, the nurse can often help patients with such problems. It takes time to develop good elimination habits. But success has been observed among patients whose cooperation has been obtained.

The nurse will sometimes note that the constipated patient complains of headache, malaise, anorexia, foul breath, and so on. Relief is usually rapid following a bowel movement. These symptoms have been produced experimentally by packing the rectum with cotton. Therefore, the belief that the symptoms are the result of poisons being absorbed from feces appears unfounded.

Measures commonly used to intervene when constipation is present are discussed later in this chapter.

Fecal Impaction. A **fecal impaction** is the retention of an accumulation of feces which forms a hardened mass in the rectum. The patient may have liquid fecal seepage in which case, small amounts of watery stool may be passing around the impacted mass. Such fecal seepage and no normal defecation almost assure the presence of an impaction. The patient is likely to say he is constipated. Usually, he experiences a frequent desire to defecate but is unable to do so. Rectal pain may be present.

Fecal impactions may be due to constipation. The impaction may result when parts of a hardened, dry stool become lodged in the tissue folds of the rectum. Certain other conditions tend to predispose to fecal impaction. Patients who are required to take constipating drugs over a period of time are likely to develop impactions. Barium used for x-ray examinations of the intestinal tract may start an impaction when care is not taken to clean the tract of barium following the examination. Investigations have shown that very fibrous foods, such as bran and fruit seeds, have been known to cause impactions. So also have certain coated pills. There is no specific time required to develop an impaction. Some have been known to develop within 24-hours.

When it has been determined that a fecal impaction is present, an oil retention enema followed by a cleansing enema may be used. These enemas are discussed later in this chapter. If they fail, it may be necessary to break up the impaction by digital means, that is, a finger is used to break up the fecal mass.

When removing an impaction, place the patient in the Sims' (lateral) position. Cover him with a bath blanket and protect the bed with appropriate material. Place the bedpan conveniently in the bed so that pieces of removed feces may be deposited in it. Use clean gloves for the procedure.

Lubricate the forefinger generously and insert it *gently* into the anal canal. The presence of the finger added to the mass already there usually causes considerable discomfort for the patient. By carefully working the finger around and into the hardened mass, it is possible to break it up and remove pieces of it. Use plenty of lubricant to limit irritation of the mucous membrane of the rectum. When a severe impaction exists, it will need to be removed at intervals. This helps avoid extreme discomfort as well as possible harm to the patient. It is often helpful to have a second person assist during the procedure. She can assure and comfort the patient while you work to break up the mass. After removing it, make every effort to eliminate the cause and prevent the formation of another impaction.

Intestinal Distention. An excessive amount of flatus in the gastrointestinal tract is known as **flatulence.** When the gas is not expelled and accumulates, the condition is called **intestinal distention,** or **tympanites.**

Any disturbance in the ability of the intestine to absorb gas or to propel it along the intestinal tract will result in distention. Irritating foods, such as beans and cabbage, often cause distention. Certain drugs, morphine sulfate being an example, tend to decrease peristalsis and thus cause distention. Swallowing large amounts of air while eating and drinking can cause distention. Persons who are tense often can be observed to be swallowing large amounts of air, especially when taking fluids. This habit can be overcome by purposely training oneself to eat and drink without swallowing air.

Distention can be seen by observing the swollen abdomen. Gentle percussion with the fingers produces a drumlike sound. Usually, the patient will complain of cramplike pain. If distention is sufficient to cause pressure on the diaphragm and the chest cavity, shortness of breath and dyspnea may result.

Acting on the cause usually brings relief. Movement in bed or walking about will often promote escape of the flatus. If activity is not possible, relief may be obtained by inserting a rectal tube.

The size of rectal tube used most frequently for the relief of distention in adults ranges from No. 22 to No. 32, Fr. Smaller sizes are used for children. The rubber or plastic tube, when well lubricated, can be introduced with relative ease beyond the anal canal into the rectum. It should be carefully inserted for approximately 4 inches. However, it may safely be inserted a bit further if no resistance is encountered and if it is noted that no flatus is being removed.

The rectal tube may be attached to a piece of connecting tubing of sufficient length to reach into a small collecting container which can be attached to the bed frame. Another method is to place the end of the tube into a urinal or a disposable container placed on the bed under the top linen near the patient.

A rectal tube should be left in place for a short period of time. Usually 20 minutes is recommended. If distention continues, there is more likelihood of stimulating the sphincters and peristalsis when the rectal tube is reinserted every two to three hours as necessary. The patient's physician may need to prescribe a medication or other therapy if distention cannot be relieved with activity and/or a rectal tube.

Diarrhea. Diarrhea is the passage of watery, unformed stools. Frequent bowel movements do not necessarily mean that diarrhea is present. However, patients with diarrhea usually pass stools at frequent intervals. Diarrhea is often associated with intestinal cramps. Nausea and vomiting and blood in the stools may also be present.

Diarrhea may be due to an allergy to certain foods and drugs. The abuse of cathartics and certain dietary indiscretions cause diarrhea. Some persons know that for them, certain foods and fluids, such as rich pastries, coffee, or alcoholic beverages, may produce temporary diarrhea. Diseases in parts of the body other than the intestinal tract may be the source of the trouble. Examples include certain cardiac and neurological disorders. Diarrhea may be caused by certain conditions existing in the intestinal tract. Examples include infections, inflammation, and tumors.

If the cause is psychological in nature, the nurse may be able to play an important part in assisting the patient to understand the cause. Situations in daily living may be disturbing him. However, diarrhea may be associated with such deep-seated problems that the help of a psychiatrist is required.

Diarrhea is often an embarrassing and usually a painful disturbance. Local irritation of the anal region and even the perineum and buttocks from frequent watery stools may occur. To help prevent irritation the nurse will wish to use special hygienic measures, such as washing the area after each movement, drying it thoroughly, and using a medicated powder or cream. Also, she uses only very soft toilet tissue and cloths.

Common problems of intestinal elimination 277

A person with diarrhea often finds it extremely difficult to delay the urge to defecate. Therefore, when a patient has diarrhea, a comment should appear on the nursing care plan. This will alert nursing personnel to watch for the patient's signal light or bell and to answer it promptly. Or, it may be necessary to place the bedpan within easy reach for the patient, yet out of sight to prevent embarrassment and accidents.

Anal Incontinence. Anal incontinence is the inability to control the discharge of feces and flatus. Usually the cause of incontinence is a disease resulting either in a condition that hinders the proper functioning of the anal sphincter or in damage to the nerve supply to the sphincters.

While anal incontinence is rarely a threat to life, incontinent patients suffer embarrassment and emotional distress. They require support and understanding as well as special nursing care to prevent odors, skin irritation, and soiling of linen and clothing.

Note if there is a time of day when incontinence is more likely to occur, such as after a meal. If so, the patient could be placed on a bedpan at such times. If there is no pattern, place the patient on a bedpan at frequent intervals, such as every two or three hours. His attempts to use the pan may be successful and may lead to better muscular control. Consult with the physician about the advisability of using suppositories or a daily enema. For some patients, the problem is so severe that moistureproof undergarments may be necessary in order to limit soiling of the patient and the bed clothing. Disposable bed pads are convenient to use. Diapering the patient should be avoided if possible to help prevent psychological distress.

Anal control is dependent ultimately on proper functioning of the anal sphincter, and nursing or medical measures depend on the cause. For some patients, functioning of impaired anal sphincters can be improved with a planned program of bowel training. Aid in regaining bowel control becomes an important part of their care. Bowel-training programs are discussed in clinical nursing courses.

Cathartics and laxatives

Cathartics and **laxatives** are preparations which induce emptying of the intestinal tract. Some of them act chemically by stimulating peristalsis. Others act by increasing the intestinal bulk which promotes stimulation on the intestinal wall. Still others act on the fecal material by softening it.

Nurses are often able to help patients understand the appropriate use and the dangers of laxatives and cathartics. Because they are available as over-the-counter remedies and because advertising promotes their widespread use, many persons take them without medical or nursing supervision. They should not be used when abdominal pain, nausea, or vomiting is present for fear of further insult to an already diseased area. Also, many persons are unaware that their habitual use is a common cause of chronic constipation. A typical problem occurs when a patient is concerned because he has not had a daily bowel movement. He then takes a cathartic. The drug's action will stimulate enough peristalsis to empty the entire intestinal tract. Since the intestine may not fill for several days and therefore no stimulation to defecate occurs, the patient often repeats taking his cathartic and continues the pattern. The habitual use very soon makes it difficult to have a normal bowel movement.

Breaking the laxative habit is not always easy. It often requires a great deal of patience, support, and teaching. The patient frequently needs to be helped to understand the importance of diet, fluid intake, activity and exercise, and good habits of elimination.

Laxatives and cathartics are important and necessary at times. Their occasional use is generally not harmful for most persons, but efforts should be taken to prevent becoming dependent on this means for stimulating defecation.

Suppositories

A **suppository** is a conical or oval solid substance shaped for easy insertion into a body cavity. It is designed to melt at body temperature. Since a certain amount of absorption takes place in the large intestine, some medications can be given by suppository. However, the most frequent use of the suppository is to aid in stimulating peristalsis and defecation. When effective, results are obtained usually within 15 to 45 minutes.

A variety of suppositories is available. Some act to soften the feces. Some stimulate peristalsis by chemical means. Others liberate carbon dioxide, thus increasing the amount of bulk to stimulate defecation.

To be most effective, a suppository should be introduced beyond the internal sphincter of the anal canal. Lubricate the suppository before inserting it to reduce irritation and possible tissue injury. A finger cot or a glove is used to protect the nurse's finger when inserting the suppository. As the patient breathes through the mouth, the anal sphincters tend to relax and the suppository can be inserted with relative ease.

Some patients are able to insert suppositories for themselves. In certain situations, family members can be taught when the patient is being cared for at home.

The enema

An **enema** is the introduction of solution into the large intestine. The most common type is the **cleansing enema** which is used to empty the lower intestinal tract of feces. The most frequently used solutions are soap solutions, normal saline, tap water, and hypertonic solutions.

Soap solutions stimulate peristalsis by chemical irritation of the mucous membrane and by distending the intestine with the solution. Too much or too strong soap can produce irritation of the mucous membrane. Concentrated liquid soaps for enemas are commercially available. They should not be used in quantities of more than 5 ml. per 1000 ml. of water. Soap solutions can be made by dissolving bland white or castile soap in water. However, estimates of the concentration are very difficult to determine. Bar soap that has been used for handwashing or bathing is not recommended because it has been found that these bars often contain organisms. Household detergents are too strong for intestinal membranes. Many physicians discourage the use of soap for enemas, especially for patients with rectal diseases and for patients being prepared for rectal examinations because of the irritating effect on the mucous membrane.

Tap water and normal saline appear to have about the same degree of effectiveness for cleansing the bowel. However, because the large intestine absorbs water, their repeated use can result in fluid and electrolyte imbalances in the body. This is especially true of tap water.

Tap water, normal saline, and soap solution enemas usually are given in quantities of 500 to 1000 ml. for the average adult patient. The quantity of solution fills the rectum and colon. This stimulates peristalsis and usually, defecation occurs within 5 to 15 minutes.

Chart 14-1 and Figures 14-2 through 14-6 describe and illustrate administering a cleansing enema.

A **hypertonic** solution is one having a greater osmotic pressure than blood plasma. Hypertonic solutions are available in commercially prepared, disposable enema units. The amount of solution is usually 4 ounces, or 120 ml. The hypertonic solution draws fluid from body tissues into the bowel by osmosis, thus creating fluid bulk in the intestine. Also, the solution acts as an irritant on the mucous membrane. The bulk and the irritation cause muscular contractions. Usually the patient defecates with good results about three to ten minutes after administering the enema. In many health agencies and in the home, these disposable enemas have become the method of choice for cleansing the intestinal tract of feces. While being very effective, they are less fatiguing and distressing to patients than are other types of enemas.

Giving the hypertonic solution enema differs from the procedure described in Chart 14-1 in the following respects:

- The equipment and solution are included in the commercial sets and therefore, no additional equipment or supplies are needed except for the bedpan.
- It is unnecessary to warm the solution. However, if it is cold, it is better to warm it to at least room temperature to prevent the patient from having intestinal cramps.
- One recommended position for the patient is the knee-chest position. The position allows for good distribution of solution in the large intestine. However, if the patient cannot assume this position, have him lie in bed on his back or either side.
- The solution is forced into the intestine by applying gentle, steady pressure to the solution container which collapses as the solution enters the intestine. It takes about a minute or two to give the solution.

A **retention enema** is one that is to be retained. Some retention enemas are intended not to be expelled at all, a nutritive enema being an example. Some are retained for a period of time. Oils, such as mineral, cottonseed, or olive oil, are usually used for retention enemas and preferably, retained for at least 30 minutes. The primary purpose of the oil enema is to lubricate and soften the stool. Usually, 100 to 200 ml. of oil is given slowly in order to avoid stimulating peristalsis and the desire to defecate. The effectiveness of oil retention enemas varies. Often, it becomes necessary to follow an oil enema with a cleansing enema before defecation occurs. Disposable oil enema units are available which ordinarily contain about 120 ml. of mineral oil.

Chart 14-1 Administering a cleansing enema

The purpose is to introduce solution into the large intestine to aid in stimulating peristalsis and removing feces

Suggested Action	Reason for Action	Figure to Illustrate
Assemble necessary equipment, according to agency procedure. Recommended size of tube for adult is No. 26 to No. 32, Fr. Prepare 1000 ml. of solution at 105 to 110°F.	For maximum stimulation, comfort, and safety, solution should enter intestine at slightly higher than normal body temperature. Adult colon is estimated to hold about 750 to 1000 ml. Size of rectal tube recommended helps produce muscular contraction by stimulating anal sphincters.	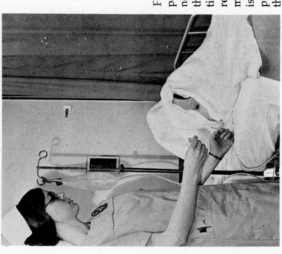 Fig. 14-2 The equipment and patient mannequin are in readiness for giving a cleansing enema: the mannequin is properly positioned and draped; the bedpan is ready; a bag containing approximately 1000 ml. of warm solution is hung on a standard at the appropriate level above anus; and the rectal tube is of a correct size.
Plan with patient where he will defecate. Have bedpan, commode, or nearby bathroom ready for his use.	Patient is better able to relax and cooperate if he knows everything is in readiness when he feels urge to defecate.	
Place container of solution so that it is no more than 18 or 20 inches above level of patient's anus, as illustrated in Figure 14-2. Plan to give solution slowly over period of five to ten minutes.	Gravity forces solution to enter intestine. Amount of pressure will determine rate of flow and pressure exerted on intestinal wall. Container placed too high and giving solution too quickly cause rapid distention and pressure in intestine, resulting in too rapid expulsion of solution and poor defecation.	
Position and drape patient on his right or left side or on his back, as dictated by his comfort as illustrated in Figure 14-2.	Patient's comfort helps him relax. Exact position of *reclining* patient has not been found to alter results of enema significantly.	

Chart 14-1   continued

Suggested Action	Reason for Action	Figure to Illustrate
Generously lubricate end of rectal tube for 2 to 3 inches.	Friction is reduced when surface is lubricated, resulting in easier insertion and less likelihood of injury to mucous membranes.	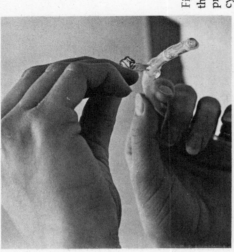 Fig. 14-3 The nurse lubricates the rectal tube generously with a prepackaged lubricant of the agency's choice.
Allow solution to fill tubing, thereby displacing air.	While allowing air to enter intestine is not harmful, it may make it more difficult to introduce solution if intestinal pressure from flatus and constipated stool is great. Filling tube with solution warms tube.	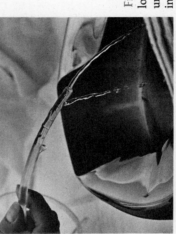 Fig. 14-4 The solution is allowed to fill the tubing so that an unnecessary quantity of air is not introduced into the patient.

Lift buttock to expose anus well. Slowly insert rectal tube 2 to 3 inches at an angle pointing toward umbilicus.

Good visualization of anus helps prevent injury to tissues. Anal canal is approximately 1 to 2 inches in length. Tube should be inserted through internal anal sphincter. Further insertion may damage intestinal wall. Suggested angle follows normal intestinal contour. Slow insertion of tube minimizes spasms of intestinal wall and sphincters.

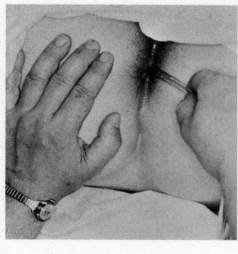

Fig. 14-5 The nurse lifts the buttock well and inserts the rectal tube at an angle pointing toward the umbilicus of the patient. From the unit "Bowel Elimination" of the multi-media *Lippincott Learning System.*

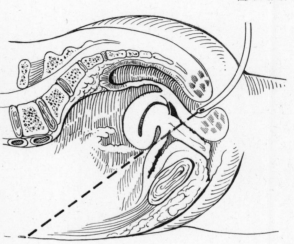

Fig. 14-6 This figure illustrates the proper angle and length for inserting the rectal tube when giving a cleansing enema.

If tube seems to meet resistance while being inserted, permit small amount of solution to enter, withdraw tube slightly, then continue to insert. *Do not force entry of tube.*

Resistance may be due to spasms of intestine or failure of internal sphincter to open. Solution may help to reduce spasms and relax sphincter, thus making continued insertion of tube safe. Forcing tube may cause injury to wall of intestine.

Chart 14-1 continued

Suggested Action	Reason for Action	Figure to Illustrate
Introduce solution slowly. Instruct patient to breathe through mouth in small, fast breaths, as if panting, and stop flow of solution briefly when patient has strong desire to defecate before sufficient solution has been given.	Stopping flow of solution and having patient pant help relax muscular contractions and allow patient to be given sufficient solution for effective defecation.	
After sufficient solution has been given, have patient retain solution until urge to defecate occurs, usually 5 to 15 minutes.	This amount of time usually allows muscular contractions to become sufficient to produce good results.	
When patient has strong urge to defecate, place him in sitting position on bedpan or assist him to commode or bathroom.	Sitting position helps in best use of body muscles to assist in act of defecation.	
Note character of stool and patient's reaction to enema. Record according to agency policy.		
Wash equipment and sterilize it before reuse. Or, discard disposable equipment properly.	There is abundant growth of bacteria in intestine which can be spread to others when equipment is not properly cared for.	
If patient is uncomfortable and unable to expell enema, siphonage may be necessary. Prepare about 100 ml. of warm water (105°F.). Attach funnel to lubricated rectal tube. Fill tube with water; kink tube and insert into patient. Allow tube to open and pour water into funnel. Before funnel empties, turn funnel upside down into bedpan at patient's side. Slow continuous flow through tube and funnel drains intestine. Repeat as necessary.		

Giving an oil retention enema differs from the procedure described in Chart 14-1 in the following respects:

- If reusable equipment is used, select a rectal tube between sizes No. 14 and No. 20, Fr. for an adult. This small-sized tube helps minimize muscular contractions at the anal sphincters.
- Give the oil at body temperature in order to minimize the muscular stimulation caused by a warmer or colder solution.
- Encourage the patient to retain the oil for at least 30 minutes before attempting to have a bowel movement.

Chart 14-2 lists some additional types of enemas. This text will not discuss them in detail since in many parts of the country, they are used infrequently. Also the nurse familiar with the procedure of giving an enema and the underlying principles discussed in this chapter will find that adapting techniques to accomplish different purposes will be relatively easy. When an enema is ordered, the nurse will wish to observe the health agency's procedures.

There are several important areas to cover when teaching patients in relation to enemas, such as the dangers of using enemas habitually. These dangers are similar to those when patients become dependent on the use of cathartics and laxatives.

When an enema is necessary, Chart 14-1 serves as a good guide to teach the patient how to take his own enema. A common misunderstanding many people have is that the enema can be given successfully while sitting on a toilet. The amount of pressure needed to force solution into the intestine while sitting is far greater than that needed while lying down. Also, the solution will tend to pool without traveling up into the intestine. This will usually cause the patient to defecate sooner than desirable and cleansing results may be poor.

As was true about cathartics and laxatives, the patient should be warned not to take an enema when nausea, vomiting, or abdominal pain is present.

Colostomy irrigation

Ostomy means the creation of an opening into the body by surgical means. Ostomy is often used as a suffix. For example, a **colostomy** is an opening into the large intestine. An **ileostomy** is an opening into the small intestine. The opening is called the **stoma.** Ostomy is also used as a noun. The word, **ostomate,** refers to a person with an ostomy.

The opening in the large intestine of the patient with a colostomy has been brought to the wall of his abdomen. Since there is no sphincter at the stoma, the patient has no voluntary control over the escape of flatus and feces. However, he can learn how to regulate discharge from the stoma. This is often done with great success by using colostomy irrigations to initiate regular bowel movements from the stoma.

A colostomy irrigation resembles an enema but differs from the procedure described in Chart 14-1 in the following respects:

- The solutions of choice are tap water and normal saline. The amount is specified by the physician.

Chart 14-2 Various types of enemas

Name of Procedure	Purpose	Comments
Harris Flush	To relieve distention	By holding container of solution about 18 inches above patient and allowing a small amount of solution (250 to 300 ml.) to enter intestine and then lowering container below level of patient, intestine alternately fills and drains. It is expected that patient will expel flatus, as well as some feces which will drain into container when it is lowered.
Colonic Irrigation	To wash out or flush large intestine	Solution is introduced and drained from intestine simultaneously by using two tubes. About 3000 to 4000 ml. of solution are used.
Carminative Enema	To relieve distention	An example of solution used is one of equal parts of milk and molasses.
Anthelmintic Enema	To destroy intestinal parasites	Usually administered as a retention enema.
Emollient Enema	To protect and soothe intestinal mucous membrane	Oils are commonly used. Enema is retained.
Nutritive Enema	To supply body with nutrients and/or fluids	Dextrose solution is commonly used. Adequate nourishment is impossible but may be used temporarily or in emergency situations. Enema is retained.

- A small tube (catheter) or a conelike appliance is inserted into the stoma for introducing the solution.
- The solution enters and leaves the large intestine more or less simultaneously. The patient, lacking sphincter control, cannot retain the solution effectively.
- The solution leaves the intestine via an irrigation sleeve which is an appliance centered over the stoma and held in place with a belt. The sleeve has an opening in the bottom. It is placed so that the opening drains into a toilet. Or, it drains into a bedpan if the patient is bedridden. If the patient is up and about, the opening at the bottom of the irrigating sleeve may be closed with a clamp so that the patient has freedom to move around while waiting for the colon to empty. When the patient does not use this sort of a sleeve, a kidney basin may be held in a manner to catch the discharge from the stoma. A second basin may be used to direct discharge downward toward the basin next to the patient, should the discharge be expelled with force.
- The catheter or cone is inserted in a way so that it follows the natural path of the colon. The surgeon is consulted to learn the path of the colon when doubt exists.
- *The tube or cone is never forced into the stoma and colon.* If resistance is met, the nurse pulls the tube or cone out slightly, releases a little water, waits a minute or so, and tries again. If another attempt fails, she discontinues the procedure and contacts her supervising nurse for further instructions.
- It usually takes about 45 minutes to one hour to complete a colostomy irrigation.

The colostomy irrigation is further described and illustrated in Figures 14-7 through 14-15.

The ileostomy is not irrigated. The discharge is liquid or the consistency of thin paste, since the large intestine is not present to absorb fluid from the stool.

More detailed discussions of the care of patients with an ileostomy or colostomy are found in clinical texts. Wound care is discussed in Chapter 18 of this text.

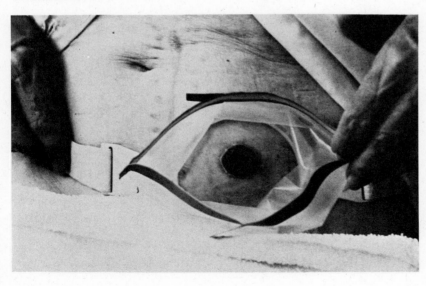

Fig. 14-7 The patient has a plastic irrigating sleeve secured with a belt around the exposed colostomy stoma.

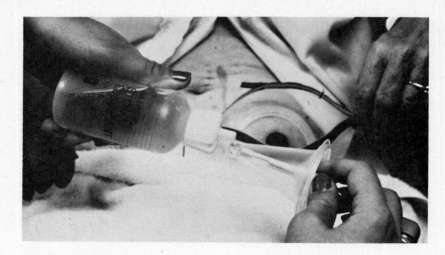

Fig. 14-8   The nurse lubricates the conelike device which this patient uses for her colostomy irrigation.

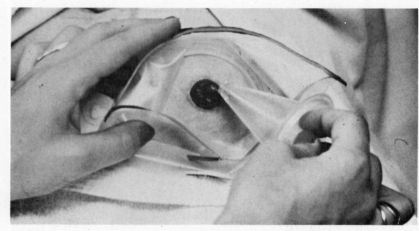

Fig. 14-9   Warm irrigating solution is allowed to fill the irrigation set so that air will not be introduced into the colon. The lubricated cone is then gently introduced into the stoma at an angle so that it follows the natural path of the colon.

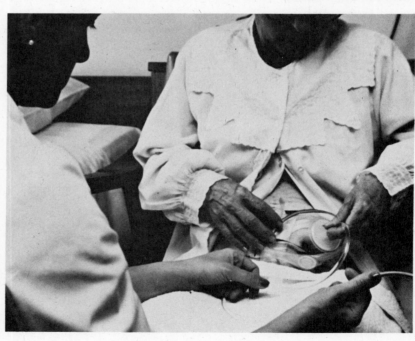

Fig. 14-10   The patient holds the cone firmly as the nurse opens the flow control valve which allows the irrigating solution to enter the colon. The valve is closed when the prescribed amount of solution has entered the colon. If the patient complains of cramps, shut off the solution until they subside. The solution may be entering the colon too fast, or, it may be too cold. Allowing the patient to assist as much as possible helps her learn to handle the equipment and gain confidence so that she will eventually be able to irrigate on her own.

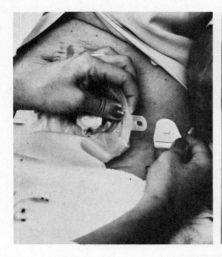
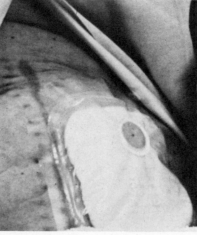

Fig. 14-11 (Left) After the cone is removed and the bowel has emptied, the belt and sleeve are removed.

Fig. 14-12 (Right) After cleaning and drying the skin around the stoma, a cap is placed over the stoma. A lightweight dressing may be used for patients who do not use a stoma cap.

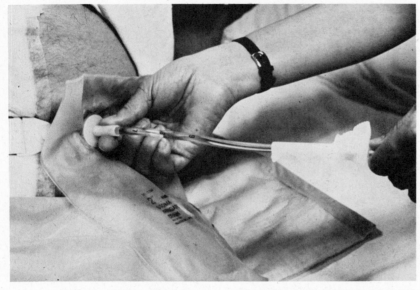

Fig. 14-13 This patient uses a calibrated catheter-type colon tube for irrigating his colostomy. The catheter is first passed through a disc and a sponge valve for the desired length and then lubricated. After filling the tube with irrigating solution, the tube is introduced through the stoma into the colon for the desired number of inches. The sponge valve rests on the stoma.

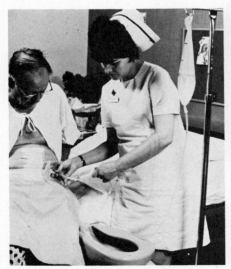
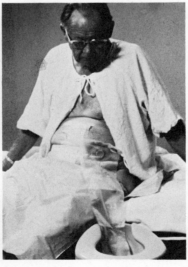

Fig. 14-14 (Left) The desired amount of solution is allowed to enter the colon. Note that a calibrated plastic bag is used for the irrigating solution.

Fig. 14-15 (Right) This patient places the irrigating sleeve in a bedpan into which bowel contents then drain. Photographs courtesy of Hollister Incorporated)

289

Obtaining a stool specimen

Stool specimens are sometimes analyzed for diagnostic purposes. For example, feces may be examined for blood, bile, parasites, parasite eggs, and so on. The nurse usually either instructs the patient in the collection of the specimen or carries out the procedure herself.

Whenever possible, it is preferable that the feces be uncontaminated with urine or other body secretions. A clean or sterile bedpan can be used for intestinal elimination. The specimen can then be transferred to the appropriate laboratory container with two clean or sterile tongue depressors or a similar disposable instrument. Care should be taken that the outside of the container remains uncontaminated.

Accurate labeling of the container is important. Depending on the examination to be performed, the specimen should either be refrigerated or kept warm. Ova and parasites cannot sustain life if the environmental temperature varies much below body temperature.

Conclusion

Intestinal elimination is an essential body process. The nurse plays an important role as she helps patients to establish and maintain normal habits of elimination. She often becomes the teacher as she helps patients and their families understand normal elimination and how it can be promoted.

A nursing problem is often met when patients become bowel conscious beyond the point of good reason. Misleading literature and advertisements, especially in relation to the frequency of having a bowel movement, have caused many people to upset normal habits unnecessarily. The nurse can assist such persons with teaching programs that include information concerning the indiscriminate use of laxatives and cathartics.

Proper elimination is as important for someone with a colostomy as for any other person. With proper teaching and care, the ostomate can lead a normal life even though elimination occurs through an artificial opening in the intestine.

References

"Are Your Patients Too Lax About Laxatives?" *Nursing '75*, 5:37, July 1975.

Baum, Mary E., "Everything You Wanted to Know About An Ostomy, **But Were Afraid to Ask," *Nursing Care*, 7:14–15, October 1974.

"Consultation: Improving Ostomy Equipment," *Nursing '75*, 5:61, June 1975.

Corman, Marvin L., et al, "Cathartics," *American Journal of Nursing*, 75:273–279, February 1975.

Jensen, Vicki, "Better Techniques for Bagging Stomas. Part 2. Colostomies," *Nursing '74*, 4:30–35, August 1974.

———, "Better Techniques for Bagging Stomas. Part 3. Ileostomies," *Nursing '74*, 4:60–63, September 1974.

Keusch, Gerald, "Bacterial Diarrheas," *American Journal of Nursing*, 73:1028–1032, June 1973.

Pike, Benjamin F., "Soap Colitis," *The New England Journal of Medicine*, 285: 217–218, July 22, 1971.

Renkun, Shirley, "Cancer of the Colon and Rectum: Cure or Crisis?" *The Journal of Practical Nursing*, 25:18–21, April 1975.

Schauder, Marilyn R., "Ostomy Care: Cone Irrigations," *American Journal of Nursing*, 74:1424–1427, August 1974.

Spitz, Martin J., "Consultation: Constipation in Aged," *Nursing '73*, 3:25, August 1973.

15 practices of surgical asepsis

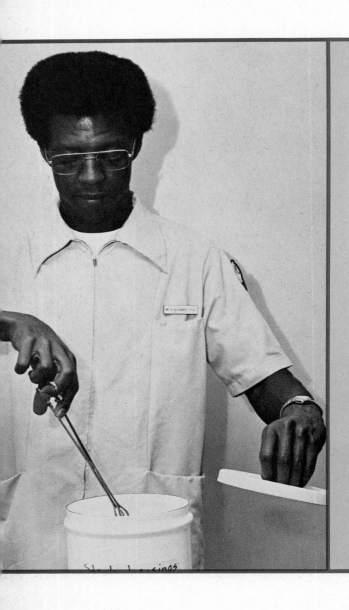

behavioral objectives

When mastery of content in this chapter is reached, the student will be able to

Define terms appearing in the glossary.

State the primary purpose and the basic principle upon which practices of surgical asepsis are based.

List at least eight practices of surgical asepsis and two basic principles upon which they are based.

Describe how to open a sterile set or tray; how to don sterile gloves; how to handle a sterile transfer forceps; and how to remove sterile equipment from a common container.

glossary

Don To put on an article of wear.

Sterile Technique Practices that render and keep objects and areas free of all microorganisms. Synonym for surgical asepsis as defined in Chapter 4.

Transfer Forceps An instrument for handling supplies and equipment.

introduction

This chapter discusses common practices of surgical asepsis. Knowledge of these practices is important in order to carry out certain nursing procedures with safety. Examples include giving a medication by injecting it into body tissues, catheterizing the patient, and applying sterile dressings to a wound.

Good preparation for studying this chapter would be to review Chapter 4 which discussed concepts basic to an understanding of both medical and surgical asepsis.

Basic principles and practices of surgical asepsis

Sterile technique is often used as a synonym for practices of surgical asepsis. Sterile technique or practices of surgical asepsis are based on several principles. The *purpose* of using these practices is based on this principle: *introducing microorganisms into the body may cause infection and disease.* For example, sterile equipment and sterile technique are used when catheterizing a patient since introducing organisms into the normally sterile bladder may cause infections in the urinary tract.

The gastrointestinal tract and the vagina ordinarily are not treated as sterile areas. Therefore, practices of medical but not necessarily surgical asepsis are observed when using procedures involving these body areas. Nevertheless, for the sake of safety, equipment used to remove and introduce substances into the gastrointestinal tract is almost always sterilized before use. Examples include the rectal tube, oral and rectal thermometers, vaginal irrigators, tubes introduced into the stomach, and solutions used for vaginal douches.

Practices of surgical asepsis are based on these principles: a sterile object or area becomes contaminated when touched by an unsterile object; and, a sterile object or area may become contaminated by microorganisms carried in air currents, dust, lint, and respiratory droplets.

The following common practices of surgical asepsis are based on the above principles:

- Do not walk away from or turn away from a sterile field. This will prevent possible contamination while the field is out of the worker's view.
- Avoid talking, coughing, or sneezing over a sterile field or object. This will help prevent contamination by droplets from the nose and mouth.
- Hold sterile objects above the level of the waist. This will help keep the object in sight, thus avoiding accidental contamination.
- Open sterile packages so that the edges of the wrapper are directed away from the worker, in order to avoid the possibility of a sterile surface touching the uniform and to avoid reaching over a sterile field. Opening a sterile tray is illustrated in Figures 15-1 through 15-3.
- Avoid spilling solutions on a cloth or paper sterile setup. The moisture will penetrate through the sterile field, carrying organisms with it, and contaminate the field. A wet field is always considered contaminated when the surface immediately below it is not sterile.
- Do not reach over a sterile field. Clothes are not sterile and could

contaminate the field by touching it or by dropping particles of lint or dust on it.

- Do not use any equipment or supplies if there is any doubt about their being sterile. It is far better to err on the safe side than to take a chance and have the patient suffer with an infection.
- Hands cannot be sterilized. Therefore, handle sterile equipment and supplies with sterile forceps or with the hands after donning sterile gloves. The use of forceps and donning sterile gloves are discussed later in this chapter.
- Avoid drafts from open windows, fans, air-conditioning units, and so on, near sterile fields. The air currents may carry organisms to the sterile field and to the patient.
- Masks and gowns are used in delivery rooms and operating rooms as part of surgical aseptic procedures in these units. These practices are discussed in other nursing courses.

Opening sterile sets or trays

Health agencies frequently provide prepackaged sterile sets or trays for procedures that require sterile equipment and supplies. For example, the catheterization set or tray contains sterile equipment and supplies needed by the nurse. Additional examples of prepackaged sterile sets or trays commonly found in health agencies include those used for the various procedures described in Chapter 20. The nurse opens a sterile set or tray as illustrated in Figures 15-1 through 15-3.

Donning sterile gloves

To **don** means to put on an article of wear. For certain procedures, the nurse will don sterile gloves. She can then safely use her hands to handle sterile equipment and supplies without contaminating these objects.

Sterile gloves are included in some sets or trays, and are also packaged in glove wrappers. Figure 15-4 illustrates how to don gloves that have been packaged and sterilized in a wrapper. The procedure is the same for gloves that have been included in sterile sets or trays.

Handling sterile transfer forceps and sterile containers

Transfer forceps are instruments used to handle supplies and equipment. Unsterile, or clean, forceps are sometimes used to handle grossly contaminated supplies and equipment in order that the hands do not become heavily contaminated. Sterile forceps are used to handle sterile equipment and supplies so that they are not contaminated by the hands. They are commonly used for such tasks as removing sterilized articles from a sterilizer, removing sterile items from a container or wrapper, and transferring sterile equipment and supplies from one area to another.

The practice of using sterile transfer forceps for handling sterile equipment and supplies is on the decrease, as is the use of common

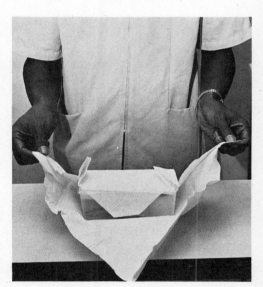

Fig. 15-1 The nurse opens a sterile set or tray by folding the top most part of the covering wrapper *away* from him. This leaves sterile equipment and supplies well covered so that they cannot be contaminated by reaching across the set or tray as he begins to open the wrapper.

Fig. 15-2 Next, the nurse opens the second layer of the wrapper to the sides of the set or tray. This still leaves sterile equipment and supplies covered with the last layer of the wrapper.

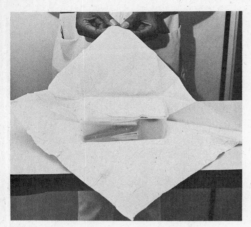

Fig. 15-3 As the last step, the nurse opens the final layer of the wrapper *toward* himself. The wrapper can now become the sterile field immediately surrounding the sterile set or tray. Note that at no time did the nurse reach across an uncovered sterile field or sterile equipment and supplies.

sterile containers for storing sterile equipment and supplies. The chances of their being accidently contaminated seems too great to use them, in the opinion of many health practitioners. More common practice is to use a forceps from a sterile package. It is used once and discarded, if disposable, or sterilized again for reuse. Likewise, rather than being stored in common containers, supplies are packaged in sterile wrappers. Each package is used only for one patient.

Despite the fact that sterile transfer forceps and sterile containers are not used as often as they once were, they are convenient in certain situations. Charts 15-1 and 15-2 were prepared for the convenience of nurses giving care in agencies where forceps and containers are standard equipment. Figures 15-5 and 15-6 on page 298 illustrate.

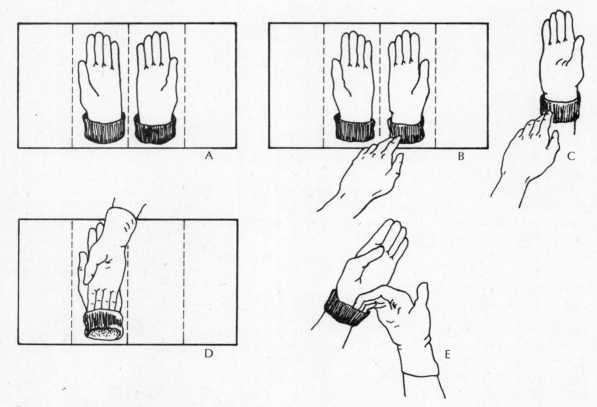

Fig. 15-4 Correct method of putting on sterile gloves. Note that the shaded portion of the glove is considered contaminated and is the only part touched by the skin as the gloves are applied.

Practices of surgical asepsis

Chart 15-1 Using sterile transfer forceps

The purpose is to use sterile transfer forceps so that neither the forceps
nor sterile equipment becomes contaminated

Suggested Action	Reason for Action
Keep only one sterile transfer forceps in container to prevent accidently touching prongs of one forceps on handle of other while removing from container.	A sterile area becomes contaminated when touched by unsterile objects. Handle of forceps is not sterile.
When removing forceps from container of solution, keep prongs together and lift forceps without touching any part of container.	Top and rim of container of solution are not sterile. A sterile area becomes contaminated when touched by unsterile object.
Hold forceps with prongs pointed downward to prevent solution from container on prongs from flowing from unsterile handle to sterile prongs.	Liquids flow in direction of gravitational pull. Liquids flowing from unsterile handle to prongs contaminate prongs.
Gently tap prongs together directly over container to remove excess solution. Do not tap prongs on rim of container.	Top and rim of container are not sterile. A sterile area becomes contaminated when touched by unsterile objects.
Keep prongs of forceps within vision while using it.	Sterile objects out of vision may accidently become contaminated and then contaminate sterile objects.
Sterilize forceps if there is danger of its not being sterile.	Using unsterile forceps will contaminate sterile objects.
Resterilize forceps and its container and fill container with fresh disinfectant of agency's choice at least daily and oftener if indicated.	To be sure of sterility after repeated use, safe practice includes regular and frequent sterilization of forceps and its container.

Chart 15-2 Managing sterile containers

The purpose is to manage sterile-covered containers so that neither
the container nor its contents become contaminated

Suggested Action	Reason for Action
Remove cover of container only as necessary and for as brief a time as possible.	Air currents may carry organisms to inside of container.
Lift cover off container so that underside of cover is facing down.	Held in this position, sterile underside of cover is less likely to become contaminated by organisms in air currents or by unsterile objects touching it.
Invert cover of container only when it is necessary to put it down.	Contact with an unsterile surface contaminates the sterile area of cover.
Consider rim or edge of cover and container to be unsterile.	Proximity of edge of cover to exposed surfaces and then to edge of container makes sterility doubtful.
Do not return unused sterile objects to container once they have been removed.	Once sterile objects are removed from container and exposed to air, sterility is doubtful.
Resterilize container and its contents at regular intervals according to agency procedure.	To be sure of sterility after repeatedly removing cover, safe practice includes regular and frequent sterilization of container and its contents.

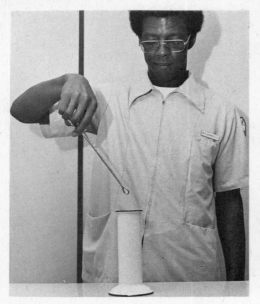 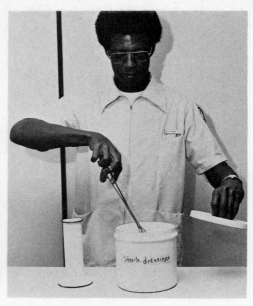

Fig. 15-5 The nurse illustrates proper handling of sterile forceps: there is only one forceps in the container; prongs of the forceps are kept together and are not allowed to touch the edge of the container; and the nurse keeps his eyes on the forceps as he handles them.

Fig. 15-6 The nurse is about to remove sterile dressings from a sterile common container: the underside of the cover is facing down; the forceps are kept well away from the edge of the container; and the nurse keeps his eyes on his work.

Chart 15-1 indicates that transfer forceps and the container in which forceps are stored should be resterilized and the solution in the container changed daily. There appears to be no demonstrated reason for this recommended daily care. However, the opportunity for contamination by means of air currents, personnel, and technique is too great to warrant less frequent precautionary measures. Actually, the more frequently the forceps and container are resterilized, the safer the practice of using transfer forceps is likely to be. Resterilizing common containers and their contents at regular and frequent intervals is equally important for the same reason, as Chart 15-2 indicates.

Conclusion

Microorganisms are naturally present in every patient environment. Some may be harmless to most people while others are harmful to many. Still others are harmless except in certain situations. An important part of nursing care is helping to prevent the patient from acquiring infections by decreasing the spread of microorganisms. One way to do this is to use sterile technique whenever indicated so that whether a particular organism is harmful or not to a particular patient, he is protected. The conscientious nurse pays constant attention to her techniques as she uses sound practices of both medical and surgical asepsis.

Practices of surgical asepsis

References

Burgess, R. E., "Aseptic Management of Disposables," *Hospital Topics*, 48:95–98, 113, January 1970.

Marinaro, Armand, "Rationale of Sterility, Sterilization and Sterility Testing," *Hospital Topics*, 49:118–120, January 1971.

Streeter, Shirley, et al, "Hospital Infection—A Necessary Risk?" *American Journal of Nursing*, 67:526–533, March 1967.

16 measures to promote elimination from the urinary bladder

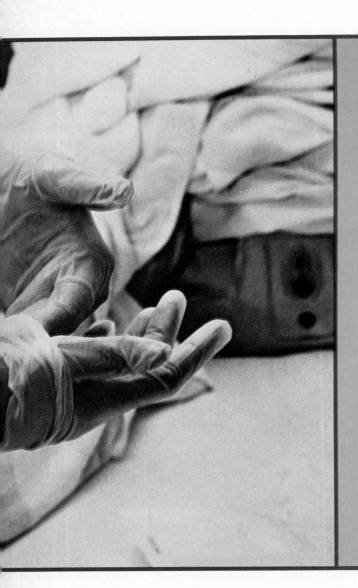

chapter outline

behavioral objectives

When mastery of content in this chapter is reached, the student will be able to

Define terms appearing in the glossary.

Explain how urine is collected in the kidneys and bladder.

Explain how voiding normally occurs.

Describe normal urine.

List common problems of urinary elimination and their common symptoms; state nursing measures that are helpful when caring for patients with these problems.

Design a teaching program for bladder training.

List common reasons for catheterizing a patient and describe common hazards of catheterization.

Describe how to catheterize a female and a male patient.

Describe how to manage an indwelling catheter.

Describe how to obtain a "clean catch" and a "midstream" urine specimen.

Explain how to test a urine specimen for sugar and for acetone, using the procedure of choice in the agency in which care is being given.

glossary

Albuminuria The presence of albumin in urine.

Anuria The lack of production of urine.

Catheter A tube for injecting or removing fluids.

Diuresis The excessive production and excretion of urine. Synonym for polyuria.

Dysuria Difficulty in voiding.

Frequency Voiding at frequent intervals.

Glycosuria The presence of sugar in urine.

Hematuria The presence of blood in urine.

Incontinence The inability to control the discharge of urine from the bladder.

Meatus The external opening of a canal of the body.

Micturition The process of emptying the urinary bladder. Synonyms are voiding and urination.

Nocturia Excessive urination during the night.

Oliguria The production and excretion of scant amounts of urine.

Overflow Incontinence The periodic involuntary escape of urine as pressure in the bladder increases.

Polyuria The excessive production and excretion of urine. Synonym for diuresis.

Pyuria The presence of pus in urine.

Residual Urine Urine remaining in the bladder after voiding.

Retention Urine is being produced but not excreted from the bladder.

Total Incontinence The inability of the bladder to store any urine; constant dribbling of urine is present.

Urinary Catheterization The introduction of a catheter through the urethra into the bladder for removing urine.

Urination The process of emptying the urinary bladder. Synonym for micturition and voiding.

Voiding The process of emptying the urinary bladder. Synonym for micturition and urination.

introduction

Excretion of waste is important for life and must continue during illness as in health. This chapter reviews briefly the process of elimination from the urinary tract and discusses measures that help to promote elimination.

Elimination from the urinary tract

Anatomy and Physiology of the Urinary Tract. The urinary tract is one of several routes from which wastes are excreted from the body. Other routes include the large intestines, lungs, and skin. Certain inorganic salts, nitrogenous waste products, and water are removed from the bloodstream and excreted through the proper functioning of the urinary tract.

The kidneys are located on either side of the spinal column behind the peritoneum and in the back part of the abdominal cavity. They carry a major responsibility for maintaining the composition and the volume of fluids normally found in body tissues. The kidneys function in a selective manner. They single out for excretion contents from the blood for which the body has no need. Despite taking in various kinds and amounts of food and fluids, tissue fluids remain relatively stable if there is proper kidney function. The waste solution which the kidneys produce is called urine. It is transported from the kidneys through the ureters to the urinary bladder.

The urinary bladder is a smooth muscle sac which serves as a reservoir for urine. There are several layers of muscle tissue in the bladder. At the base of the bladder, muscle tissue forms the internal sphincter which guards the opening between the urinary bladder and the urethra. The urethra carries urine from the bladder to the exterior of the body.

The bladder normally contains urine under very little pressure. As the volume of urine increases, the pressure increases only slightly. The adaptability of the bladder wall to pressure is believed to be due to the characteristics of the muscle tissue in the bladder. This makes it possible for urine to continue to enter the bladder from the ureters against low pressure. When the pressure becomes sufficient to stimulate stretch receptors located in the bladder wall, the desire to empty the bladder becomes noticeable.

In men, the urethra is common to both the excretory and the reproductive systems. It is approximately 5½ to 6½ inches in length. The external urethral sphincter is located near the place where the urethra leaves the body and enters the penis. The external sphincter is under voluntary control.

The female urethra is about 1½ to 2½ inches long. Its only function is to carry urine from the bladder to the exterior of the body. The external sphincter is located approximately midway in the urethra. It is under voluntary control. No portion of the female urethra is external to the body as is true in the male.

A **meatus** refers to an external opening of a canal in the body. The opening at the end of the urethra in both the male and female is called the meatus.

The process of emptying the urinary bladder is known as **micturition.** Synonyms are **voiding** and **urination.** As noted above, when urine collects in the bladder, eventually the stretch receptors are stimulated, and the desire to void becomes noticeable. Usually this occurs when about 100 to 200 ml. for the child and 200 to 300 ml. for the adult have collected. The act of micturition is normally painless and without strain.

Normal Urine. Healthy adults excrete approximately 1000 to 1700 ml. of urine in each 24-hour period. The color of normal urine is golden yellow or amber. If the urine is scant and concentrated, the color will be darker. If it is dilute, the color will be lighter. The first voided urine of the day is usually more concentrated than urine excreted during the remainder of the day.

Urine has a characteristic odor. Some foods, such as asparagus, and certain drugs will alter the odor.

The urine of a person on a normal diet is slightly acid. Vegetarians excrete a slightly alkaline urine. Normally the urinary tract is sterile. Therefore, urine is free of bacteria. Bacteria are normally found at the end of the urethra. If they are washed into a urine specimen, they will usually be identified by laboratory examination.

Normal urine is clear. On standing and cooling, cloudiness and a sediment may occur which are due to precipitation of certain normal contents in the urine as it changes from an acid to an alkaline. Normal urine will clear rapidly if acid is added and the urine is heated to body temperature. Table 16-1 gives laboratory findings when urine is normal.

Table 16-1 Normal urine laboratory values	
Urea	20–35 Gm. per 24 hours
Uric acid	0.4–1 Gm. per 24 hours
Urea clearance	54 ml. blood per minute
Chlorides (Na)	10–15 Gm. per 24 hours
Penolsulfonphthalein P.S.P.	60–75 per cent in 2 hours
Average amount in 24 hours	1000–17000 ml.

Factors Normally Influencing Urinary Elimination. The amount of urine normally excreted will vary with fluid intake. The greater the amount of fluid intake, the larger will be the amount of urine, and vice versa. If large amounts of fluid are being excreted by the skin, lungs, or intestine, the amount excreted by the kidneys will decrease. Persons on high-protein diets will produce more urine than those on a regular diet. Children and infants excrete more urine in proportion to their weight than adults do.

The frequency of voiding depends on the amount of urine being produced. Normally from two-thirds to three-fourths of the urine output is voided during the day. Unless the fluid intake is large, most healthy adults do not void during their sleeping hours.

Some persons normally void small amounts at frequent intervals. This is usually due to the habit of responding to the first early urge to void. The habit is insignificant and is not necessarily an indication of disease.

Increased abdominal pressure, such as occurs with coughing and sneezing, sometimes forces the escape of urine involuntarily. This is especially true in women because the urethra is short. Strong psychological factors, such as marked fear, may also result in involuntary urination. Under certain conditions, it may be difficult to relax muscles sufficiently to void. This occurs sometimes when a urine specimen is requested from a person who is embarrassed or shy.

Women find it easier to void in the semisitting or sitting position than in the back-lying position. For the bedridden patient, elevating the head of the bed and the knees is helpful when this is permitted. Or, if allowed, the patient may be assisted to a commode or to the bathroom. Men find it easiest to void when standing and this position is preferable when the patient's condition allows.

Common problems of urinary elimination and suggested nursing care

There are terms used to describe abnormal symptoms that are related to urinary tract problems. The following are common ones with which the nurse will wish to be familiar:

Anuria refers to a lack in the production of urine. Since the kidneys do not produce urine, the bladder remains empty.

Oliguria refers to the production of only scant amounts of urine. Anuria and oliguria are serious symptoms and should be reported promptly.

Diuresis means an excessive production and excretion of urine. **Polyuria** is a synonym. Certain fluids act as diuretics and will cause an increase in the production of urine. Examples include coffee, tea, and cocoa. Some drugs also produce diuresis.

Retention means that urine is being produced but it is not being excreted from the bladder.

Residual urine is urine retained in the bladder after voiding. The patient may say that he still feels as though he needs to void. Normally all but 1 to 3 ml. is excreted.

Incontinence is the inability to control discharge of urine from the bladder. If the bladder is unable to store any urine and urine dribbles constantly, the condition is called **total incontinence.** If urine accumulates in the bladder and there is periodic dribbling when the bladder becomes overdistended, the condition is called **overflow incontinence.**

Hematuria refers to urine that contains blood. When blood is present in large enough quantities, the urine becomes reddish brown in color.

Pyuria means pus in the urine. The urine appears cloudy. This should not be confused with the cloudiness that may occur when normal urine stands and cools.

Albuminuria means there is albumin in the urine.

Glycosuria refers to sugar in the urine. It may normally occur after a large intake of sugar or after a marked emotional disturbance.

Dysuria means difficult voiding. It may or may not be associated with pain. However, pain is usually present. A feeling of warmth and of local irritation occurring during voiding is called burning.

Frequency refers to voiding at very frequent intervals.

Nocturia is present when there is excessive voiding during night hours, especially when it is not associated with a large fluid intake.

Urinary Incontinence. Urinary incontinence may be either permanent or temporary, depending on the cause. It is a problem faced by many elderly patients. Family members often need the nurse's help on ways to deal with it in the home.

Nursing measures should be directed toward helping restore normal function if there is a possibility of success. As with fecal incontinence, urinary incontinence should not be a condition to which everyone becomes resigned. The value to the patient of knowing that effort is being made to help him cannot be overestimated.

It is sometimes helpful to suggest a routine for taking fluids followed shortly by an effort to void. Voluntary efforts either to control or to induce voiding may be sufficiently stimulating to help restore function for some patients. For others, especially the chronically ill and the elderly, it may be simply a matter of taking them to the bathroom or offering a bedpan every two to three hours. Perineal exercises may help. These exercises consist of contracting the muscles as though urination is to be halted. This is followed by relaxing muscles in the area, as though about to start to void. This can be done 10 to 15 times daily.

Additional nursing measures for the incontinent patient include keeping him dry, clean, and comfortable. Often, great skill is required to prevent discomfort from wet clothing and linens. The ammonia of the urine and lying on wet linen can quickly irritate the skin, and soon lead to the development of bedsores.

Various types of collection appliances are available for male patients. These devices fit over the penis and are secured by straps. A collection bag is usually attached to the patient's leg to permit him to be up and about. Collection bags must be applied carefully to prevent skin irritation, cleansed regularly to avoid odor, and emptied at regular intervals to prevent spilling. Since a man's trousers can cover the entire appliance, his independence and activity can be maintained with no embarrassment.

The nurse will wish to demonstrate tact and understanding while caring for incontinent patients. Offering emotional support and allowing the patient to talk of his problem and to assist with decisions about his care are often helpful. Whenever possible, the patient should be consulted about measures to collect and absorb urine, such as the use of absorbent pads, urinary appliances, and waterproof undergarments. Incontinent patients often limit their fluid intake. They need to be helped to understand the relationship between adequate fluid intake and total body functioning.

Bladder Training. More extensive training than that just described is sometimes used. This training usually requires the physician's consent.

To start the patient on a bladder-training program when there is little or no possibility of his achieving results could be unfortunate. Even if he is likely to succeed, he must be helped to understand that it will be a slow process and the gains may be slight and very gradual. As in any situation, it is poor policy to permit the patient to set unrealistic goals for himself.

The management of the patient's fluid intake is especially important. Because of the relationship between drinking and the occurrence of urine in the bladder, it is best to plan a drinking schedule that will permit convenient occasions for the patient to attempt to void. Most persons urinate shortly after awakening. This is usually the first and a good time for the patient to attempt to empty the bladder. Drinking some water upon awakening is helpful. Other fluids can be spaced throughout the day according to the patient's wishes. Fluids should be limited in the late evening hours, thus limiting the risk of incontinence during the night.

If there has been any regularity to the patient's incontinence, these times should be considered in the scheduling. For example, if the patient notes that a frequent wetting time is at 10:30 AM, he should attempt to void about 10:00 AM.

The times selected for attempting to empty the bladder need not be spaced regularly, such as every four hours. However, they should be at the same time each day.

Any sensation that precedes voiding should be noted. The usual kind of stimulus produced by a full bladder may or may not be present. Common sensations include chilliness, perspiring, muscular twitching, and restlessness. It is important that the patient understand these signs and use them as clues for a need to void.

When the patient attempts to start bladder training, he should be comfortable and relaxed. Adjustments should be made so that a good sitting or standing position may be maintained. If the patient is not able to be out of bed and is going to use the bedpan or urinal, the head of the bed should be raised and the patient well supported with pillows. The knees may be slightly flexed, especially for the female patient. A toilet or commode may be used if the patient is able to be out of bed.

It is often helpful if the patient bends forward in a slow, rhythmic fashion. This creates pressure on the bladder. It also helps if the patient applies light pressure with the hands over the bladder. The pressure should be directed toward the urethra. Other helpful measures include listening to running water, drinking fluids while attempting to void, and placing the hands in a basin of water.

It is possible for the patient to void during the attempt without knowing of it or without specific stimulus or control. This is still considered involuntary voiding. Not until the patient is able to use a specific method to stimulate and empty the bladder is the bladder-training program considered successful.

As a means of gauging the success of the attempts, examination for residual urine may be included as a part of the training program. Using slight percussion over the lower part of the bladder may indicate whether the bladder is empty. Or, a catheter may be inserted into the bladder to determine if there is residual urine present.

Urinary Retention. When retention is present, the bladder continues to fill and may distend until it reaches the level of the umbilicus. The height of the bladder can be determined by palpating with light pressure on the abdomen.

Retention is often temporary. It is common following surgery, especially if the patient cannot be up and about. Any obstruction will cause retention. Swelling at the meatus that often occurs following childbirth is an example.

Nursing measures should be instituted as soon as the patient feels that he cannot void, even if the interval since the last voiding was only a few hours. This is particularly true if the patient has been having a normal fluid intake.

The following common nursing measures often help the patient to void:

- Place the patient in a semisitting or sitting position, if this is permitted. Sometimes, voiding will begin if the patient sits at the edge of the bed on a bedpan or with a urinal in place while supporting the feet on a chair.
- If the female patient is allowed out of bed, have her sit on a bedpan placed on a chair, use a commode, or go to the bathroom.
- If the male patient is allowed out of bed, have him stand while he uses the urinal, use a commode, or go to the bathroom.
- Offer the patient fluids, especially warm drinks.
- Warm the bedpan.
- Allow water to run from a tap within hearing distance of the patient.
- Place the patient's hands in warm water.
- Pour water over the perineal area.

Urine retained in the bladder increases the likelihood of urinary tract infections, and is also painful and unpleasant. The patient often becomes worried and tense, which, unfortunately, makes matters worse.

When all measures fail it becomes necessary to catheterize the patient.

Catheterization

A **catheter** is a tube for injecting and removing fluids. **Catheterization** of the urinary bladder is the introduction of a catheter through the urethra into the bladder for removing urine.

The dangers of introducing a catheter into the bladder are injury and infection. An object forced through a stricture, an irregularity, or a curve from the wrong angle can cause injury to mucous membranes. Microorganisms can enter the bladder by being pushed in as the catheter is inserted. The procedure of catheterization is used as infrequently as possible in view of these two hazards.

There are various reasons for catheterizing a patient. It was once common practice to obtain a urine specimen by catheterization. Occasionally, in order to obtain a specimen free of contamination, the procedure may be used. However, much more commonly today, a voided or a "clean catch" specimen is requested. The voided specimen was discussed in Chapters 9 and 10. The "clean catch" technique will be discussed later in this chapter.

Catheterization may be used before surgery to empty the patient's bladder completely. It is commonly recommended that the catheterization be performed in the aseptic conditions of the operating room in order to help prevent infections. Catheterization is used postoperatively when patients are unable to void and when nursing measures to induce voiding have failed. It is used before and after delivery for the same reason. It is also used in some situations when the patient is incontinent and when residual urine is present.

Catheterization may be used to remove urine from a greatly distended bladder. It is generally agreed that gradual emptying of the bladder is a safer procedure than rapid removal of all urine. For patients with severe retention, if as much as 2000 ml. is suspected, a special apparatus may be used to empty the bladder over a period of 24 hours or more. At other times, the nurse will need to use her judgment. Some authorities believe that safe procedure is to remove no more than approximately 100 ml. of urine at one time from a greatly distended bladder.

In most agencies, disposable sterile catheterization sets are provided. These sets include the catheter, a receptacle to receive the urine, materials to clean the area at the meatus, a lubricant, and sterile gloves. For the female patient, sizes No. 14 and No. 16, Fr. catheters are used. No. 16 and No. 18, Fr. are usually used for male patients, and No. 8 and No. 10, Fr. are appropriate for children. The catheters are ordinarily made of plastic or rubber.

The preparation of the patient includes explaining that usually there is a sensation of pressure when the catheter is inserted rather than one of pain. In addition, the patient is assured that every measure to avoid exposure and embarrassment will be taken. The more relaxed the patient is, the easier it will be for the nurse to insert the catheter.

The most frequently used position for the female patient is the dorsal recumbent, preferably on a firm mattress or on a treatment table. A soft mattress into which the patient sinks makes seeing the meatus difficult. Also, sinking into the mattress may cause the patient's bladder to be lower than the outlet of the catheter. The buttocks are supported on a firm cushion if the patient must be in a bed with a soft mattress.

The Sims' position can also be used for the female patient. It often provides better visualization for a nurse of short stature. In addition, it is usually more comfortable for the patient who finds it difficult to hold knees and hips in place for the dorsal recumbent position. The patient may lie on either side. However, for the right-handed nurse, having the patient lie on her left side is generally preferred. The patient's buttocks are placed near the edge of the bed with her shoulders near the opposite edge. Her knees are drawn toward her chest. The nurse lifts the upper buttock and labia to expose the meatus. Figure 16-1 illustrates alternate positions for catheterizing the female patient.

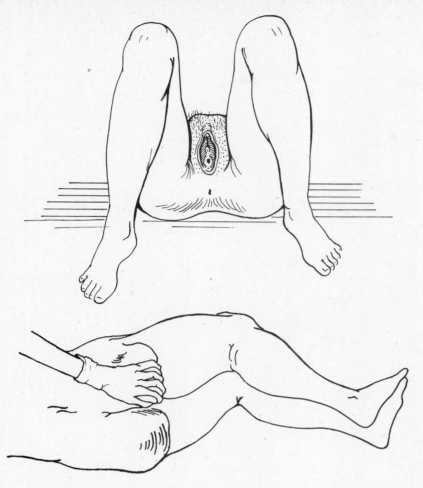

Fig. 16-1 Alternate positions for female urinary catheterization. (Top) The patient is in the dorsal recumbent position. (Bottom) The patient is in the lateral position. Drapes are omitted in the sketches to more clearly show positioning of the patient.

Good positioning and lighting are especially important for the female patient so that the nurse can locate the meatus quickly and easily. Artificial light is almost always necessary for this procedure. The patient is properly draped to protect her from unnecessary exposure and from drafts.

The male patient is usually positioned flat on his back. The knees may be flexed a bit and the legs separated.

Proper positioning of the patient allows sufficient area for the nurse to prepare and to maintain a sterile working field. If the dorsal recumbent position is used, the sterile area is generally between the patient's legs near the perineum. When the lateral position is used, the sterile area is next to the lower buttock and thigh. In the supine position, the sterile area is between the edge of the bed and the patient's thighs; the receptacle for collecting urine is placed between the patient's legs. Placing the sterile working area properly helps prevent having to reach across the sterile field. Chart 16-1 and Figures 16-2 through 16-10 describe and illustrate catheterization of the male and female patient.

The procedure for catheterization suggested in this book recommends the use of sterile gloves. However, there may be some occasions when gloves are not worn. Sterile equipment must then be handled with sterile forceps. The nurse must wash her hands *thoroughly* immediately

Catheterization

Chart 16-1 Catheterization of the urinary bladder
(Male and Female)

The purpose is to remove urine from the bladder

Suggested Action	Reason for Action	Figure to Illustrate
Assemble equipment; a sterile catheterization set is used in most health agencies. Position and drape patient appropriately.	Good visualization of meatus is important to introduce catheter. Embarrassment, chilliness, and tension can interfere with introduction of catheter. Comfort of patient will promote relaxation.	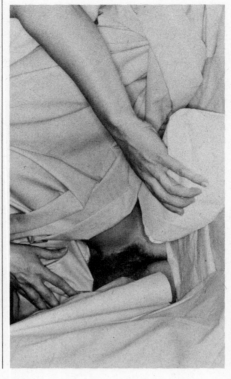 Fig. 16-2 The female patient has been positioned and properly draped for catheterization in the dorsal recumbent position. From the unit "Urine Elimination" of the multi-media *Lippincott Learning System*.
If patient is soiled, wash area around meatus well with soap or detergent and water, rinse well, and dry.	Having area as clean as possible decreases likelihood of introducing organisms into bladder.	
Place catheter set conveniently and open as described in Chapter 15.	Reaching across sterile items increases risk of contamination.	

Don sterile gloves as described in Chapter 15.

Sterile equipment can be handled without contamination when sterile gloves are worn.

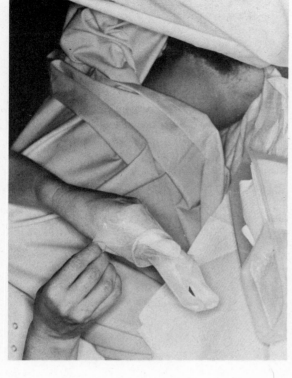

Fig. 16-3 The nurse has opened the catheterization set, which she had placed conveniently near her work area, and dons sterile gloves. From the unit "Urine Elimination" of the multi-media *Lippincott Learning System.*

Arrange equipment to provide convenience and to avoid having to reach over sterile field.

Placing equipment in order of use increases speed of performance. Reaching over sterile items increases risk of contamination.

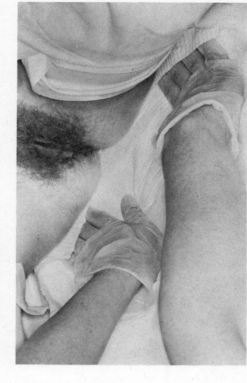

Fig. 16-4 Note how the nurse wraps the edges of a sterile towel around her gloved hands to protect them from contamination while placing the towel near the edge of the patient's buttocks. From the unit "Urine Elimination" of the multi-media *Lippincott Learning System.*

Chart 16-1   continued

Suggested Action

Generously lubricate catheter for about 1½ to 2 inches, being careful not to plug eye of catheter. For male, generously lubricate catheter for about 6 or 7 inches.

For female, place thumb and finger between labia minora, spread, and then pull upward. Hand separating labia is now considered contaminated.

Reason for Action

Lubricant reduces friction and facilitates insertion of catheter. For male, generous lubrication is especially important because of length and tortuousness of urethra.

Stretching tissue irons out area and makes meatus visible for easy insertion of catheter. Touching labia contaminates gloved hand.

Figure to Illustrate

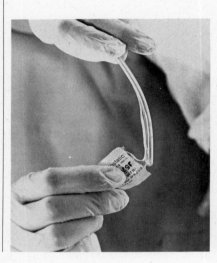

Fig. 16-5   The nurse lubricates the catheter generously with a pre-packaged lubricant of the agency's choice.

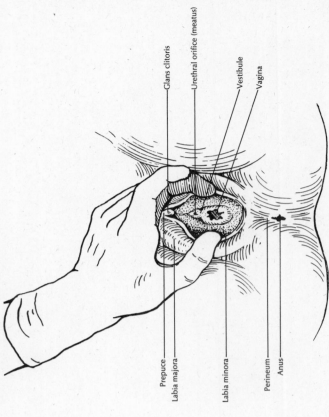

Glans clitoris

Urethral orifice (meatus)

Vestibule

Vagina

Prepuce

Labia majora

Labia minora

Perineum

Anus

Fig. 16-6   The labia minora are well separated and then the nurse exerts pressure toward the symphysis pubis. This helps to expose the area for cleansing and for locating the meatus for inserting the catheter.

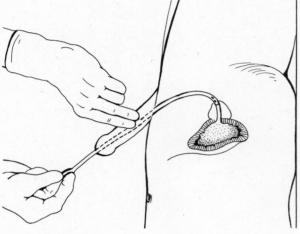

Fig. 16-7 The penis is elevated nearly perpendicular to the body and held in position in order to straighten the urethra well.

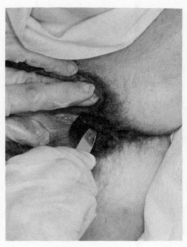

Fig. 16-8 The nurse cleanses by holding cotton balls, soaked in an antiseptic of the agency's choice, with forceps. She uses one cotton ball for each stroke over the area, moving from above the meatus downward toward the rectum. From the unit "Urine Elimination" of the multi-media *Lippincott Learning System.*

For male, lift penis upward nearly perpendicular to body. In uncircumcised male, retract foreskin. Meatus should be visible at tip of penis. Hand holding penis is now considered contaminated.

Lifting penis helps straighten its long and curved urethra for easier and safer insertion of catheter. Organisms may harbor under foreskin. Good visualization of meatus makes easy insertion of catheter possible. Touching penis contaminates gloved hand.

Cleanse exposed area at meatus *thoroughly* using solution of agency's choice. For female, move cotton ball held in forceps from above meatus down toward rectum. For male, start at meatus; use circular motion, moving from tip toward base of penis.

Be prepared to maintain separation of labia, or position of penis, until urine is flowing well and continuously or until bladder is empty.

Moving from area where there is likely to be less contamination to an area where there is more helps prevent spread of organisms. Thorough cleansing helps reduce possibility of introducing organisms into bladder.

Allowing labia to drop back into position during procedure, or penis to drop down, may contaminate area around meatus as well as catheter when it is in place.

Chart 16-1 continued

Suggested Action	Reason for Action	Figure to Illustrate

Pick up catheter with uncontaminated gloved hand and insert into meatus 2 to 3 inches for female and 6 to 8 inches for male.

Female urethra is approximately 1½ to 2½ inches long. Male urethra is about 5½ to 6½ inches long.

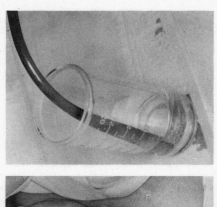

Fig. 16-9 The catheter is inserted while the nurse continues to hold the labia apart. From the unit "Urine Elimination" of the multi-media *Lippincott Learning System.*

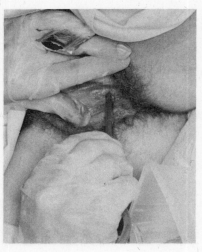

Hold catheter securely while bladder empties. Avoid pushing and pulling catheter in and out as bladder drains. Place end of catheter into receptacle or into specimen container if specimen is required.

Withdrawing and reinserting catheter increases chances of contaminating catheter.

When flow of urine begins to decrease, withdraw catheter slowly about ½ inch at a time until urine barely drips and then withdraw catheter.

Tip of catheter passes through urine remaining in bladder as catheter is slowly withdrawn.

Fig. 16-10 Once the urine is flowing well, the nurse can allow her left hand to hold the catheter in place securely while collecting a urine specimen. From the unit "Urine Elimination" of the multi-media *Lippincott Learning System.*

Remove no more than 750 to 1000 ml. of urine at one catheterization.

Removing more than 750 to 1000 ml. of urine at one time may cause bladder damage and shock.

Reduce foreskin of uncircumcised male following catheterization.

Failing to reduce foreskin of uncircumcised male will cause discomfort, swelling of penis, and possible serious complications.

Care for equipment and urine specimen as required. Record results.

Agency policy is observed.

before starting the procedure. When a sink is in the patient's room, it is recommended that the handwashing be done after the patient has been positioned and draped, if at all possible. This means that the patient must keep the knees flexed in the dorsal recumbent position, but it eliminates having the nurse handle linens and other objects before handling sterile equipment.

Slight resistance may be met as the catheter encounters the external sphincter. Pausing briefly and asking the patient to breathe deeply will generally result in sufficient relaxation for the catheter to be passed readily. Rotating the catheter gently may also be helpful. Under no circumstances should force be used to insert the catheter for either the male or female. In the male, when resistance is encountered, the nurse straightens the penis slightly more. If resistance continues, a stricture in the urethra may be present; or, lower in the penis, an obstruction may be present due to an enlarged prostate gland. If the male or female patient seems to be experiencing unusual discomfort, the procedure is discontinued and the situation reported promptly.

Immediately following the insertion of the catheter, some patients react by tightening the muscles in the area. The flow of urine may be delayed momentarily until the patient is able to relax. If the nurse waits for a short time after she believes the bladder has been entered, she may save the patient and herself the necessity of repeating the procedure.

Following catheterization, the nurse records according to agency policy. Most often, she records the time the patient was catheterized, a description of the urine, the amount of urine obtained, and the patient's reaction to the procedure. If a specimen was prepared and sent to the laboratory, this also is recorded.

Management of the indwelling catheter

If a catheter is to remain in place, usually an indwelling or retention catheter is used. The catheter is designed so that it does not slip out of the urethra.

One type of catheter has a portion that expands after the catheter is in place in the bladder. It is called a mushroom catheter.

Another type has a balloon which can be inflated after the catheter is inserted. There are several types available but the principle on which they operate is similar. The catheter has a double lumen. One lumen is connected directly with the balloon. The other is the portion through which the urine drains. When the balloon is inflated, the sidepiece through which the solution was introduced is clamped. There are also catheters which are self-sealing. Equipment for inflating the balloon is usually included in the agency's indwelling catheter set.

The basic procedure for inserting the catheter is the same as that for catheterization. As soon as the bladder has been emptied of urine, the balloon of the indwelling catheter is filled with solution. Sterile water or normal saline is usually used. The balloons are designed to hold from 5 to 30 ml. of solution. The nurse follows the agency's procedure on the amount of solution to use and the method for injecting it. One type of an indwelling catheter is illustrated in Figure 16-11.

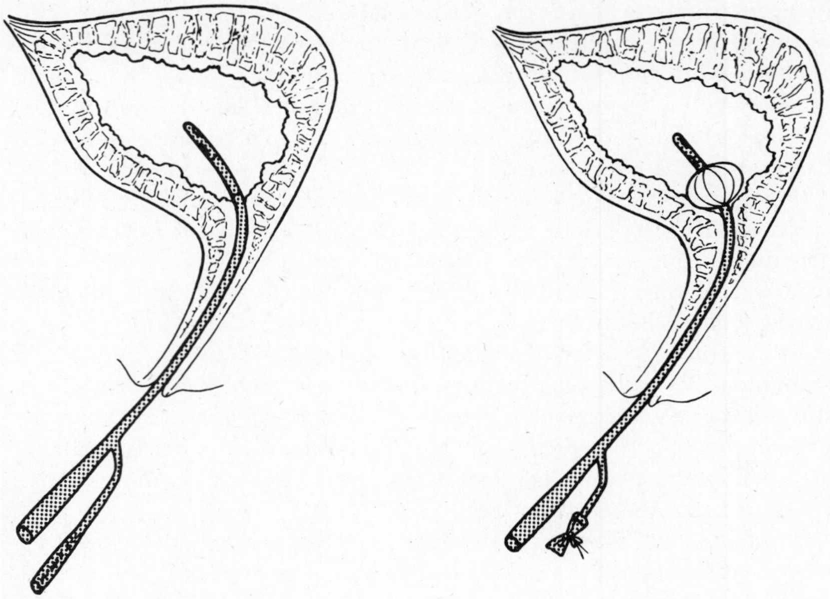

Fig. 16-11 (Left) An indwelling (Foley) catheter has been inserted into the urinary bladder. (Right) The bag is inflated to prevent the catheter from slipping from the urinary bladder. The inner tube of the catheter is tied to prevent air from leaving the bag.

After the balloon has been inflated, the nurse tests the catheter to see that it is secure. *Slight* tension on it will indicate whether or not it is well located in the bladder. Also, the catheter may be irrigated. The catheter is properly located if the irrigation solution returns. If the patient complains of pain or discomfort while the balloon is being filled, the nurse withdraws the fluid and inserts the catheter farther. The balloon may be in the urethra.

An indwelling catheter is attached to a receptacle to collect urine by tubing so that drainage occurs by gravity. The tubing should be of sufficient length to reach the collecting container and still give the patient freedom to move about. If the drainage tubing is too short, the patient's movements in bed will be restricted. If it is too long, urine tends to pool in the tubing. This may interrupt the drainage from the bladder.

The tubing may be attached to the patient's catheter with a glass or plastic rod. This makes it possible to examine drainage from the catheter. The tubing is generally taped to the patient's leg. It may be secured to his clothing or to the bed linen. It is important that the tubing be placed so that it cannot be compressed by the weight of any part of the patient's body.

Placing the drainage tubing over the patient's thigh may cause urine to collect in the bladder. Drainage will not occur until the urine is forced over the thigh, and then suction empties the bladder. If this occurs rapidly, there may be damage to the mucous membrane of the bladder.

The receptacle to collect urine should be placed lower than the catheter's entry into the bladder to prevent urine from re-entering the bladder. Attaching it to the bed frame is common practice when the patient is in bed, as Figure 16-12 illustrates. Calibrated containers have several advantages. Amounts of drainage can be determined readily, and measuring when emptying the container is eliminated.

The closed drainage system has a continuous sterile passageway leading from the bladder to the collecting container. Most containers are disposable. A special air filter permits air to escape from the container as

Elimination from the urinary bladder

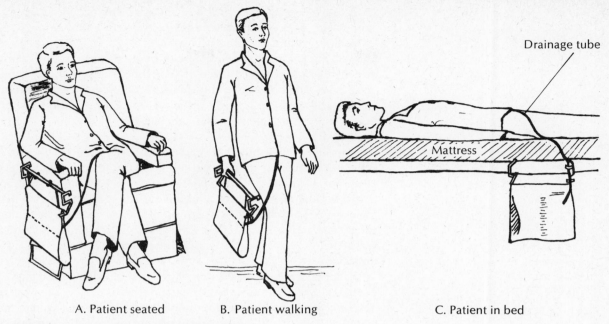

A. Patient seated B. Patient walking C. Patient in bed

Fig. 16-12   Urine collection receptacle for an indwelling catheter. Note that whether the patient is seated, ambulatory, or in bed, the tube is free of kinks and pressure, and lower than the bladder.

it fills with urine. The catheter, tubing, and container are not disconnected from each other in some setups. This prevents the introduction of microorganisms. When the patient's catheter is changed, the entire setup is changed. Other setups allow for disconnecting the catheter from the drainage tubing.

The open drainage system allows the catheter, tubing, and collection container to be disconnected from each other; in addition, the collecting container has an open top. The risk of infection is great with this system since organisms can easily enter the system. However, in home situations, when cross-infection from other patients does not exist, open drainage containers are sometimes used. If the equipment is not disposable, the patient and the family will need instruction on its care.

To irrigate a catheter means to flush it with solution. An irrigation is used when blood clots or other debris threaten to block the catheter. In the past, this procedure was done routinely for almost all indwelling catheters. Because it is another possible way of introducing microorganisms, the current recommendation is that an irrigation be done only when there is demonstrated need. "Natural" irrigation through an increased fluid intake by the patient is thought to be better.

A physician's order is usually required for catheter irrigation. The physician also specifies the solution to be used. Strict sterile technique must be followed. Sterile equipment consisting of a bulb syringe, solution, and a collecting basin are necessary. The ends of both the catheter and the tubing must be handled carefully to prevent contamination. Sterile tube protectors and catheter plugs are commercially available. When it is necessary to use these items, they should be discarded after each use. It is recommended that when catheter irrigations are done at home using nondisposable equipment, the syringe should be boiled for at least ten minutes before it is used.

Varying amounts of solution may be used for irrigation. Thirty ml. per instillation, repeated three or four times, usually is sufficient. The solution should be instilled and allowed to return by gravity. Milking the tubing *away* from the bladder may be necessary if it is obstructed. Suction should not be used routinely because the mucous membrane of the bladder may be injured.

Careful handwashing between the care of patients with indwelling catheters cannot be emphasized too strongly. Special body hygiene is urged for all patients with indwelling catheters. Complete and at least daily cleaning of the area around the meatus is recommended for both male and female patients. Organisms allowed to accumulate in this area can ascend and cause infection. Provisions and reminders for patients to wash their hands, especially following a bowel movement, are also important.

Patients who have indwelling catheters should have the benefit of full explanation on how the system functions and on how they can assist. Teaching includes keeping the tubing free from kinks, maintaining an adequate fluid intake, keeping a record of the output, and preventing contamination. The patient may be allowed out of bed, as Figure 16-12 illustrates.

When an indwelling catheter is in place, the nurse notes any comments the patient may make about it, such as irritation, burning sensations, or annoyances with it. She also notes the volume and character of the urine. Any signs of infection should be reported promptly. After an indwelling catheter is removed, it should be noted on the patient's nursing care plan. There is still need for observation. Frequency, burning on voiding, interference with the ability to start urination, and cloudy urine may be part of the aftermath of an indwelling catheter. Too often, patients endure the discomfort because they believe that it is to be expected.

Obtaining urine specimens

Obtaining voided or catheterized urine specimens has already been discussed. Some situations may require a "clean catch" specimen. This is especially true if a urinary tract infection is suspected and a urine culture is desired.

In the "clean catch" technique, the external meatus area is cleansed thoroughly with soap or detergent and water or an antiseptic solution. In the uncircumcised male, the foreskin or prepuce should be retracted to expose the glans penis before cleaning. In the female, the labia are well separated before cleansing and kept apart until the specimen is collected. In many agencies, it is recommended that a sterile glove be worn during the cleaning and collection. The patient voids directly into a sterile container.

Some agencies catch the specimen "midstream." Cleansing the

Elimination from the urinary bladder

meatus is carried out as described above. The patient voids a bit, about 30 ml., and this urine is discarded. Then the collection of urine begins. The patient voids directly into a sterile container. It is expected that any additional organisms harbored at the meatus will have been flushed out by the stream of urine. A patient who can be adequately instructed and expected to carry out the aseptic precautions may collect his own "clean catch" and "midstream" specimens and often prefers to do so. Following the specimen collection the foreskin of the male patient should be returned to its reduced position.

If a patient finds it difficult to void directly into a sterile container, he may void into a sterile bedpan or urinal. The urine is then poured into an appropriate container. In some situations, sterile containers, bedpans, and urinals are not required for a "clean catch" and "midstream" specimen. Thoroughly clean equipment is used instead.

In some health agencies, "clean catch" and "midstream" are used synonymously. In other words, an order for a "clean catch" urine specimen automatically also means that the specimen is to be collected "midstream," and vice versa. Agency policy concerning the use of these two terms should be observed.

Twenty-four hour specimens are required for some types of laboratory studies. Instructing the patient about the importance of collecting *all* urine for a period of 24 hours is important. The collection is begun at a specified time by having the patient empty his bladder. This specimen is discarded. All urine for the next 24 hours is saved. The urine from each voiding may be kept in a separately marked container, indicating the time of urination. Or, all voidings may be put into a common receptacle. The specimens are ordinarily kept cold. Sometimes a preservative is added to retard decomposition of the urine.

Children who are too young to cooperate in urine specimen collection often require the use of special techniques and apparatus. They are described in texts dealing with the care of children.

Common test for sugar and acetone in the urine

The nurse may be asked to test the patient's urine for sugar and acetone content, sometimes abbreviated S and A. She also may need to teach the patient how to do these tests. They are used for patients with diabetes. The results help to determine the amount of insulin the patient requires.

Several different types of tests are available. Some require using a tablet which is dropped into a urine specimen. After a recommended period of time, the color of urine is compared with a color chart provided by the manufacturer. Others use a strip of treated paper as illustrated in Figure 16-13. The strip is held in a specimen of urine for a recommended period and then its color is compared with a color chart. The particular test used will be the one of the agency's or physician's choice.

These tests are relatively simple to do and manufacturers' instructions are easy to follow. However, *accuracy is essential.* Instructions must be followed with care.

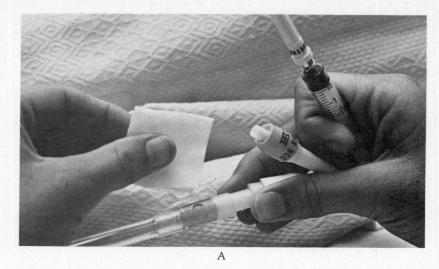

A

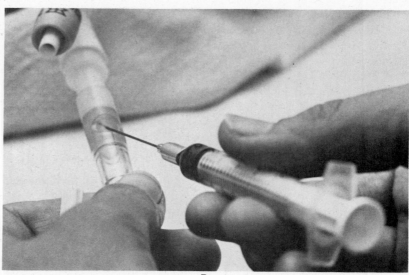

B

Fig. 16-13 The nurse obtains a urine specimen from a patient with an indwelling catheter and tests the specimen for sugar and acetone. To obtain freshly voided urine, this health agency's policy is to remove urine with a sterile needle and syringe from the drainage tube at a point near that at which the tube and catheter connect. (A) The nurse first thoroughly cleanses the area on the drainage tube into which she will insert the needle. (B) She aspirates the amount of urine she will need for testing. (C) She places a strip of specially treated paper into the urine specimen for the number of seconds specified by the manufacturer of the testing equipment. (D) The color of the strip is compared with the color chart provided by the manufacturer to determine the amounts of sugar and acetone present in the urine.

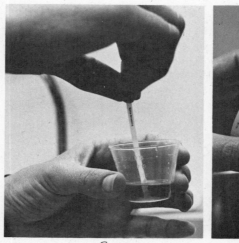

C

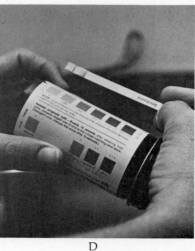

D

320   Elimination from the urinary bladder

Conclusion

Urinary elimination is an essential body process. Procedures involving the urinary tract carry a great risk of infection. Therefore, these procedures must be carried out while continuously using sound practices of surgical asepsis. An infection of the urinary tract can be serious. Using every nursing measure to help avoid the introduction of a catheter into the bladder is part of high-quality nursing care.

References

Beaumont, Estelle, "Product Survey: Urinary Drainage Systems," *Nursing '74*, 4:52–60, January 1974.

Beaumont, Estelle and Claypool, Shirley, eds., "Innovations in Nursing: How to Prevent Catheter-Related Urinary Tract Infections," *Nursing '75*, 5:36–37, January 1975.

Beaumont, Estelle and Wiley, Loy, eds., "Innovations in Nursing: Successful Bladder Training for Geriatric Patients," *Nursing '74*, 4:68–69, May 1974.

Castle, Mary and Osterhout, Suydam, "Urinary Tract Catheterization and Associated Infection," *Nursing Research*, 23:170–174, March-April 1974.

Clark, Cheryl Lee, "Catheter Care in the Home," *American Journal of Nursing*, 72:922–924, May 1972.

Degroot, Jane and Kunin, Calvin M., "Indwelling Catheters," *American Journal of Nursing*, 75:448–449, March 1975.

Eppinik, Henrietta, "Catheterizing the Maternity Patient," *American Journal of Nursing*, 75:829, May 1975.

Garner, Julia S., "Urinary Catheter Care," *Nursing '74*, 4:54–56, February 1974.

Khan, Abdul J. and Pryles, Charles V., "Urinary Tract Infection in Children," *American Journal of Nursing*, 73:1340–1343, August 1973.

17

the preparation and administration of drugs and the intravenous infusion

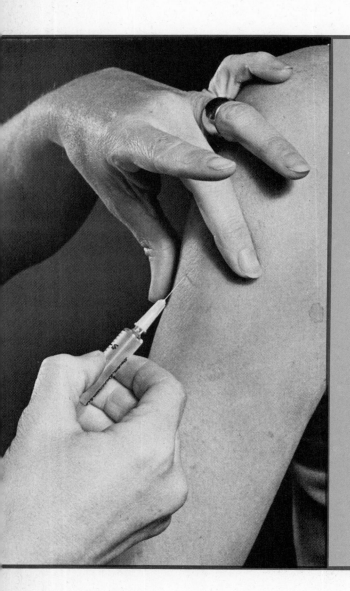

behavioral objectives

When mastery of content in this chapter is reached, the student will be able to

Define terms appearing in the glossary.

Describe methods commonly used to safeguard drugs, including narcotics.

Interpret abbreviations commonly used when prescribing and administering drugs.

List the parts of a medication order and specify what is included in each part.

List five common types of orders and describe each one.

State three types of situations in which a patient's medication orders are ordinarily discontinued automatically.

Describe basic guides given in this chapter for preparing and administering drugs and explain the importance of each.

Describe how the label of a drug container is checked with the medication order.

List the five RIGHTS of preparing and administering drugs.

Describe how to give an oral medication.

Describe how to give a sublingual and a buccal medication.

Explain why sterile technique is used for parenteral drug administration.

Indicate the size of the syringe and how it is calibrated, and the size of the needle commonly used for subcutaneous, intramuscular, intradermal, and insulin injections; list factors that influence the selection of the size of the needle and syringe.

Explain how drugs for injection are placed into a syringe when the drug is in powder form in a vial; in an ampule; in a single-dose vial; in a multiple-dose vial.

Discuss why an air bubble is often left in the syringe when a drug is prepared for injection.

Explain how the skin at the site of injection is prepared.

behavioral objectives cont.

List eight or nine practices that help reduce pain when giving an injection.

Explain why some agency policies specify that a needle should be broken before it is discarded.

Describe areas used for intramuscular injections, how the site of injection is located, and give advantages and disadvantages of each site.

Describe sites commonly used for subcutaneous and intradermal injections.

Describe how to give an intramuscular injection; a subcutaneous injection; an intradermal injection.

Describe how to give an intravenous infusion, including the selection of a vein, the equipment commonly used, how the solution is selected and checked, the preparation of the patient, and the insertion of the needle into the vein.

Explain why a vein low on an extremity is selected whenever possible when an intravenous infusion is to be given.

Demonstrate how the nurse determines the number of drops the patient shall receive intravenously each minute when the physician orders the number of milliliters the patient should receive each hour; when the physician orders the number of milliliters the patient should receive in a 24-hour period.

Discuss briefly the dangers of giving an intravenous infusion more slowly or more rapidly than ordered.

List three or four symptoms the patient receiving intravenous therapy may present that should be reported promptly and that may mean the infusion must be halted because of the patient's undesirable reaction to it.

List four symptoms that suggest to the nurse that the intravenous solution is infiltrating.

List two symptoms that suggest to the nurse that phlebitis may be present.

Explain how drugs and additional solution may be added to an intravenous infusion with the equipment used in the agency where the nurse gives care.

Describe how to discontinue an intravenous infusion.

List seven areas where drugs are given by topical administration and describe the manner in which a drug is usually given at each site.

Design a program for patients who are to be taught how to give themselves medications by injection at home; for patients who are to be taught how to take oral medications at home.

Discuss briefly the nurse's role in relation to discouraging drug abuse.

glossary

Air Embolism Relatively large quantities of air circulating in the bloodstream.

Buccal Administration Placing a drug between the cheek and gum.

Hypodermic Injection Introducing solution into subcutaneous tissue. Synonym for subcutaneous injection.

Infiltration The escape of intravenous infusion solution into surrounding tissues.

Intracutaneous Injection Introducing solution into the upper layers of the skin. Synonym for intradermal injection.

Intradermal Injection Introducing solution into the upper layers of the skin. Synonym for intracutaneous injection.

Intramuscular Injection Introducing solution into muscular tissues.

Intravenous Infusion Introducing relatively large amounts of solution into a vein.

Inunction Rubbing substances into the skin.

Oral Administration Giving a drug by mouth.

Parenteral Administration Giving a drug by routes other than the oral route; usually refers to injection routes.

Phlebitis Inflammation of a vein.

Prescription The physician's order for a drug.

PRN Order A directive to be followed at the nurse's discretion.

Single Order A directive to be carried out one time.

Standing Order A directive to be carried out until canceled by agency policy or by the physician.

Stat Order A directive to be carried out immediately.

Subcutaneous Injection Introducing solution into subcutaneous tissue. Synonym for hypodermic injection.

Topical Administration A drug applied directly to a body site; usually given for its local action.

introduction

Among the nurse's most important duties is administering drugs to her patients. In most situations, she not only gives drugs, but she is also usually in the best position to observe the effects of drugs on her patients.

This chapter discusses preparing drugs for administration and giving them. It is assumed that you have studied or are currently studying pharmacology. Therefore, information concerning specific drugs and their desired effects, symptoms of undesirable effects of drugs, average safe dosages and how they are calculated, mathematical calculations necessary for preparing proper dosages, and so on, will not be included.

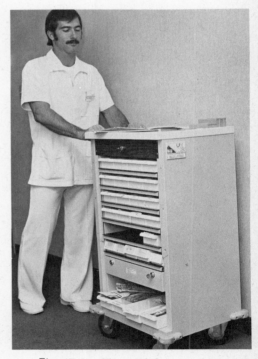

Safeguarding drugs

In each health agency, there is at least one area where drugs are stocked and kept in readiness for dispensing to patients. To protect persons from unsafe drug use, the cabinet or room is locked, and only authorized personnel members have access to the key.

Drugs may be kept in a central area for all patients or they may be kept separately for individual patients. Some hospitals have locked wall cupboards for drug storage near the entrance to each patient's room. Other agencies have mobile cupboards. An example of one is illustrated in Figure 17-1. Whatever the setup, the nurse is expected to observe the agency's policy carefully to help in preventing accidents and drug abuse.

Narcotics are kept in a double-locked drawer, box, or room. Narcotics may be ordered only by physicians who are currently registered with the Department of Justice, Bureau of Narcotics and Dangerous Drugs. According to federal law, a record must be kept for each narcotic that is administered. The following information is generally required: (1) the name of the patient who received the narcotic; (2) the amount of the narcotic used; (3) the hour the narcotic was given; (4) the name of the physician who prescribed the narcotic; (5) the name of the nurse who administered it. It is common practice to check narcotics daily at specified times. For example, most hospitals have narcotics checked at each change-of-shift time. A narcotic count that does not check should be

Fig. 17-1   This mobile cart, along with the Kardex, is moved to the patient's room when medications are given. Note that there are locked drawers on the cart. Each patient's medications are stored in a separate drawer, numbered according to the patient's room number. The entire cart is stored between uses in a locked area of the nurses' station.

reported immediately. These special precautions are used to help control drug abuse. The nurse administering narcotics has a responsibility to see that the federal law is observed.

The medication order

The physician is responsible for planning the patient's drug therapy. He prepares an order or **prescription** which the nurse follows. Safe practice is to follow only a *written* order to help avoid misunderstandings and errors. The physician writes his order on a special form provided by the agency, an example of which was illustrated in Chapter 7.

The physician's prescription will state the dosage of the drug in either the apothecaries' or metric system, depending on the agency's policy. Approximate equivalents of these two systems are given in Table 17-1. Common abbreviations for measures are given in Table 17-2, and other common abbreviations used for prescribing drugs are given in Table 17-3.

Table 17-1 Approximate equivalents of fluid and weight measures

Weights (approximate)

Metric	Apothecaries'	Metric	Apothecaries'
0.2 mg.	$\frac{1}{300}$ grain	60.0 mg.	1 grain
0.3 mg.	$\frac{1}{200}$ grain	0.12 Gm.	2 grains
0.4 mg.	$\frac{1}{150}$ grain	0.2 Gm.	3 grains
0.5 mg.	$\frac{1}{120}$ grain	0.3 Gm.	5 grains
0.6 mg.	$\frac{1}{100}$ grain	0.5 Gm.	$7\frac{1}{2}$ grains
1.0 mg.	$\frac{1}{60}$ grain	0.6 Gm.	10 grains
3.0 mg.	$\frac{1}{20}$ grain	1.0 Gm.	15 grains
6.0 mg.	$\frac{1}{10}$ grain	4.0 Gm.	60 grains (1 dram)
10.0 mg.	$\frac{1}{6}$ grain	6.0 Gm.	90 grains
15.0 mg.	$\frac{1}{4}$ grain	10.0 Gm.	$2\frac{1}{2}$ drams
25.0 mg.	$\frac{3}{8}$ grain	15.0 Gm.	4 drams
30.0 mg.	$\frac{1}{2}$ grain	30.0 Gm.	1 ounce

Liquid Measure (approximate)

Metric	Apothecaries'	Household	Metric	Apothecaries'
0.06 cc./ml.	1 minim	1 drop	30 cc./ml.	1 fluid ounce
0.5 cc./ml.	8 minims		250 cc./ml.	8+ fluid ounces
1.0 cc./ml.	15 minims		500 cc./ml.	1+ pint
4.0 cc./ml.	1 fluid dram	1 teaspoon	1,000 cc./ml. (1 liter)	1+ quart

Adaptation courtesy of Becton, Dickinson and Company, Rutherford, New Jersey.

Table 17-2 Common abbreviations for measures

Abbreviation	Unabbreviated form
cc.	cubic centimeter
℥	dram
gtt.	drop
gr.	grain
Gm.	gram
mg. or mgm.	milligram
ml.	milliliter
m.	minim
℥	ounce
tbsp.	tablespoon
tsp.	teaspoon

Table 17-3 Common abbreviations used in
prescribing drugs

Abbreviation	Meaning
a.a.	of each
a.c.	before meals
ad lib.	freely
Aq.	water
b.i.d.	twice each day
c̄	with
h	hour
h.s.	at bedtime
IM	intramuscular
IV	intravenous
OD	right eye
OS	left eye
OU	both eyes
p.c.	after meals
PO	by mouth
p.r.n.	according to necessity
q3h, q4h, and so on	every three, four, and so on hours
q.d.	every day
q.h.	every hour
q.i.d.	four times each day
q.o.d.	every other day
q.s.	a sufficient amount
Rx	take
s̄	without
S.O.S.	if necessary
ss.	one half
stat.	at once
subq	subcutaneous
t.i.d.	three times a day
tinct.	tincture

It is usual to discontinue drugs the patient has been taking before surgery. After surgery, the physician writes new orders he wishes the nurse to follow. This practice is common also when patients are transferred to another service within a hospital or to another health agency. Upon admission to a hospital, drugs that the patient had been taking at home are not continued unless the physician so orders. Agency policies vary concerning allowing the patient to keep drugs at his bedside and taking them as he would at home. The nurse will observe the policies of the agency in which she is giving care. Chart 17-1 describes the medication order.

Basic guides for preparing and administering all drugs

There are certain basic guides the nurse will follow whenever she prepares and administers drugs. Additional guides that apply specifically to the preparation and administration of drugs given orally and of those given by injection are described later in this chapter.

• When preparing drugs for several patients, time your work so that medications are given within approximately 15 to 30 minutes of the time at which they were ordered to be given. Agency policy generally states the time leeway allowed. Ordinarily, a medication given before or after this time limit is considered a drug error.

Chart 17-1 The medication order

Item	Description	Example
Type of Order		
Standing order without termination date	Drug given until discontinued by physician's order. Or, in some agencies, standing orders are automatically discontinued after a stated period of time; order must be written again by physician to continue medication.	Lanoxin 0.5 mg. daily
Standing order with termination date	Drug given for stated number of days or times as ordered.	Diuril 0.25 Gm. b.i.d. × 5 days premenstrually
PRN order	Drug given only when, in nurse's judgment, patient needs it.	Seconal 100 mg. h.s. p.r.n.
Single order	Drug given only once, at earliest convenience or at specified time.	Milk of Magnesia, at bedtime
Stat order	Drug given only once and immediately.	Sus-phrine 1:200 0.2 ml. subq stat.
Part of Drug Order		
Name of patient	Full name, including middle initial, is recommended to avoid confusing patients.	Jerome T. Black
Date and time order is written	This information is needed when discontinuation date and time are calculated and to help prevent oversights and errors.	11/12/76 10:15 AM

Name of drug	Official or proprietary name of drug is usually used. Generic name may be required in some agencies.	Morphine sulfate
Dosage	Dosage is stated in either apothecary or metric system, depending on agency policy. For home use, household measures are commonly used.	4 ml, or 1 ʒ, or 1 tsp. See Tables 17-1 and 17-2 for approximate equivalents and abbreviations.
Route	If route is not specified in order, it is general policy that drug is given by mouth. Since some drugs may be given by several routes, it is important that route to be used is clear. Question order if there is any possibility of confusion.	Demerol 100 mg. IM. See Table 17-3 for commonly accepted abbreviations for route of administration.
Time and frequency	Time and frequency medication is to be administered are usually written in standard abbreviations.	t.i.d., q.d. See Table 17-3 for commonly accepted abbreviations for time and frequency of administration.
Signature of person who has written order	Authority is given to certain persons for prescribing drugs by law. If there is a question about order, signature indicates whom to contact.	David R. Slope, M.D.
Questioning Order	Nurse questioning order or any part of it should omit giving drug and check with physician or other authorized person. Check in same manner if order is difficult to read.	Demerol 500 mg. DOSAGE COULD BE FATAL! Route is not given; this drug can be given orally, intramuscularly, or subcutaneously.

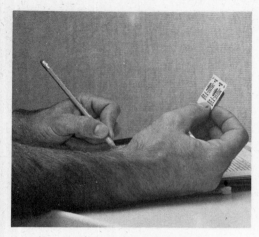

Fig. 17-2   The hospital in which this nurse gives care uses a Kardex system for checking medication orders. The nurse is checking a single-dose pre-packaged medication with the patient's medication order on the Kardex.

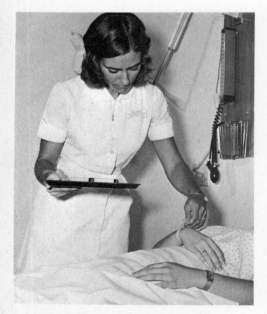

Fig. 17-3   The hospital in which this photo was taken uses a card system for preparing and administering medications. The patient's name on her identification bracelet is checked with the name on the medication card which is on the medication tray in this instance. Whatever procedure is used for administering medications, an essential step is to check the patient's identification bracelet carefully to avoid errors.

- Check the medication order. Procedures differ among health agencies. Some use a card system; others may have a Kardex system. Checking in some cases may include reading the original order. A computer printout may be used. Errors are minimized when medication orders are carefully checked according to agency policy. Figure 17-2 illustrates a nurse checking the order on the Kardex with a unit-dose medication.
- Know the patient and the drug he is to receive. The nurse should know the patient's diagnosis, his plan of care, and the expected results of drug therapy. To observe the patient intelligently, and administer drugs safely, she should know the drug's common average dosage, desired action, undesirable side effects, symptoms of toxicity, and the common route of administration.
- Prepare drugs while using a good light and work alone without interruptions and distractions. Also, allow sufficient time so that you do not have to leave during the preparation of drugs you will administer. These practices help eliminate errors.
- When using an agency's or patient's stock supply of drugs, check the label of the drug container *three* times for safety and accuracy: (1) when reaching for the medication; (2) immediately prior to pouring the medication; and (3) when returning the container to its storage place.
- Do not use medications from containers when the label is difficult to read or when it has come off. Return the container to the pharmacy.
- Do not return medications to a container or transfer medications from one container to another. This prevents mixing drugs and placing the wrong ones in a container.
- Do not use a medication that has a sediment at the bottom of the container unless the medication is to be shaken well before using. Do not use one that appears cloudy or has changed color. The medication may have lost its sterility and usefulness. Or, the characteristics of the drug may have changed.
- Prepare medications in the order in which you will give them. This practice helps save time as you go from patient to patient.
- Plan to give medications last to patients who will require help. This avoids delaying medications for patients as you assist others.
- Transport drugs from the area of preparation to the patient carefully and safely. Use the method of transporting provided by the agency. Keep identification information and the drug together to avoid confusing drugs and patients.
- To prevent contamination, protect needles for injecting drugs according to the method of the agency's choice. Most disposable needles have their own sterile protective cover to prevent contamination. If the needle is reusable, it may be protected with a *dry* sterile cotton ball or gauze while transporting it. If wet, the needle will become contaminated.
- To prevent others from disturbing or taking the medications, do not leave medications out of eyesight.
- Identify the patient by checking the medication card with the patient's identification bracelet, as illustrated in Figure 17-3. Call the patient by name accurately and distinctly or have him tell you his name. Be very careful when you do not know the patient well, when the patient has a language handicap, or when he is confused.

- Omit giving a drug if the patient has symptoms suggesting an undesirable reaction to the drug and report your observation immediately.
- If the patient states he is allergic to a drug, do not give the drug without further checking. An allergic reaction can be serious.
- If the patient indicates that what you are about to give him is different from what he has been receiving, do not give the medication without further checking. An error may have been made.
- Report immediately when the patient refuses a drug so that necessary adjustments in his care can be taken.
- Report drugs inadvertently omitted as soon as it is discovered so that necessary adjustments in the patient's care can be taken.
- Report errors in administering drugs immediately so that proper measures can be taken promptly. It is customary practice to complete an accident or incident form that describes the error in full. The form, more fully discussed in Chapter 7, becomes a permanent part of the patient's record.
- After the drug is given, record the date, time, name of the drug, dose, and route by which it was given in the appropriate place on the patient's record. Indicate the site you used when the drug was injected. Place your signature or initials in this entry according to agency policy. The following information is recorded when intravenous solutions have been given: the date and time the infusion was started and completed; the kind and amount of solution given; the name and amount of any drugs added; and the name or initials of the person who started and discontinued the infusion. In addition, the amount of solution infused is ordinarily recorded on the patient's intake form.
- Record the administration of medications as soon after giving them as possible. This is especially important for a stat order. It helps other members of the nursing and the health team to know that the patient has had the prescribed drug and eliminates the chance of the drug being given again.
- When drugs are omitted intentionally, as for example, when the patient is being prepared for surgery, record the omission and its reason on the patient's record.
- Do not give medications that have been prepared by another person. If an error was made in preparation, the person administering the drug is responsible.
- Check to see that you have observed the five RIGHTS of preparing and administering drugs. These are giving the *right* drug of the *right* dosage at the *right* time, using the *right* route, to the *right* patient. Figure 17-4 illustrates these five RIGHTS.

Oral drug administration

Chart 17-2 describes the administration of **oral** medications, that is, those given by mouth. The suggested actions in the chart are in addition to those given in the previous section. Figures 17-5 and 17-6 illustrate several correct actions (see p. 333–335).

There are certain drugs given by mouth that are not to be swallowed. The tablet is placed under the tongue where it dissolves. The thin

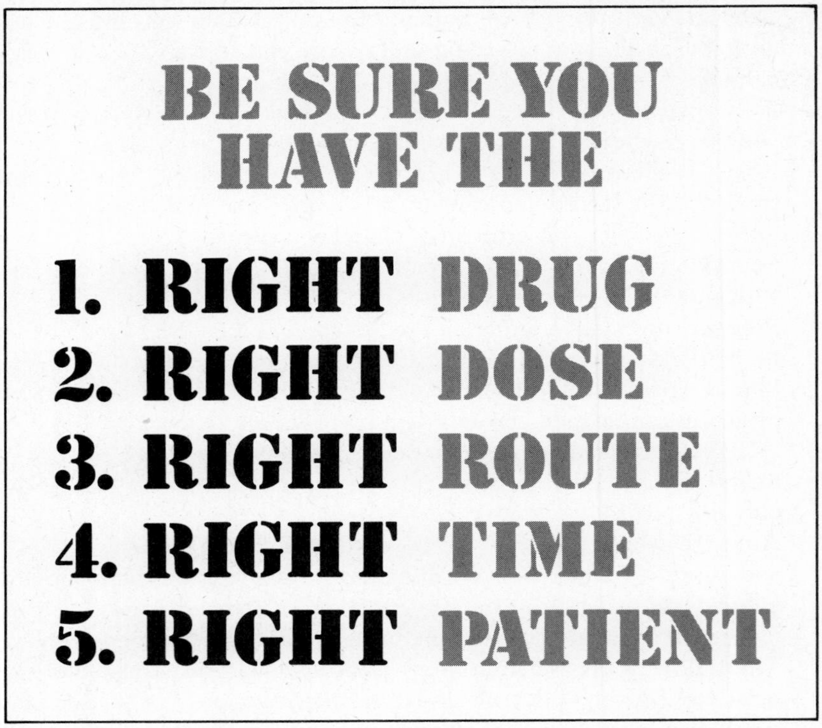

BE SURE YOU HAVE THE

1. RIGHT DRUG
2. RIGHT DOSE
3. RIGHT ROUTE
4. RIGHT TIME
5. RIGHT PATIENT

Fig. 17-4. The 5 RIGHTS of giving medications.

mucous membrane and abundant capillaries in the area make absorption and rapid action of the drug possible. This is called **sublingual administration.** An example of a drug given sublingually is nitroglycerine, commonly used in the management of the patient with the heart disease, angina pectoris.

There are a few times when **buccal administration** is used, that is, the drug is placed between the cheek and the gum. An example is streptokinase-streptodornase (Varidase), an agent used to help in the relief of such symptoms as pain, swelling, and tenderness associated with infection and tissue damage.

Parenteral drug administration

The term **parenteral** refers to routes other than oral. However, the term is used most commonly to indicate injection routes. It is used in that manner here. Table 17-4 describes the various parenteral routes, as well as other routes for administering drugs (see p. 336).

Use of Sterile Technique. Practices of surgical asepsis as described in Chapter 15 are observed when injections are given. Using sterile technique minimizes the danger of injecting organisms into body tissue.

Figure 17-7 illustrates a syringe and needle. Note the marked areas that are kept free of contamination. The same areas are to remain sterile for any size or type of syringe and needle (see p. 336).

When a reusable syringe and needle are used, they are sterilized in the manner of the agency's choice, usually in autoclaves. A small sterile

Chart 17-2 Administering oral medications

The purpose is to prepare and administer oral medications safely and accurately*

Suggested Action	Reason for Action	Figure to Illustrate
Observe practices of medical asepsis when preparing and administering oral medications.	Organisms on medications and medication containers can be spread from person to person.	
Pour capsules and tablets into cap of stock container and then pour proper amount into medication cup.	Pouring medication into hand contaminates capsule or tablet.	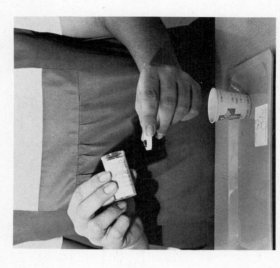 Fig. 17-5 The correct number of tablets ordered for the patient is poured into the container's cap and then into the medication cup.
Prepackaged single-dose medications are opened at patient's bedside when patient is given medication.	If patient refuses medication, it can be used at another time when package has not been opened.	

Chart 17-2 continued

Suggested Action	Reason for Action	Figure to Illustrate
Pour liquids from side of bottle opposite label to prevent liquids from running onto label.	Liquids spilled onto label make reading label difficult.	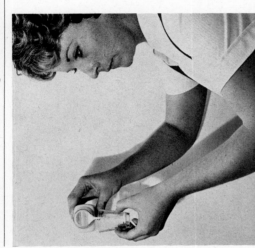 Fig. 17-6 For a liquid medication, the nurse places her thumbnail at the marking on the medication glass which indicates the dosage ordered for the patient. She holds the glass and medication bottle at a level so that she can clearly see the meniscus.
Use appropriate measuring device when pouring liquids and read amount at bottom of miniscus, as illustrated in Figure 17-6.	Accuracy is possible when appropriate and calibrated measuring device is used and then read accurately.	
Place each medication, tablet or liquid, in separate container. Assist patient to sitting position and offer drugs separately.	If a drug is spilled or refused, or if a p.r.n. drug is found to be unnecessary, positive identification of drugs can be made when they are not mixed. Mixing liquids may produce a chemical change. Swallowing is easier when patient is in sitting position.	
Offer water or other permitted fluids with capsules, tablets, and most liquid medications.	Liquids help patient to swallow solid drugs. Cough mixtures are examples of liquid medications that should not be followed by fluids. Fluid washes medication from area where it is intended for local action.	

Offer drugs irritating to gastric mucosa well dissolved and diluted. Or, offer them with food or after meals. Certain iron preparations are examples.

There is less irritation of stomach lining when drug is well diluted or well mixed with food.

Dilute medication well if it is likely to discolor or damage enamel of teeth. Have patient use drinking tube and offer fluids generously, if permitted, after he has taken medication.

Diluting medication and using drinking tube minimizes drug's contact with teeth.

Have patient suck on ice chips before taking medications with objectionable taste.

Ice numbs taste buds.

Use vehicles to disguise medications with objectionable taste. Fruit juice, milk, applesauce, and bread are examples. Use judgment with this practice.

A vehicle disguises objectionable taste. Patient may learn to dislike food used to disguise taste.

Offer oily medications after they have been refrigerated.

Cold oil is less aromatic and hence, less objectionable than oily preparations at room temperature.

Stay with patient until drug is swallowed. Do not leave drugs with patient to take later without an order to do so.

Patient may dispose of drug he does not want to take. Or, he may accumulate drugs and harm himself by taking many at one time. It is an inaccuracy to record that patient was given medication when nurse did not observe him taking it.

If patient is to have fluid intake recorded, record amount of fluids patient took with medication.

All fluids are to be recorded when patient's fluid intake is measured.

*This chart assumes that the nurse will also observe suggestions offered in the section of this chapter entitled Basic Guides for Preparing and Aministering All Drugs.

Table 17-4 Routes for administering drugs

Route	How drug is administered	Term used to describe route
Given by mouth	Having patient swallow drug	Oral administration
Given via respiratory tract	Having patient inhale drug	Inhalation
Given by injection	Injecting drug into 1. Subcutaneous tissue	Parenteral administration 1. Hypodermic or subcutaneous injection
	2. Muscle tissue	2. Intramuscular injection
	3. Corium (under epidermis)	3. Intracutaneous injection
	4. Vein	4. Intravenous injection
	5. Artery	5. Intra-arterial injection
Given by placing on skin or mucous membrane	Inserting drug into 1. Vagina	1. Vaginal administration
	2. Rectum	2. Rectal administration
	Placing drug under tongue	Sublingual administration
	Placing drug between cheek and gum	Buccal administration
	Rubbing drug into skin	Inunction
	Placing drug into direct contact with mucous membrane	Instillation
	Flushing mucous membrane with drug in solution	Irrigation

forceps may be used to attach the needle to the syringe. Or, the fingers can be used to hold the needle at the hilt or hub. The nurse must be sure that the hilt does not touch a sterile needle holder or sterile gauze or cotton ball when she transports the syringe and needle to the patient's bedside. The needle should be well secured so that it does not slip off. This is best done by twisting the needle as it is being attached until it is well anchored.

To help reduce discomfort, needles should be sharp and free of burrs. If a needle has been bent, it should not be forced back into position for reuse. This weakens the needle and it may break off in the patient's

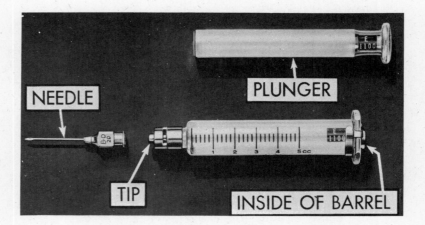

Fig. 17-7 The parts of a needle and syringe to be kept free of contamination are marked in this illustration. (Courtesy of Becton, Dickinson and Company, Rutherford, N. J.)

Preparing and administering drugs and IV's

tissue. Reusable needles usually are sterilized with a stylet in place. This is a small wire that keeps the needle lumen open. It is removed before assembling the syringe and needle. Chipped, cracked, or ill-fitting syringes are also dangerous to use and should be discarded.

Most health agencies now use prepackaged, disposable, sterile needles and syringes. This type of equipment eliminates the handling of the needle and syringe described above.

Selection of Syringe and Needle. The sizes of needles will vary. Needles with large lumens are needed when the material to be injected is thick or oily. Short sizes are used for children and for adults with little fat tissue. For patients with considerable fat tissue, longer needles may be necessary in order to be sure that the needle reaches subcutaneous or intramuscular tissue. These are common sizes of syringes and needles used for various injections:

Type of Injection	Size of Syringe	Size of Needle
Subcutaneous	2, 2½, or 3 ml. calibrated in 0.1 ml.	25 gauge, ½ or ⅝ inch
Intramuscular	5 ml. calibrated in 0.2 ml.	20 or 22 gauge, 1½ inch
Intradermal	1 ml. calibrated in tenths or hundreths of a ml. and/or in minims	26 or 27 gauge, ½ to ¾ inch
Insulin	2 ml. calibrated in units	25 gauge, ½ or ⅝ inch

Placing the Drug into the Syringe. Some medications are available in syringes or cartridges that are prefilled by the manufacturer. An example of one is illustrated in Figure 17-8. In addition to the name of the drug, drug companies give the dose contained in the syringe or cartridge, and the parenteral route intended. The drug should not be administered by any route other than the one for which it is specified.

Drugs that deteriorate in solution may be dispensed in a vial in powder form. One ml. or so of normal saline, in which the powder dissolves, is added to the vial and then the medication is drawn up into the syringe.

Some drugs are dispensed in glass ampules. Most of these ampules have a constriction in the stem which facilitates opening. Since the drug tends to trap in the stem, it is important to make certain that all of the drug is in the ampule. The ampule should be tapped several times to help bring the solution down. Ampules without a constriction do not present this problem.

Some agency procedures specify that the ampule be cleansed with an antiseptic solution before it is opened. Although some persons have questioned this procedure, local policy should be observed.

Gauze is used to hold the ampule as it is being opened. This protects the nurse's fingers. Sterile material is used since it is held close to the opening of the ampule filled with sterile solution. A saw-toothed file is used to scratch the glass gently on the stem, well above the level of the medication. Scratching it on opposite sides helps to insure a quick, even break, as Figure 17-9 illustrates. After the scratch marks have been made, the ampule is held in one hand and the other is used to break off the stem. Prescored ampules make filing unnecessary. But the nurse's fingers should still be protected to prevent injury. A commercial ampule opener with a protective flange is available in some agencies.

After the stem is removed, the medication is in an open vessel. The

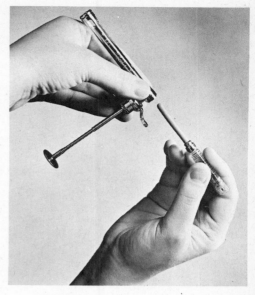

Fig. 17-8 The cartridge in the nurse's right hand has been prefilled with a drug in solution by the manufacturer. The name of the drug, dosage, and route of administration are marked on the cartridge. The needle on the cartridge is protected from contamination by a rubber needle sheath. The cartridge is inserted into the barrel of the syringe and the plunger is locked into place. The medication is then ready to be transported to the patient with the sheath still in place to protect the needle from contamination. (Courtesy of Wyeth Laboratories, Philadelphia, Pennsylvania)

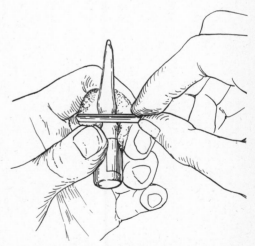

Fig. 17-9 The nurse's fingers are protected with sterile cotton or gauze when the stem of the closed glass ampule is scored with a file and then broken off.

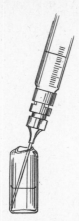

Fig. 17-10 When the stem of a glass ampule is removed, the drug is drawn up into the syringe easily because air displaces the fluid. The needle must not touch the rim of the ampule for fear of contaminating the needle.

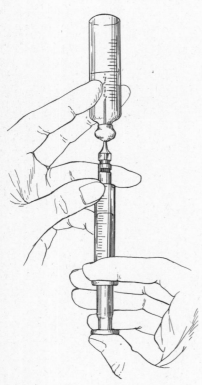

Fig. 17-11 An amount of air equal to the amount of solution to be withdrawn is injected. Pressure within the vial is increased and the drug is removed easily and accurately.

nurse inserts the needle into the ampule and withdraws the solution. To avoid contaminating the needle, she is careful not to touch the edge of the glass with the needle. Figure 17-10 illustrates removing the solution from an ampule. With skill, it will be possible for the nurse to pick up the ampule and hold it between two fingers of one hand and to hold the syringe in the other hand. When removing the drug in this manner, the trick lies in keeping the needle in the solution at all times, even as the ampule is inverted.

The single-dose rubber-capped vial usually is covered with a soft metal cover. After removing the cover, the rubber cap is entered with the needle. At the time of preparation, this rubber is sterilized. Nevertheless, many agency procedures specify that the cap be cleansed with an antiseptic before the needle is inserted. Use friction when cleansing. The rubber cap should be entered with slight lateral pressure on the needle to prevent a core of the stopper from entering the vial.

To make removal of the drug from the closed container easy, the nurse injects an amount of air comparable to the amount of solution to be withdrawn. This increases the pressure within the vial, making withdrawal of solution from an area under pressure easy. If air is not injected first, a partial vacuum is created in the vial as fluid is withdrawn. This makes it difficult to withdraw solution. Figure 17-11 illustrates removing a drug in solution from a vial.

Some drugs are dispensed in vials containing several or multiple doses. An example is an insulin vial. These are managed in the same manner as the single-dose vial. Care should be taken to inject no more air than the amount of solution to be withdrawn. If too much air is injected, the pressure in the vial will force solution into the syringe. This makes accurate dosage difficult to obtain.

There are times when a rather large amount of solution will be removed from a multiple-dose vial. Or, several doses will be removed in succession. A simple practice is to insert a separate sterile needle through the cap. This allows air to enter and replace the fluid as it is being withdrawn.

Air may enter the syringe when it is being filled with solution. Small amounts for subcutaneous and intradermal injections will do no harm and are sometimes recommended. The air will force medication remaining in the needle into the tissue. When giving an intramuscular injection, an air bubble of 0.2 to 0.3 ml. is also sometimes recommended, as illustrated in Figure 17-12. Solution allowed to remain in the needle is in danger of draining into superficial tissue as the needle is being withdrawn. If the drug is irritating, this causes pain and may result in tissue damage. Many disposable syringes are constructed so that they dispense the medication very effectively, making the air bubble unnecessary.

Make certain air does not cause an error in the measurement of the proper dosage of drug. All or excessive amounts of air are removed by holding the syringe in a vertical position and pushing gently on the plunger. Figure 17-13 shows a patient removing excess air from her syringe.

When the drug is ready to be administered, it is transported to the patient. Care is taken to prevent contamination, as described earlier. Materials for cleansing the patient's skin are also transported with the medication.

Cleansing the Skin. Usual procedure is to cleanse the area where the injection is to be made with a cotton ball or piece of gauze dampened with an antiseptic of the agency's choice. The purpose is to clean the skin as much as possible in order to minimize injecting organisms into body tissues. If the patient's skin is soiled with drainage or discharge, the area should be washed with soap or detergent and water before using the antiseptic.

When cleansing the skin, move the cotton ball or gauze in a circular motion. Use firm pressure, thus creating friction, to help remove soil. Begin at the point of injection and move outward. This carries material away from the site of injection. Haphazard up-and-down movements and superficial swipes accomplish little.

Reducing Discomfort. Skill in giving an injection can greatly reduce discomfort. These practices help to decrease pain:

* Use a sharp needle free of burrs.
* Use a needle of the smallest gauge that is appropriate for the site of injection and the solution to be injected.
* Insert and withdraw the needle without hesitation.
* Inject solution slowly, especially when the amount is sizeable. This allows solution to spread into surrounding tissues.
* Select a skin site that is free of irritation.
* Rotate sites of injection so that an area recently used is not injected again. The pattern of rotating sites should be described on the nursing care plan. The patient as well as the nurse may forget where he was last injected. When the nurse records having given the injection, she indicates the site she used.
* After injecting the drug and removing the needle, use firm pressure and massage the area of injection with a cotton ball or gauze to help spread the solution into surrounding tissues. Move the tissue as you massage, not the cotton ball or gauze.
* Applying a cold compress or an ice cube over the area to be injected, before the skin is cleansed, numbs the skin receptors and helps reduce pain.
* Gently tapping the site of injection with the fingers several times, before cleansing the skin, also helps to decrease discomfort.
* An anesthetic, such as ethyl chloride, may be sprayed over the area of injection. Or, a small amount of anesthesia, such as procaine hydrochloride, may be added to a medication to be injected intramuscularly if the drug is very irritating. These practices ordinarily require the approval of the patient's physician.

After Care of Equipment. Reusable equipment is handled according to agency procedure.

Agencies provide proper receptacles for discarding disposable equipment. The danger is in discarding the needle. Persons with drug abuse problems have recovered discarded needles. Therefore, many agencies require that the needle be broken off at the hilt so that reuse is not possible. This is illustrated in Figure 17-14.

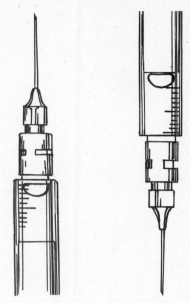

Fig. 17-12   A small amount of air, 0.2 to 0.3 ml., is drawn into the syringe as final preparation for intramuscular injection. When the syringe and the needle are inverted, as during injection, the bubble rises in the syringe. The air serves to push the solution trapped in the shaft of the needle into the tissues.

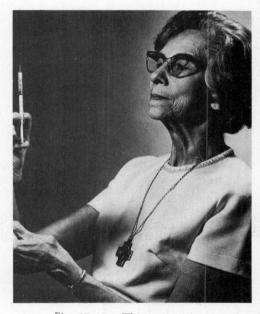

Fig. 17-13   This patient is removing excess air from her syringe in preparation for administering her insulin. (Courtesy of Bectoin, Dickinson and Company, Rutherford, N. J.)

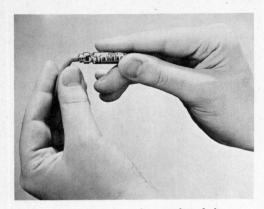

Fig. 17-14   The nurse has replaced the sheath on the needle and then bends and breaks it before discarding it in the proper receptacle provided by the health agency. The needle cannot be used by another person. (Courtesy of Wyeth Laboratories, Philadelphia, Pa.)

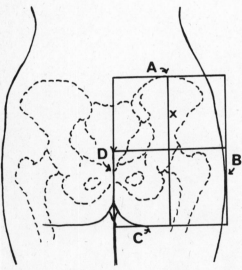

Fig. 17-15   One site for an intramuscular injection is the inner portion of the upper outer quadrant. This area is obtained by using the following guides. The upper line is determined by the iliac crest, A; the outer lines by the division of the buttocks and the outer surface of patient's body, D and B. The lower line is determined by the lower edge of the buttock, C. This area is then divided into equal parts vertically and horizontally. The injection is given 2 to 3 inches below the top of the iliac crest in the upper outer quadrant.

Intramuscular injection

An **intramuscular injection** introduces solution into muscular tissue. Ordinarily, approximately 2 to 5 ml. of solution is given. When as much as 4 or 5 ml. is required, judgment is recommended concerning whether the dose should be divided with half given in one site and half in another. Giving as much as 4 or 5 ml. in one site usually is very uncomfortable. When it is necessary to do so, the solution is injected very slowly to allow solution to spread well into surrounding tissues.

The site of injection should be one where large nerves or blood vessels are unlikely to be struck by the needle. Various sites are available, as described below. When the patient is receiving intramuscular injections regularly, rotating the site is especially important to avoid discomfort for the patient and possible tissue damage. Therefore, it is important for the nurse to be familiar with the various sites and the landmarks which identify them so that she can safely rotate sites as necessary.

Gluteus Muscles. Several sites in the gluteal muscle group are used. One site is used to introduce medication into the gluteus maximus muscle. Figure 17-15 illustrates and describes how the site is located. As the figure shows, the fleshy part of the buttock is an incorrect site. Also, many incorrectly include the fleshy portion of the upper thigh, especially in obese patients, as part of the buttock. Selecting the site is so important to prevent injury that no injection should be made without good visualization of the area. This requires removing undergarments to expose the entire buttock. A common error is made when the landmarks are merely identified by eye. The result is that the injection is often given too low and there is then danger of striking the sciatic nerve. Because of this, many persons are no longer recommending this site and prefer the sites about to be described.

When injecting into gluteus muscles, it is recommended that the patient lie on his abdomen with toes pointed inward. This position helps to promote maximum exposure and muscle relaxation. In the standing position, the exposure is not as good and the muscles are usually tense, adding to discomfort.

A second site located on the buttock is used to introduce medication into the gluteus medius muscle in the posterior and lateral aspect of the gluteal region. The injection is given above and outside of a diagonal line drawn from the greater trochanter of the femur and the posterior superior iliac spine. The patient should be lying on his abdomen, as described above. Bending over a table and the standing position with the area partially covered with clothing are not recommended because of the danger of missing the correct site. The landmarks and manner of locating this injection site in an adult are illustrated in Figure 17-16. Figure 17-17 illustrates the site in a child (see p. 342).

A third site, often called the ventrogluteal site, may be used. Palpate for the greater trochanter of the femur, the anterior superior iliac spine, and the iliac crest. Injection is made within a triangular area formed by these landmarks. The site and method of locating it are illustrated in Figure 17-18. This site is well removed from major nerves and blood vessels. Fatty tissues are relatively small, and good muscle tissue is present for injection. The site is often recommended for children since

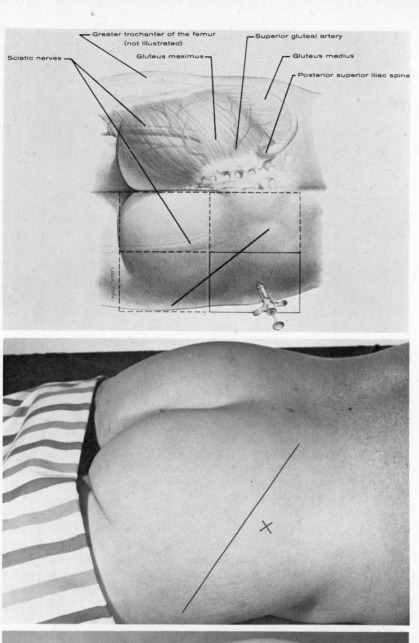

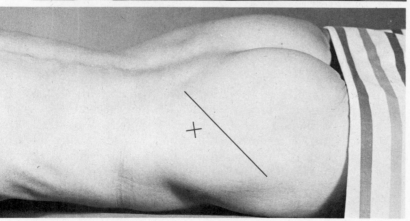

Fig. 17-16. (Top) The needle is in the proper place for an intramuscular injection into the gluteus medius muscle. It is above and outside of a diagonal line drawn from the greater trochanter of the femur to the posterior superior iliac spine. Note how this site avoids entering an area near the sciatic nerve and the superior gluteal artery. (Center) The area is identified on a patient weighing 190 pounds. (Bottom) The area is identified on a patient weighing 120 pounds. (Drawing courtesy of Wyeth Laboratories, Philadelphia, Pa.)

341

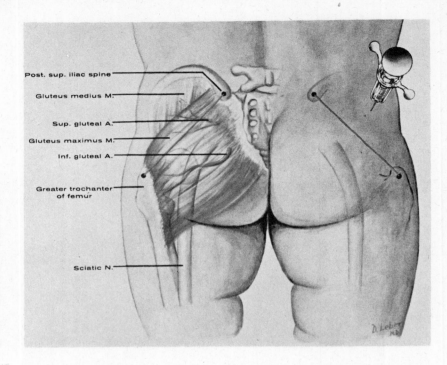

Fig. 17-17. Precautions observed when giving adults an intramuscular injection also apply to infants and children—except the margin of error is critically narrower. Note the same landmarks are used for a child when locating the site of injection to enter the gluteus medius as are used for the adult. No injection should be given into the gluteal prominence of the buttocks for any patient because of the danger of striking the sciatic nerve or gluteal artery. (Courtesy of Wyeth Laboratories, Philadelphia, Pennsylvania)

the landmarks are easily identified. The patient usually is placed on his abdomen. However, with this site, the side-lying or the back-lying position may also be used.

The Vastus Lateralis Muscle. This muscle, on the side of the leg, is being recommended more frequently than in the past. It is a thick muscle and there are no large nerves or vessels nearby. Nor does it cover a joint. Figure 17-19 illustrates and describes how the site is located (see p. 344).

The Deltoid Muscle. The deltoid muscle forms the prominence at the shoulder. In general, this muscle is selected infrequently because it is relatively small. Only a small amount of solution can be given and the area in one arm should not be used repeatedly. Many patients experience more pain and tenderness in this area than in others. A misplaced needle may injure the radial nerve in the triceps muscle. The advantages of the site are that it is easily located and the patient may be in a standing, sitting, or lying position. The site is illustrated and described in Figure 17-20 (see p. 345).

The Rectus Femoris Muscle. This muscle is on the anterior part of the thigh. The site is used only when others are not available. Many patients find it an uncomfortable site. Patients who must give themselves intramuscular injections commonly use this site since it is easy for them to see what they are doing.

Chart 17-3 and Figures 17-21 through 17-29 illustrate and describe how to give an intramuscular injection (see pp. 346–350).

The Z Technique. The Z or zigzag technique is used to inject medications that cause superficial irritation or staining when the drug leaks through the path of injection. The tissue is displaced laterally before giving the injection. Immediately following removal of the needle, the tissue is allowed to assume its normal position, thus preventing the escape of the drug from its intramuscular site.

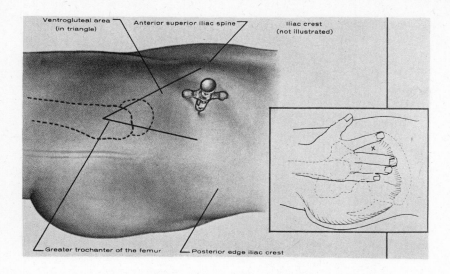

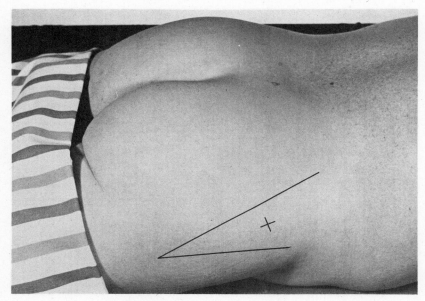

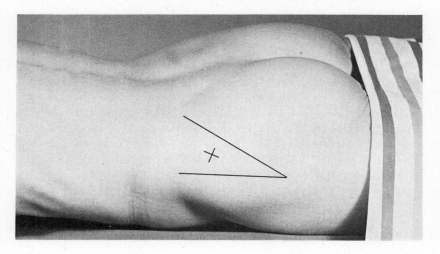

Fig. 17-18. (Top) The needle in position has been injected into the ventrogluteal area. Note how the nurse's palm is placed on the greater trochanter and the index finger, on the anterior superior iliac spine. The middle finger is spread posteriorly as far as possible along the iliac crest. The injection is made in the middle of the triangle formed by the nurse's fingers and the iliac crest. (Center) The area is identified on a patient weighing 190 pounds. (Bottom) The area is identified on a patient weighing 120 pounds. (Drawing courtesy of Wyeth Laboratories, Philadelphia, Pennsylvania)

343

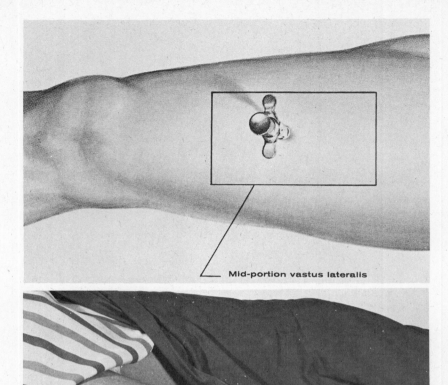

Mid-portion vastus lateralis

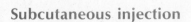

Fig. 17-19. (Top) The needle in position has been injected into the vastus lateralis. It is generally easier to have the patient lying on his back. However, the patient may be in the sitting position when using this site for intramuscular injections. It is a suitable site for children when the nurse grasps the muscle in her hand to concentrate the muscle mass for injection. (Bottom) The area is identified on a patient. (Drawing courtesy of Wyeth Laboratories, Philadelphia, Pennsylvania)

Subcutaneous injection

A **subcutaneous injection** introduces a solution into subcutaneous tissues. **Hypodermic injection** is a synonym.

The site for giving a subcutaneous injection is usually the upper arm. Another common site is the thigh. The abdomen and the back may also be used. Figure 17-30 illustrates these areas on the body (see p. 351).

When a patient must receive repeated subcutaneous injections, it is important to rotate the sites of injection to avoid discomfort and possible tissue damage. For example, for the diabetic patient who is receiving insulin subcutaneously regularly, it is recommended that a sketch of the body be used, such as the one in Figure 17-30. Each time an injection is given, the nurse indicates on the sketch exactly where she has injected the patient. When teaching the patient how to inject his own insulin, the

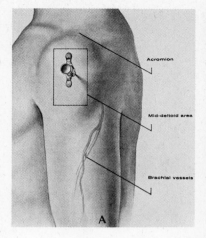

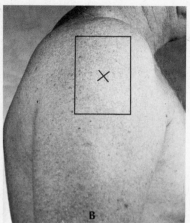

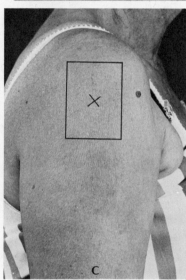

Fig. 17-20 (A) The needle in place has been inserted into the deltoid muscle. The area for injection is bounded by the lower edge of the acromion on the top to a point on the side of the arm opposite the axilla on the bottom. The side boundaries of the rectangular site are parallel to the arm and one-third and two-thirds of the way around the side of the arm, as illustrated. (B) The area is identified on a patient weighing 190 pounds. (C) The area is identified on a patient weighing 120 pounds. (Drawing courtesy of Wyeth Laboratories, Philadelphia, Pennsylvania)

nurse must be sure to stress the importance of rotating the site. The patient can also use a sketch so that he can keep an accurate account of the site of every injection.

Recommendations differ concerning the angle at which a subcutaneous needle should be held for injection. The goal is to inject into subcutaneous tissue and the nurse needs to use judgment concerning the angle to use for each patient. Figure 17-31 illustrates needles being introduced at different angles. A shorter needle must be injected at a 90° angle in order to reach subcutaneous tissue, while a longer needle is injected at a 45° angle. Figure 17-31 also illustrates a nurse preparing to inject patients who are of different weights. For a large patient, the nurse uses a 90° angle while for the patient with little fat tissue, she uses a smaller angle (see p. 352).

Opinion also differs concerning whether the nurse should grasp the patient's tissues between her thumb and fingers or whether she should stretch the skin at the site of injection. The decision depends on the length of the needle and also on the patient. For a dehydrated or very thin patient and for most children and infants, grasping the tissue is

Chart 17-3 Administering an intramuscular injection

The purpose is to inject a medication into muscular tissue*

Suggested Action	Reason for Action	Figure to Illustrate
Select appropriate site for injection. (Nurse demonstrating this procedure chose posterolateral aspect of gluteal region.)	Selection of appropriate site decreases discomfort for patient and possible damage to body tissue.	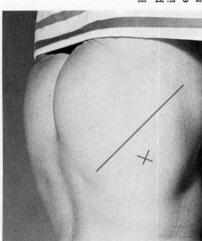 Fig. 17-21 The buttock is exposed and the area of injection is identified, in this case, the posterolateral aspect of the gluteal region.
Using friction, cleanse skin *thoroughly* at intended site of entry.	Cleansing area of injection minimizes danger of forcing organisms into tissues.	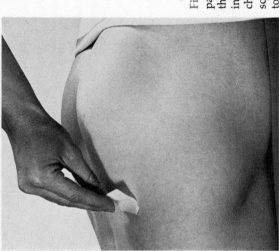 Fig. 17-22 The site is being prepared for injection by cleansing it thoroughly with a swab containing an antiseptic of the agency's choice. An area at least 2 inches square is prepared around the site to be injected.

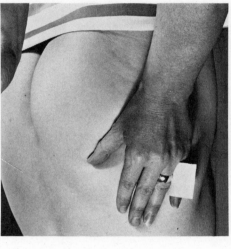

Fig. 17-23   The thumb and fingers spread the skin at the injection area. The nurse is careful not to contaminate the site of entry.

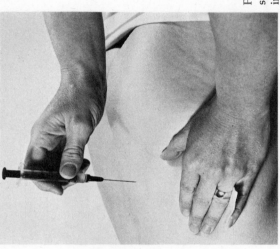

Fig. 17-24   The nurse holds the syringe as she would a dart and introduces the needle quickly.

Using thumb and first two fingers, press tissue down firmly.

Compression of tissue helps insure having needle enter muscle tissues.

Hold syringe vertically, like a dart, and quickly thrust needle into tissue at 90° angle.

Thrust and angle help insert needle into muscular tissue.

Chart 17-3 continued

Suggested Action	Reason for Action	Figure to Illustrate
Continue to insert needle firmly and steadily for almost its full length.	Sufficient penetration of needle places it in muscular tissue.	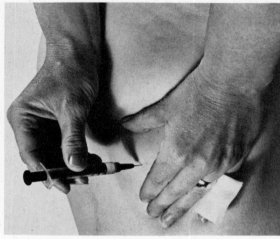 Fig. 17-25 After entering the skin, the needle is introduced for almost its full length. Unless the patient is very thin, the nurse continues to hold the skin firmly.
When needle is in place, pull back gently on plunger of syringe to determine whether needle is in bloodstream. If blood is noted, remove, replace needle, and select new site.	Drugs injected directly into bloodstream are absorbed immediately. Drugs injected intramuscularly are intended for slower absorption and may be dangerous if placed in bloodstream.	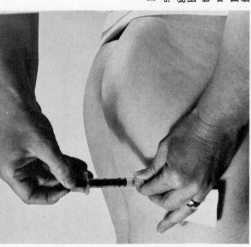 Fig. 17-26 While steadying the syringe, the nurse pulls back gently on the plunger to see if blood can be brought back into the syringe. If blood returns, the nurse withdraws the needle, re-places it, and selects another site for injection.

Inject solution slowly followed by air bubble.

Rapid injection of solution creates pressure in tissues, resulting in discomfort. Slow injection allows solution to disperse into surrounding tissues. Air bubble will force solution through needle and prevent dribbling of solution in muscle and subcutaneous tissue as needle is withdrawn.

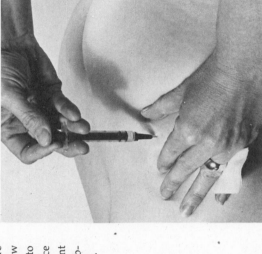

Fig. 17-27 The nurse holds her fingers in a manner to push the plunger its entire length. This forces the solution and the air bubble through the needle and into muscular tissue.

Withdraw needle quickly while applying pressure against injection site.

Quick withdrawal of needle reduces discomfort, and reduces risk of medication leaking into subcutaneous tissue.

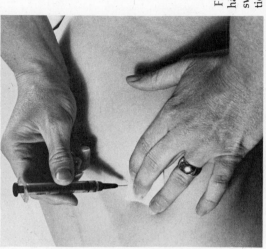

Fig. 17-28 After the solution has been injected, pressure on the swab is applied against the injection site.

Chart 17-3 continued

Suggested Action	Reason for Action	Figure to Illustrate
Massage area, as long as two minutes if rapid absorption is desired.	Massaging area of injection helps spread medication in muscular tissue and hastens absorption by increasing blood supply to area.	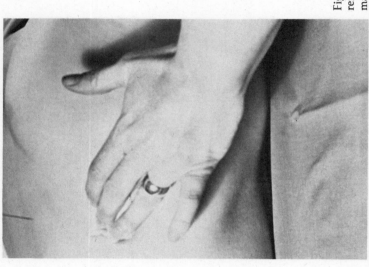 Fig. 17-29 After the needle is removed, the injection site is massaged.

*This chart assumes that the nurse will also observe suggestions offered in the sections of this chapter entitled Basic Guides for Preparing and Administering All Drugs and Parenteral Drug Administration.

preferred to stretching the skin. The nurse injecting patients in Figure 17-31 did not grasp the sites of injection. She judged that by changing the angle at which she injected the needle into two adult patients of different weights, the needle would readily reach subcutaneous tissue. But the teenager injecting insulin into her thigh found that a relatively short needle could best reach subcutaneous tissue if she injected it at almost a 90° angle while grasping her tissues between her thumb and fingers. Chart 17-4 describes how to give a subcutaneous injection.

Intradermal injection

Solutions injected into the upper layers of the skin are referred to as **intradermal injections.** The phrase **intracutaneous injection** is synonymous. A common site is the inner aspect of the forearm, although other areas are also satisfactory. Small amounts of solution are used— usually no more than several minims. The needle and syringe are held almost parallel with the forearm. The needle is injected very super- ficially, bevel side up. The lumen should hardly be concealed by the skin. After the solution is injected, it will form a small raised area or wheal. The area is not massaged after the injection. Intradermal injections are commonly used for diagnostic purposes. Examples include the tuber- culin test and tests to determine the patient's sensitivity to various substances.

Intravenous infusion

Policies and practices vary concerning who may introduce fluids and drugs into the vein. This section was prepared to help those nurses who will be responsible for administering fluids and drugs intravenously. Nevertheless, it is still recommended reading for nurses who will not be responsible for these procedures. They are often asked to help and a clear understanding of what is done is necessary for the assisting nurse. Also, nurses who do not start intravenous therapy are still responsible for monitoring the solution, for observing the patient, and for discon- tinuing the therapy.

An **intravenous infusion** is the injection of relatively large amounts of solution into a vein. The physician is responsible for ordering the kind of solution, the amount to be used, and the rate at which it is to be introduced on the basis of the patient's individual needs. The variety of solutions on the market is almost without limit. Should the nurse have questions concerning the particular solution that is ordered, two good sources usually are readily available. The physician in charge of the patient generally is glad to explain his selection. The pharmaceutical companies have excellent literature explaining the nature and common indications for the various solutions they prepare.

Selecting a Vein for Intravenous Therapy. The selection of the vein will vary with each patient. These factors influence selection: acces- sibility and condition of veins; type of fluid to be given; and anticipated duration of the infusion.

Accessibility of the vein is partially determined by the patient's

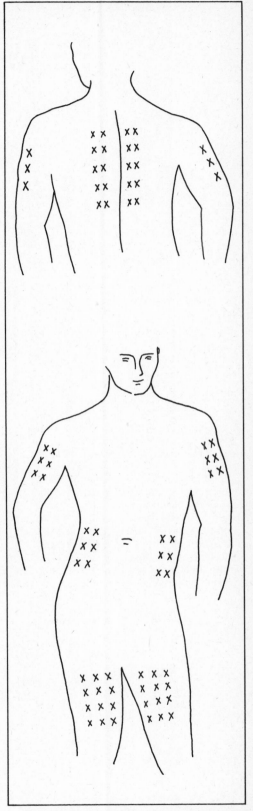

Fig. 17-30   Sites on the body where subcutaneous injections can be given.

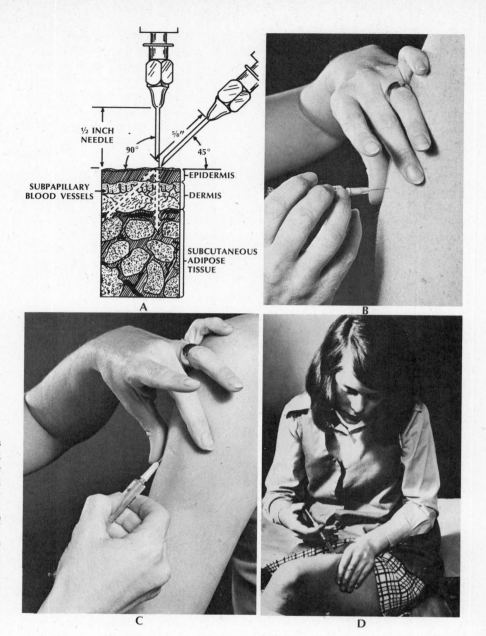

A

B

C

D

Fig. 17-31   (A) The sketch illustrates that a ½-inch needle at a 90° angle and a ⅝-inch needle at a 45° angle will be located in subcutaneous tissue. (B and C) The nurse is using a ½-needle. She holds the syringe and needle at a 90° angle to inject a patient weighing 190 pounds (B) but at approximately a 45° angle to inject a patient weighing 120 pounds (C). (D) This teenager grasps tissue between her thumb and fingers and is about to inject the needle at a little less than a 90° angle to reach subcutaneous tissue when giving herself insulin.

In the sketch (A): ½ INCH NEEDLE — 90° — ⅝" — 45° — EPIDERMIS — DERMIS — SUBPAPILLARY BLOOD VESSELS — SUBCUTANEOUS ADIPOSE TISSUE

condition. For example, a person with severe burns of both forearms will not have vessels in these areas available. Veins in a surgical area should not be used, nor usually even those veins adjacent to the area. For example, infusions in the arm should not be given on the same side as recent extensive breast surgery because of possible problems with circulation in the area.

In general, when the arm is used, it is best to select a vein as low as possible on the back of the hand or on the forearm. If the vein is damaged during therapy, another vein higher on the arm can be selected. The anticubital veins located on the inner side of the elbow are usually very accessible and relatively easy to enter. But damage to these vessels may limit later use of the lower arm and hand veins. Also, using the

Chart 17-4 Administering a subcutaneous injection
The purpose is to inject a medication into subcutaneous tissue*

Suggested Action	Reason for Action
Select appropriate site of injection, as illustrated in Figure 17-30, p. 351.	Selection of appropriate site decreases discomfort for patient and possible damage to body tissues.
Using friction, cleanse skin *thoroughly* as for an intramuscular injection, as illustrated in Figure 17-22, p. 346.	Cleansing area minimizes danger of forcing organisms into tissues.
Hold skin taut over injection site, or grasp area surrounding site of injection and hold in cushion manner, the decision depending on patient's condition and length of needle, as illustrated in Figure 17-31, p. 352.	Holding tissue taut helps nurse to be sure that subcutaneous tissue is being entered in most well-nourished, hydrated persons. Grasping tissue helps nurse to be sure that subcutaneous tissue is being entered when person is very thin, dehydrated, or small.
Inject needle almost its full length at angle of 45 to 90°, angle depending on amount and condition of tissue and length of needle, as illustrated in Figure 17-31.	Subcutaneous tissue is abundant in well-nourished persons. It is usually sparse in very thin, dehydrated, or small persons.
When needle is in place, release grasp if you are cushioning tissue.	Injecting solution into relaxed tissue allows solution to enter without discomfort.
Pull back gently on plunger of syringe to determine whether needle is in bloodstream, as for an intramuscular injection, as illustrated in Figure 17-26, p. 348.	Drugs injected directly into bloodstream are absorbed immediately. Drugs injected subcutaneously are intended for slower absorption and may be dangerous if placed in bloodstream.
Inject solution slowly, as for an intramuscular injection, as illustrated in Figure 17-27, p. 349.	Rapid injection of solution creates pressure in tissues, resulting in discomfort. Slow injection allows solution to disperse into surrounding tissues.
Withdraw needle quickly while applying pressure against injection site, as for an intramuscular injection, as illustrated in Figure 17-28, p. 349.	Rapid withdrawal of needle reduces discomfort.
Massage area as for an intramuscular injection, as illustrated in Figure 17-29, p. 350.	Massaging area of injection helps spread medication in subcutaneous tissues and hastens absorption by increasing blood supply to area.

*This chart assumes that the nurse will also observe suggestions offered in the sections of this chapter entitled Basic Guides for Preparing and Administering All Drugs and Parenteral Drug Administration.

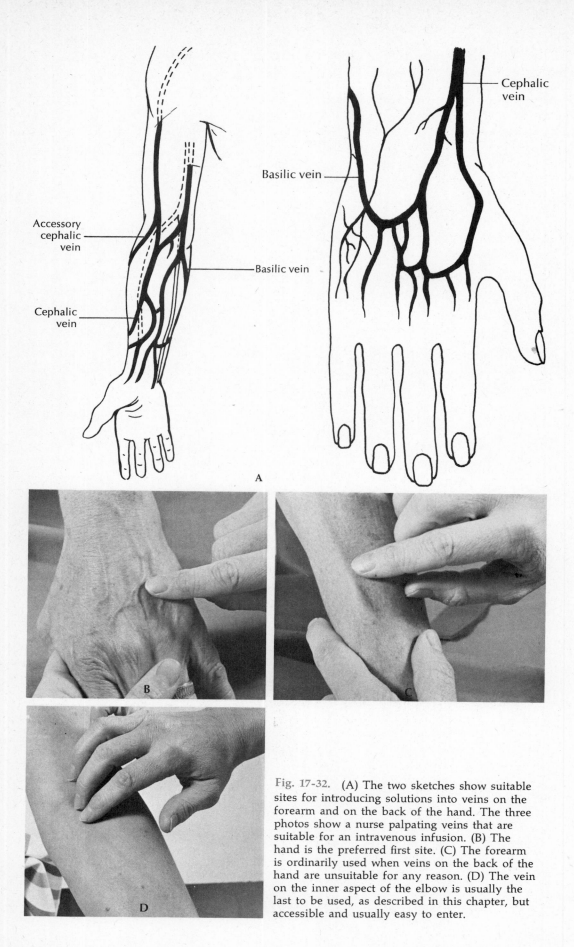

Cephalic vein

Basilic vein

Accessory cephalic vein

Basilic vein

Cephalic vein

A

B

C

D

Fig. 17-32. (A) The two sketches show suitable sites for introducing solutions into veins on the forearm and on the back of the hand. The three photos show a nurse palpating veins that are suitable for an intravenous infusion. (B) The hand is the preferred first site. (C) The forearm is ordinarily used when veins on the back of the hand are unsuitable for any reason. (D) The vein on the inner aspect of the elbow is usually the last to be used, as described in this chapter, but accessible and usually easy to enter.

anticubital veins limits the patient's ability to flex his arm. This may prove to be very uncomfortable if the infusion is to take several hours' time.

The metacarpal, basilic, and cephalic veins are good sites. Figure 17-32 includes a schematic drawing of these veins, and also illustrates a nurse palpating for suitable veins on the patient's hand and arm.

Veins of the legs are generally not recommended, unless other sites are not accessible, because of the danger of interfering with circulation and possible serious complications. Scalp veins are often used, especially for infants. They are usually readily accessible and the needle is less likely to be dislocated than it would be if other areas of the infant's body were used.

Thin-walled and scarred veins, especially in elderly patients, may be difficult to enter. Experience will help the nurse acquire skill in palpating veins to determine their general condition.

The type of solution to be given influences vein selection. Hypertonic solutions, those containing irritating medications, those administered rapidly, and thick, sticky solutions should be given in a large vein. Generally, the forearm veins are preferred over those on the back of the hand for the types of solutions just mentioned.

The duration of the therapy influences vein selection. Comfort of the patient is easier to attain when he is restricted as little as possible. When a joint is immobilized for a long period of time, discomfort is common. When intravenous therapy is given frequently, sites should be changed, starting with sites low on the arms and moving toward the body, as explained earlier.

Either arm may be used. If the patient is right-handed and both arms appear to be equally usable, usually the left arm is selected so that the right arm will be free for the patient's use.

Equipment Commonly Used for Intravenous Infusions. Because a vein is being entered, sterile technique is used. Most health agencies use disposable infusion tubing and needles, thus eliminating possible sources of contamination from reusable equipment.

For most intravenous infusions for adults, a 20-, 21-, or 22-gauge needle with a short bevel, 1 to $1\frac{1}{2}$ inches long, is used. Needle gauge determines the size of the inner diameter or lumen. The bevel of the needle is sloped. Figure 17-33 illustrates these characteristics. Whenever possible, the needle size should be appreciably less than the vein in order to reduce possible tissue damage when it is introduced. A short bevel also tends to reduce tissue damage. Butterfly needles, which are short-beveled, thin-walled needles with plastic flaps, are also used extensively because of the ease of handling and stabilizing them. The nurse in Figures 17-35 through 17-43 is using a butterfly needle.

If an infusion is to run for an extended period of time, an intravenous catheter may be used. Catheters are little plastic tubes which have been mounted on a needle for insertion. They are very flexible, yet strong, which adds to the patient's safety as he moves about. An example of a needle with a catheter is illustrated in Figure 17-34.

Normally, the pressure in the patient's vein is higher than atmospheric. The solution is placed on a standard at a level approximately 18 to 24 inches above the level of the vein. At this height, gravity is sufficient to allow the solution to enter the vein. The height of the

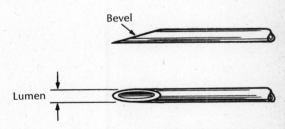

Fig. 17-33   Bevel and lumen of a needle.

Fig. 17-34 (Top) A catheter-threaded needle. The needle's protective sheath, above the needle in this photo, has been removed. (Center) After the needle and catheter have been introduced into the vein, the needle and syringe are carefully withdrawn, leaving the catheter in place in the vein. (Bottom) After the needle is withdrawn completely, the tubing from the intravenous solution is connected to the catheter.

solution will affect the rate of flow. The higher the solution, the faster it will run. As the bottle is lowered, the flow will become slower.

The rate of flow of the solution is also manually controlled by a clamp or a constricting device of some type. A dripmeter along the tubing permits the nurse to count the number of drops entering the patient's vein each minute.

The Solution. The kind and amount of solution are ordered by the physician, as indicated earlier. When there are electrolytes or drugs to be added to the solution, it is generally recommended that this be done by the pharmacist, preferably under a laminar airflow hood. The danger of contamination has been shown to be reduced by the use of this air-filtering device. Because certain substances added to solutions may be incompatible with others, having pharmaceutical personnel prepare solutions also decreases the likelihood of administering undesirable combinations. Any substance added to solutions should be clearly labeled on the bottle.

Before the infusion is started, a final check should be made to make sure the solution is clean and contains no particles of any kind. Since some substances create a precipitate, this check is especially important. Filters in the setup are available and may be used to filter the solution immediately before it enters the patient's vein.

Preparing the Patient for Intravenous Infusion. The procedure should be explained to the patient and he should be told how he can best cooperate. Since an infusion usually takes several hours to complete, or may even be continuous for days, the patient should be made comfortable. The arm to be used is abducted slightly from the body and placed on an armboard, if necessary. Cooperative and alert patients often do not require an armboard. When the armboard is secured, if one is used, attention should be given to keeping it in good position. Very often, it is possible to have the forearm and palm of the hand placed downward, as illustrated in Figure 17-35. The hand can then grasp the edge of the armboard. This more nearly resembles the normal position and is therefore, usually very comfortable. Hyperextension of the elbow causes fatigue for the patient. The nurse may need to flex and extend the arm after therapy to help the patient regain "feeling" if the elbow has been extended. If the injection site is hairy, it may be best to shave the area. Chart 17-5 and Figures 17-35 through 17-43 describe and illustrate starting an intravenous infusion.

Monitoring the Infusion. Monitoring the infusion is the nurse's responsibility and involves maintaining the rate of flow while assuring the comfort and safety of the patient. The physician indicates the milliliters to be given within a period of time, such as for a 1-, 8-, or 24-hour period. The rate is then calculated by the nurse on the basis of drops of solution to be given each minute.

There is no standard size drop, or drop factor as it is called. The size of the drop varies with the commercial company preparing the product. Most health agencies use the products of a single company. The nurse should familiarize herself with the products used in the agency in which she gives care. The more common drop factors are 15 drops per ml., 20 drops per ml., and 60 drops per ml. There are adapters for some equipment which makes it possible to reduce or increase the drop size.

If the physician orders 3000 ml. of solution to be infused over a period of 24 hours and the drop factor is 20 drops per ml., the rate of flow would be determined as follows:

First, determine the number of milliliters to be given every hour:

$$\frac{\text{Total number of ml. to be given}}{\text{Period of time to be infused}} = \frac{3000 \text{ ml.}}{24 \text{ hr.}} = 125 \text{ ml. to be given every hour}$$

Then, determine the number of drops to be given every minute:

$$\frac{\text{Number of ml. to be given each hour} \times \text{drop factor}}{60 \text{ minutes}} = \frac{125 \text{ ml.} \times 20 \text{ drops}}{60}$$

$$= \frac{2500}{60} = \frac{\text{Approximately 41–42 drops}}{\text{per minute}}$$

Assume that the physician orders that 125 ml. of solution are to be given each hour and the drop factor is 15 drops per ml. The number of drops to be given each minute is determined as follows:

$$\frac{125 \text{ ml.} \times 15 \text{ drops}}{60 \text{ min.}} = \frac{1875}{60} = \frac{\text{Approximately 31–32 drops}}{\text{per minute}}$$

Many factors can alter the rate of flow of an intravenous infusion, such as the height of the container in relation to the patient, the patient's blood pressure, and the patient's position. The nurse needs to know the ordered rate and then make adjustments as necessary to maintain that rate. Her task can be simplified when she marks points on the container at which the solution should be for each hour. An example of a marker that can be placed on the solution bottle is illustrated in Figure 17-44. The nurse should check the marker at frequent and regular intervals. As she checks, she can tell at a glance whether the solution is being infused at the proper hourly rate. If it is not, she again regulates the drops per minute (see p. 362).

Maintaining the proper rate of flow is important. Too slow a flow may not meet the patient's needs for the solution. Infusing fluid too rapidly

Chart 17-5 Administering an intravenous infusion
The purpose is to inject solution into a vein*

Suggested Action	Reason for Action	Figure to Illustrate
If possible, have patient in back-lying position and bed in semi-Fowler's position.	Back-lying position permits either arm to be used and allows for good body alignment. Semi-Fowler's position usually is most comfortable for patient.	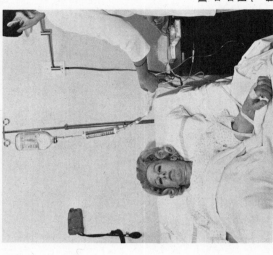
Select appropriate site by looking and palpating accessible veins, as illustrated in Figure 17-32, p. 354.	Selection of appropriate site decreases discomfort for patient and possible damage to body tissues.	Fig. 17-35 The patient has been made comfortable for an intravenous infusion and her arm has been secured on an armboard. The nurse allows solution to fill the tubing.
Place arm on a support as necessary with tourniquet under arm a few inches above site of entry. Secure arm to support with tape or bandage. Fix arm only snugly enough to hold it securely. Allow solution to fill tubing. Figure 17-35 illustrates.	Arm motion may move needle and dislodge it. Circulation of blood in arm will be impaired if arm is secured too tightly. Emptying tubing of air prevents introducing air into vein.	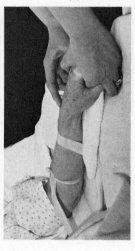
Tie tourniquet to obstruct venous flow. Direct tourniquet ends away from site of entry.	Interrupting blood flow causes veins to distend. Distended veins are easy to see, palpate, and enter. Ends of tourniquet could contaminate area of entry if allowed to all over site of entry.	Fig. 17-36 The nurse has secured the tourniquet with its ends directed away from the site of entry. She then palpates for a suitable vein.
Ask patient to open and close his fist. Observe and palpate vein, as illustrated in Figure 17-36.	Contraction of muscles of lower arm forces blood along in veins, thus distending them further.	

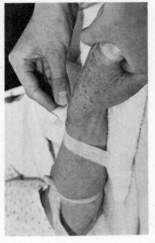

Fig. 17-37 After locating a suitable vein, the nurse cleanses the area thoroughly at and around the site of entry with a swab moistened with an antiseptic.

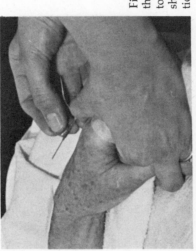

Fig. 17-38 Note the nurse's thumb holding the patient's vein to prevent its moving about as she readies her needle for insertion.

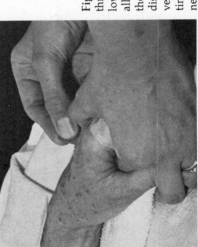

Fig. 17-39 The needle is through the skin. The nurse allows the needle, now nearly parallel with the skin, to slide along the side of the vein for a short distance. She then pierces the vein with the needle and continues to insert it into the vein for nearly its entire length.

Using friction, cleanse skin *thoroughly* at and then around site of entry.

Organisms on skin can be introduced into tissues or blood with needle.

Use thumb to retract down on vein and soft tissue about 2 inches below intended site of entry.

Pressure on vein and surrounding tissue helps prevent movement of vein as needle is being introduced.

Hold needle at a 30 to 45° angle with bevel up, in line with vein at point about ½ inch away from intended site of entry into vein.

Pressure needed to pierce skin can be sufficient to force needle into vein at improper angle and possibly through opposite wall of vein.

When needle is through skin, lower angle of needle until nearly parallel with skin, following same course as vein, and then insert into vein.

Following course of vein briefly prevents needle from leaving vein at another area because of pressure needed to puncture skin and vein simultaneously.

When blood comes back through needle into tubing, insert needle farther into vein for almost its full length.

Pressure of patient's blood is usually greater than pressure in tubing, causing automatic backflow. Having needle placed well into vein helps prevent easy dislocation of needle. "Riding" needle into vein while it is distended helps prevent pushing it through vein wall.

Chart 17-3 continued

Suggested Action	Reason for Action	Figure to Illustrate
Release tourniquet.	Closed off vein prevents solution from entering circulatory system.	
Start flow of solution by releasing clamp on tubing, as illustrated in Figure 17-40.	Patient's blood can clot readily in needle if solution flow is not started promptly.	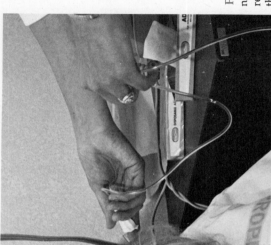 Fig. 17-40 As soon as the needle is in the vein, the nurse releases the tourniquet and begins the flow of solution.
Support needle with small piece of dry gauze if necessary to keep needle in proper position. A protective shield may be placed over site of entry.	Pressure of wall of vein against bevel of needle will interrupt flow of solution. Wall of vein can be punctured easily by improperly placed needle.	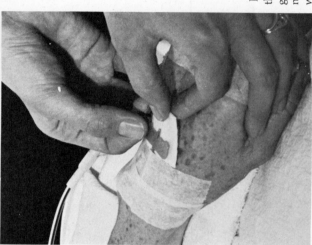 Fig. 17-41 The nurse supports the needle with a small piece of gauze so that the bevel of the needle does not rest against the wall of the vein.

Provide loop of tubing near site of entry and anchor loop with tape.

Weight of tubing and movement of patient may pull needle out of vein when tubing is not well anchored.

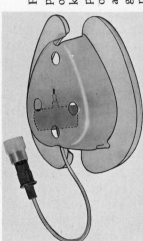

Fig. 17-42. This transparent, protective shield can be placed over a needle in a vein to help keep the needle in place. It is especially helpful when a scalp vein on a child has been entered for an intravenous infusion. (Photograph courtesy of the Posey Company)

Adjust rate of flow according to physician's order.

Physician specifies rate of flow.

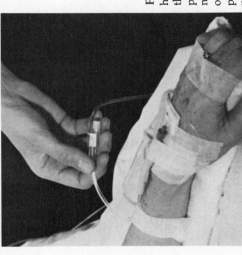

Fig. 17-43. A loop of the tubing has been brought around and then the tubing is fastened to the patient's skin with tape. The nurse demonstrates that pulling on the tubing will not exert pressure on the needle and possibly dislodge it.

* This chart assumes that the nurse will also observe suggestions offered in the sections of this chapter entitled Basic Guides for Preparing and Administering All Drugs and Parenteral Drug Administration.

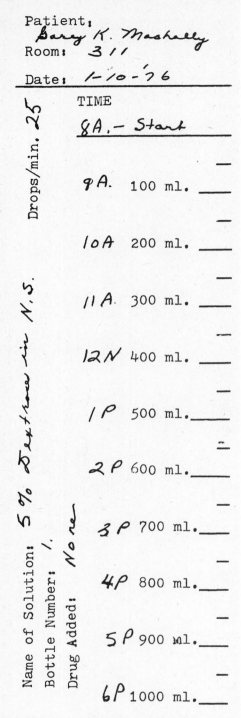

Patient:
Gary K. Marshally
Room: 3 1 1

Date: 1-10-'76

Drops/min. 25

Name of Solution: 5% Dextrose in N.S.
Bottle Number: 1.
Drug Added: None

TIME

8A. – Start

9A.   100 ml. ____

10A   200 ml. ____

11A. 300 ml. ____

12N   400 ml. ____

1P   500 ml. ____

2P   600 ml. ____

3P   700 ml. ____

4P   800 ml. ____

5P   900 ml. ____

6P   1000 ml. ____

Fig. 17-44 Marker placed on bottle of solution so that flow rate can be easily determined. 100 ml. of solution is to be given each hour until 1000 ml. is infused. With drip factor of 15, solution is introduced at 25 drops per minute for a total of 10 hours.

may overtax the body's ability to adjust to the increase in the fluid volume or the electrolytes it may contain. Nurses who allow infusions to fall behind schedule and increase the rate too much to catch up may be seriously harming the patient's well-being.

Devices which limit the amount of fluid which can be infused at any one time are available. There are also battery-operated rate meters which quickly calculate the milliliter per hour rate of a solution as it is infusing. In addition, a device is available that automatically regulates the number of drops the patient will receive. The nurse sets the dial at the number of drops to be administered each minute. The device shuts off the infusion automatically and emits a signal when the drip chamber is empty. This device is especially useful when the patient is to receive a drug in an intravenous solution at a very slow rate, as for example, ten or less drops per minute.

Care and Observation of the Patient. After it has been started, the infusion should not create discomfort for the patient. If the patient is uncomfortable, the nurse should check to see that the infusion is entering the vein, that the rate of flow is as ordered, and that the patient's position is satisfactory.

If the patient is allowed out of bed, the nurse hangs the infusion container on a portable standard and assists the patient out of bed, as described in Chapter 12. Figure 17-45 illustrates a nurse helping a patient walk about while the patient is having an infusion.

The patient's personal hygiene needs are met as described in Chapter 10. The patient's gown may be removed by slipping it off the body except for the arm in which the solution enters the vein. Then the sleeve is slipped over the needle, tubing, and solution container while the nurse holds the container temporarily in her hand. The reverse technique is used to replace the gown, beginning with slipping one sleeve of the gown over the solution container and then down over the tubing and needle and into place.

Any unusual symptoms the patient may have, such as difficult or noisy breathing, nausea, chills, or a headache, should be reported promptly. They may indicate serious complications that mean the infusion must be stopped.

A dislodged needle or a needle that has penetrated the wall of the vein can cause the fluid to pass into the subcutaneous tissue. The escape of solution into tissues is called **infiltration.** The symptoms are swelling in the area, pallor (whitish color) of the skin, coldness, or pain at the site. Lowering the solution bottle below the infusion site so the vein pressure is higher than the pressure in the tubing, and then looking for blood to enter the tubing is not a foolproof way to decide if the needle is in the vein. The needle may have penetrated only partially through the vessel wall. A backflow of blood in the tubing can then occur even though fluid is passing into the tissue. The needle bevel can be lodged against the vessel wall, and therefore, no blood backflow will occur when the bottle is lowered even though the needle is in the vein.

The needle should be removed when infiltration occurs and a new site should be selected for introducing additional solution.

Phlebitis is an inflammation of the vein. It is another potential danger of intravenous infusions. There will be painful inflammation along the course of the vein. Further use of the vein should be avoided.

Air can circulate in the blood. When there are large quantities, it is called an **air embolism.** Normally, well-handled infusions do not permit air to enter the vein. It has occurred, for example, when the patient's blood pressure was very low or when a solution bottle was allowed to become empty. The quantity of air which would be fatal to humans is not known, but animal experimentation indicates that it is much larger than usually thought. The average infusion tubing holds about 5 ml. of air, an amount not ordinarily considered dangerous. Patients, however, are often frightened when they see air, and every effort should be made to avoid this from happening. On certain equipment, air can often be removed at a juncture in the tubing with a sterile needle and syringe.

If more than one bottle of solution is ordered for the patient, the nurse ordinarily attaches additional bottles. The method by which this is done will depend on the agency's equipment and procedures. Figure 17-46 illustrates how additional bottles may be attached to the infusion setup (see p. 364).

Because infusions often are continued after the responsibility for a patient's care changes from one nurse to another, it is a good practice to agree on one common method for managing infusions. This helps to avoid errors and valuable time is not lost when checking and rechecking becomes necessary.

Adding Drugs to an Intravenous Infusion. When drugs the physician orders are not added to the bottle of solution in the pharmacy, the nurse may be required to add them while the infusion is being given. Most intravenous setups allow for a place where a drug can be added, either to a special chamber, as illustrated in Figure 17-47, or at a bifurcation in the intravenous tubing (see p. 364). The method of giving the drug will be determined by the agency's equipment and procedures.

Occasionally, a drug is to be given intravenously at regular intervals, such as four times a day, but the patient does not require intravenous solutions. Rather than puncture the patient repeatedly, equipment is used in some agencies that allows the needle to remain in place; the drug is then given through a short tubing attached to the needle. The drug heparin is sometimes administered in this manner. The equipment is illustrated in Figure 17-48 on page 365.

When a single dose of drug is to be administered intravenously, the drug is prepared for injection in the same manner as for an intramuscular or subcutaneous injection. The size of the syringe will depend on the amount of solution; a 20- or 22-gauge needle is commonly used. A tourniquet is used as for an intravenous infusion. Since the procedure is of short duration, the arm is not ordinarily secured to an armboard. After the drug in solution is given, the site of entry is cared for as after an intravenous infusion. This procedure is also used for injecting dyes prior to certain examinations, as for example, x-ray studies of the kidneys, ureters, and bladder.

Discontinuing the Infusion. When the total amount of solution ordered for the patient has been given, the nurse discontinues the infusion. First, she removes the tape or shield which has held the needle in place, and gently presses a sponge with antiseptic solution over the needle and site of entry. Then, she removes the needle by pulling it out quickly, following the course of the vein as she does so. If the needle is removed by twisting, raising, or lowering it, it could damage vein tissue. The nurse applies pressure with the sponge for a short time until bleeding stops and then applies a small pressure bandage.

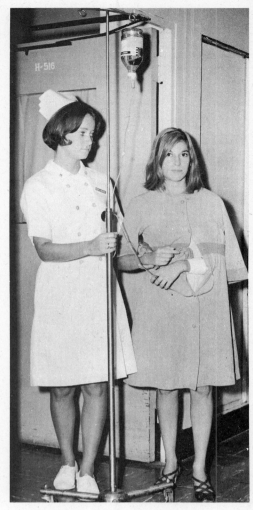

Fig. 17-45.   The patient's infusion solution is hung on a pole that is easily pushed ahead of the nurse as she supports the patient.

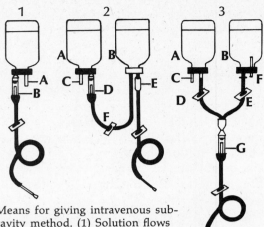

Fig. 17-46 Means for giving intravenous substances by gravity method. (1) Solution flows through drip-meter B (which also may be a filter if blood is given) at rate that can be controlled by clamp on tubing. A provides air inlet so air may enter bottle to displace fluid that leaves. It has a one-way valve to prevent fluid from running out. (2) A tandem setup. Fluid leaves bottle B if clamp F is open. As fluid leaves B, area of lesser pressure is created in B. Lesser pressure exerts its influence on bottle A and draws fluid from it. The system will operate only if air vent C, is open and permits air to displace fluid that leaves A. D is a drip-meter and filter. E is a drip-meter. In this setup, A always empties before B. If F is clamped off, no fluid is able to leave B. (3) Solution may leave either bottle, depending on regulation of clamps D and E. In this setup, A is blood and B is normal saline. If D stops blood flow from A, saline will flow from B if clamp E and clamp below filter are opened. Reverse also can happen. Thus, both bottles must have air inlet, C and F, so air can enter to displace fluid as it leaves. In this setup, G is a filter and drip-meter.

Topical drug administration

When a drug is applied directly to a body site for its local action, it is called a **topical administration.**

Skin Applications. The drug is incorporated into a vehicle, such as oil, lotion, or ointment, and rubbed into the skin. This procedure is referred to as an **inunction.** The drug is absorbed by the lining of the sebaceous glands. The skin has limited ability to absorb drugs. The skin is cleansed well with soap or detergent and water before the oil, lotion, or ointment is rubbed onto the skin. This removes debris and oil from the skin, both of which retard absorption. Applying local heat to the area increases blood circulation which also helps absorption.

The use of medicated skin applications in the treatment of skin diseases is described in clinical nursing textbooks.

Eye Instillations. The eyelids are lined with mucous membrane which forms two conjunctival sacs, one under the upper eyelid and the other under the lower eyelid. The cornea is the transparent structure on the eyeball. It is very sensitive and easily injured. Therefore, direct application of a solution or ointment onto the eyeball is rarely recommended for fear of injuring the cornea. Rather, drops and ointments are instilled into the lower conjunctival sac. For maximum safety for the patient, equipment used and solutions and ointments introduced into the eye should be sterile.

The lids and lashes are wiped clean as necessary prior to instillation. Normal saline and a cotton ball are usually used. One cotton ball is

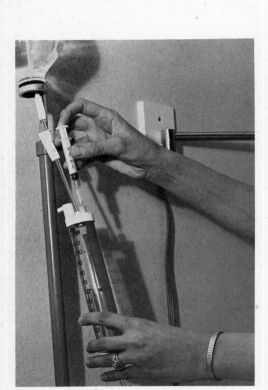

Fig. 17-47 This nurse is using equipment that allows a drug to be injected with a needle and syringe into a chamber that is located between the bottle of solution and the patient. The patient will receive the medication more quickly in this manner than had the drug been mixed with the entire amount of solution in the bottle. Also, introducing the drug into the chamber eliminates needing to open the bottle of solution, thereby decreasing the danger of contaminating the solution with airborne organisms.

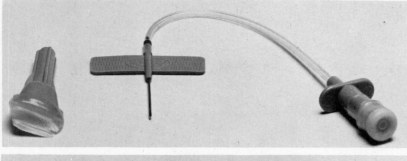

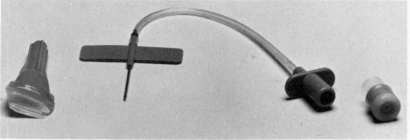

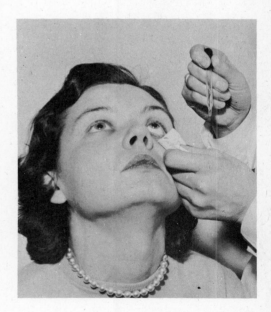

Fig. 17-48   (Top) The needle sheath has been removed to show an intravenous butterfly needle. The needle is inserted into the patient's vein and the short tubing is then anchored to his skin with tape. (Bottom) A sterile plug has been removed which now makes it possible to attach a syringe with a drug in solution to the tube. The drug is then injected. After injection, the plug is replaced until the next time the intravenous drug is to be introduced. This equipment makes it unnecessary to puncture the patient every time a regularly ordered intravenous medication is to be given.

used for one wipe. The cotton ball is moved from the area of the eye near the nose, called the inner canthus, outward toward the side of the head or outer canthus.

To expose the conjunctiva of the lower lid, the nurse asks the patient to look up while she places her thumb near the margin of the lower lid immediately below the eyelashes. She then exerts pressure downward over the bony prominence of the cheek. As the lower lid is pulled down and away from the eyeball, the conjunctival sac is exposed. It is important to work carefully and gently to prevent injuring the eye or eyelids. This is of particular importance when the lids are swollen, inflamed, and tender.

Ointments are dispensed in tubes. The ointment is pushed from the tube with the fingers and allowed to fall into the conjunctival sac. An eyedropper is used to instill solutions. It is unsafe practice to return unused solution to a stock bottle. Therefore, no more solution than is needed should be drawn into the eyedropper. Once the solution has been drawn into the dropper, it is held with the bulb uppermost. Allowing the solution to enter the bulb may result in contaminating the solution with fine particles of rubber.

The dropper or ointment tube is held close to the eye but not touching the eyelids or the eyelashes. This prevents injury should the patient become startled by the sensation and move quickly. The ointment or the prescribed number of drops of solution are allowed to enter the center of the exposed sac. After instillation, the patient should be asked to close his eyelids and move the eye. This helps to distribute the solution or ointment over the conjunctival surfaces and eyeball. Figure 17-49 illustrates instillation of eye drops.

Ear Instillations. In adults, the canal of the external ear is directed inward, forward, and downward. In an infant, the canal is almost straight. In order for solution to reach all parts of the canal, the top of the ear should be pulled downward and backward for infants, and upward and backward for adults.

The outer ear is not a sterile cavity. Practices of medical asepsis are

Fig. 17-49   The nurse uses a wipe to protect her finger from slipping while instilling eye drops. The patient is asked to look up, and the lower lid is everted so that the conjunctival sac is exposed.

Topical drug administration   365

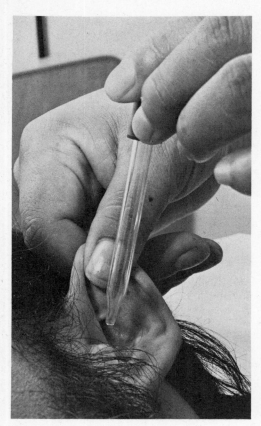

Fig. 17-50   To instill ear drops in this adult patient, note that the nurse pulls the ear upward and backward and drops the solution along the side of the ear canal.

used when instilling solutions into the ear. However, if the tympanic membrane on the base of the canal is not intact, sterile technique is used.

It is more comfortable for the patient if the solution is warmed to approximately body temperature. The ear canal is straightened and the drops are allowed to fall on the side of the canal. The patient lies on his side with the ear being treated uppermost. He remains in this position following instillation to prevent the drops from escaping. Figure 17-50 illustrates a nurse giving ear drops to a patient. Occasionally, a loose cotton wick is inserted into the canal. A wick should not be packed into the ear. It may interfere with the outward movement of normal secretions and could create undue pressure in the ear canal.

Nose Instillations. The nose is not considered a sterile cavity. However, because it connects with the sinuses, caution should be observed when placing solutions in the nose.

Most physicians recommend using a drug in normal saline solution for nose drops. Oily solutions may be aspirated into the lungs and possibly cause infection.

The patient is assisted to a sitting position with his head tilted back. Or, he lies in bed with his head tilted back over a pillow. This position allows the solution to flow back into the nose. Sufficient solution for both nares is drawn into a dropper. The dropper is placed just inside the nose and the prescribed number of drops is instilled. Touching the dropper to the nose may create a desire to sneeze. The patient should be instructed to keep his head tilted back for several minutes to prevent the escape of solution from the nose. He usually will wish to expectorate solution that runs down into the back of the mouth and should be provided with tissues for this purpose. Figure 17-51 illustrates a nurse about to instill nose drops.

When instilling drops into the nose of an infant or an irrational patient, the tip of the dropper should be protected with a piece of soft rubber or plastic tubing to minimize the danger of injury.

Solutions may be instilled with a spray. A small atomizer generally is used. The end of the nose is held up. The tip of the nozzle is placed just inside the nose and directed backward. Only sufficient force is used to bring the spray into contact with the membranes. Too much force may drive the solution and contamination into the sinuses and the eustachian tubes.

Throat Applications. Lozenges may contain drugs that are used for local treatment of the throat. Cough drops are an example. When sucked, the lozenge liberates the drug. The throat is then bathed in the solution. The patient should be instructed to suck the lozenge. Chewing or swallowing it renders it largely ineffective. The patient should not take fluids during or after having a lozenge. The fluids will flush away the drug and decrease its effectiveness.

Throat irrigations, sprays, and paints are very rarely used. The agency's procedures should be observed on those occasions when they may be ordered.

Vaginal Applications. Medicated creams are ordinarily applied by using a narrow tubular applicator with an attached plunger. Suppositories that melt when exposed to body heat are also prepared for vaginal insertion. They are placed into the vagina with gloved fingers. Practices of medical asepsis are used since the vagina is not considered sterile.

Rectal Applications. Rectal suppositories are used primarily for their local action. Insertion of the rectal suppository was described in Chapter 14. Occasionally, a drug in solution may be given rectally for its systemic effect. The solution is instilled as a retention enema. The procedure was described in Chapter 14.

Teaching the patient to take his own medications

The nurse usually is responsible for teaching the patient how to take his own medications. Or, if this is not possible, she teaches a family member to do so. It is recommended that in addition to demonstration, the patient or family member practice in the presence of the nurse until skill for safe administration is reached.

Studies have shown that the most frequent cause of errors when patients take their own medications is lack of understanding about the dose and the frequency of taking them. Written instructions are best. Color-coded systems or other reminders can also be used effectively.

The patient needs to be aware of what effect is desired from the drug and what the signs of undesirable effects are. Prompt reporting of untoward symptoms should be emphasized.

Patients who will administer their own injections need to be taught surgical asepsis. They should understand why sterile technique is important.

If the patient is using a reusable needle, he should test for burrs by running it along a piece of cotton or the back of the hand before sterilizing it. Keeping the needle sharp and free of burrs can be accomplished with an emery stone. But the patient should be taught not to reuse needles that are worn and may have lost their strength. The danger of a needle breaking off in tissue is serious.

Cross-contamination between patients is not a problem at home. Therefore, boiling cleaned syringes and needles is usually the recommended method of sterilization. A good practice is to boil the needle and separated syringe in a sieve in a pot with sufficient water to cover the equipment well. A small forceps may be included for assembling the sterile syringe and needle. The handle of the forceps should be so placed that the patient can grasp it without contaminating the water and equipment. Or, after lifting the sterilized equipment out of boiling water in the sieve, some patients quickly learn how to assemble the equipment by hand without contaminating it or burning themselves.

Disposable equipment is recommended whenever possible so that sterilizing and caring for needles and syringes are not necessary. The patient will need to be taught how to dispose of this equipment carefully to prevent its use by others.

For home technique, cotton used to cleanse the skin need not necessarily be sterile as long as the patient is instructed not to cover the needle with it. Usually, the patient learns to place the syringe on a table with the needle over the edge while he prepares his skin for injection. The syringe and needle should be so placed that the patient cannot touch it accidentally while he cleans the skin.

The technique for self-administration of an injection is the same as that used by the nurse when she gives an injection. The preferred site is the thigh so that the patient can readily see what he is doing. The

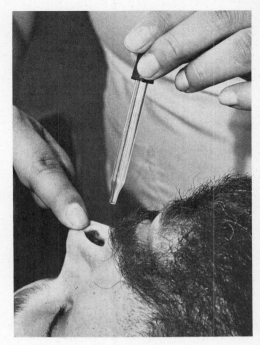

Fig. 17-51   The nurse is about to place the dropper at the opening to the nose. The patient's head is resting over a pillow. In this case, the nurse lifts the tip of the nose slightly for best visualization of the nares.

abdomen can also be used for subcutaneous injection. Some patients become sufficiently skilled to inject their upper arm subcutaneously or intramuscularly.

Patients often need to be taught the importance of safeguarding drugs at home. Keeping all medications out of the reach of children is especially important. The number of children who are poisoned from drugs every year is alarmingly high.

Self-medication is the treating of oneself with drugs. Occasional treatment of minor problems is a common practice with over-the-counter (OTC) drugs. However, repetitious or long-term self-medication can be dangerous. The Food and Drug Administration attempts to protect the public by requiring truthful advertising, proper labeling, and directions on OTC drug use. As an attempt to protect the individual from harm, the Food and Drug Administration has given the following recommendations which the nurse will wish to share with her patients:

- Don't be casual about taking drugs.
- Don't take drugs you don't need.
- Don't overbuy and keep drugs for long periods of time.

- Don't combine drugs carelessly.

- Don't continue taking OTC drugs if symptoms persist.

- Don't take prescription drugs not prescribed specifically for you.

- Do read and follow directions for use.
- Do be cautious when using a drug for the first time.
- Do dispose of old prescription drugs and outdated OTC medications.
- Do seek professional advice before combining drugs.
- Do seek professional advice when symptoms persist or return.
- Do get medical checkups regularly.

Conclusion

The careful administration of drugs is of utmost importance. Safe practice does not allow for automatic habits. Constant thinking, purposeful action, and repeated checking for accuracy are essential. This also holds true for administering intravenous solutions and drugs.

Drug abuse has become a major national problem. The nurse can play an important role through her teaching and nursing practice to help prevent abuse. She can share information concerning the dangers and problems when drugs are used carelessly. Drugs can be a blessing. They can destroy when used improperly.

Literally thousands of drugs are available and new ones are being added constantly. Therefore, knowledge about drugs is an area where the nurse's education never ends.

References

Bahruth, April, "Keeping Track of Injection Sites," *Nursing '73*, 3:51, June 1973.

Chezem, Joanne L., "Consultation: Aspirating Before IM Injections," *Nursing '74*, 4:87, September 1974.

———, "Locating the Best Thigh Injection Site," *Nursing '73*, 3:20–21, December 1973.

Egan, Alphonsine, "Perfecting Piggyback Techniques," *Nursing '74*, 4:28–33, January 1974.

Feld, Lipman G., "The Nurse's Liability for Faulty Injections," *Nursing Care*, 7:25, April 1974.

Geolot, Denise H. and McKinney, Nancy P., "Administering Parenteral Drugs," *American Journal of Nursing*, 75:788–793, May 1975.

Harris, Barbara, "Are You Ready for the Switch to the Metric System?" *Nursing Care*, 8:12–14, March 1975.

Hays, Doris, "Do It Yourself the Z-Track Way," *American Journal of Nursing*, 74:1070–1071, June 1974.

McGill, Docia, "Giving I. V. Push," *Nursing '73*, 3:15–18, June 1973.

Rodman, Morton J., "Drug Therapy Today: Dangers of Unsupervised Medications," *RN*, 37:51, 52, 59, 62, 64, 66, 68, July 1974.

Smola, Bonnie Ketchum, "Stop: Read Before You Pour One More Medication," *Nursing Care*, 8:26, January 1975.

Snider, Malle Avolaid, "Helpful Hints on I. V.'s," *American Journal of Nursing*, 74:1978–1981, November 1974.

Wiley, Loy, ed., "Innovations in Nursing: How Many of Your Patients Are Taking Their Medicines?" *Nursing '73*, 3:3–16, April 1973.

18

measures to promote tissue healing

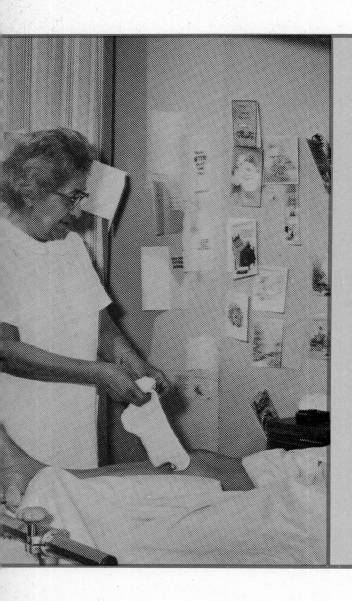

370

behavioral objectives

When mastery of content in this chapter is reached, the student will be able to

Define terms appearing in the glossary.

Discuss how the body reacts to injury and how healing occurs.

List five reasons why a wound may be ordered to be left undressed.

List four purposes of a dressing.

Describe how to change a dressing when drainage is present and discuss various methods for securing a dressing.

Describe how the skin can be protected when adhesive is applied.

List three common symptoms of the patient who is allergic to adhesive.

Discuss several purposes of elasticized stockings and describe how such stockings are applied.

Describe 15 measures to promote safety and comfort when applying a bandage or binder.

Describe the five basic turns used to apply roller bandages and explain when each is most appropriately used; explain two ways to remove a roller bandage.

Describe the proper application of the T binder, the four-tailed binder applied to the chin, the scultetus binder, the straight binder applied to the chest, the sling, and the cravat.

Discuss six factors that guide the nurse when she uses applications of heat and cold and list common purposes for using such applications.

Describe how to apply an ice bag and cold compresses and how to give an alcohol or cold sponge bath.

Describe how hypothermia is commonly accomplished.

Explain how to use a heating pad and a hot-water bag; how to give a hip or sitz bath and a soak; and how to apply hot packs and compresses.

List two common purposes of irrigations.

behavioral objectives cont.

Describe how to irrigate the eye, the ear, the vagina, and a wound.

Design a teaching program for the patient who will change dressings on a draining wound; who will use hot and cold applications at home; and who will give herself a vaginal irrigation at home.

glossary

Abscess A circumscribed collection of pus.

Bandage A length of material applied in a manner to fit a part of the body.

Binder A type of bandage designed to fit a large body part, such as the abdomen or chest.

Circular Turn A bandage turn that encircles a part; each turn completely overlaps the previous turn.

Closed Wound A wound without a break in the skin or mucous membrane.

Contusion A bruise.

Cravat Binder A binder made by folding a triangular binder over and over upon itself, starting at the apex, until the desired width is obtained.

Débridement A method of cleaning a wound of debris.

Douche An irrigation of the vagina.

Figure-of-Eight Turn A bandage turn consisting of oblique overlapping turns that ascend and descend, forming a figure eight.

Granulation Tissue New tissue formation over a wound.

Hypothermia Lowered body temperature.

Inflammation The defensive local response of the body to injury.

Insulator A substance that is a poor conductor.

Open Wound A break in the skin or mucous membrane.

Recurrent Turn A bandage turn in which an area is covered by carrying the bandage back and forth over a rounded surface.

Roller Bandage A continuous strip of material wound on itself to form a roll.

Scultetus Binder A many-tailed binder.

Sling A triangular binder.

Spiral Turn A bandage turn that only partly overlaps the previous turn.

Spiral-Reverse Turn A spiral turn in which reverses are made halfway through each turn.

Straight Binder A rectangular piece of material, usually 6 to 8 inches wide and long enough to more than circle the body.

T Binder A binder shaped like the letter T.

Tailed Binder A rectangular piece of material which has vertical tails, each about 2 inches wide, attached to its sides.

Trauma Injury to tissue.

introduction

This chapter discusses ways in which the healing process can be helped. The body has a remarkable ability to recover when tissue is damaged. Nevertheless, there are some actions that can be taken to support or assist the healing mechanism. These may be especially necessary when the patient is ill and his normal body defenses and recuperative abilities are decreased.

In some health agencies, measures described in this chapter require a physician's order. In others, some of them may not. The nurse should observe the policies of the agency in which she gives care. Agency policy is also followed when nursing care described in this chapter is recorded.

The body's reaction to injury

Trauma is a general term referring to an injury. An **open wound** means there is a break in the skin or mucous membrane. Such a wound may have been caused by an accident, or it may be an intentional wound, such as the one made by the surgeon when he cuts tissue to enter the field of operation. In a **closed wound** there is no break in the skin or mucous membrane. The most common closed wound is a bruise, often called a **contusion.** The escape of blood into subcutaneous tissues at the site of a contusion gives the characteristic bluish color to the site of injury.

Both open and closed wounds can be invaded by microorganisms and an infection can result. The entrance of organisms in an accidental wound can easily occur as a result of contamination from the instrument causing the injury. Pathogens in a surgical wound usually result from poor aseptic technique or an accidental break in the technique. An infection in a closed wound is usually the result of the presence of pathogens in the blood.

The body's normal reaction to a wound is an inflammatory process. An **inflammation** is a defensive response of the body to injury. It works to limit the tissue damage, remove the injured cells, and repair damaged tissues.

The healing process normally occurs in stages. Blood serum and cells form a network in the wound. The edges of the wound are "glued" together by this network which becomes the scab. Fragile, pinkish-red tissue, called **granulation tissue,** then forms. This is gradually replaced by normal-appearing skin and a scar. The strength of the wound is slight until a scar begins to develop. A scar is strong but does not have the elasticity that normal skin does.

The body's ability to handle trauma is affected by the extent of the damage and the patient's condition. If the injury is overwhelming and the body is unable to cope with it, even with assistance, death occurs. When this is not the case, the patient's general state of health plays an important role in the healing process. The promotion of high-level wellness helps the body deal with trauma. Adequate rest, relief from emotional tensions, a nourishing diet, and adequate fluid intake are particularly important for persons undergoing a response to injury.

An adequate blood supply is necessary for healing. Certain heart and blood vessel diseases, anemia, and extensive blood loss at the time of injury, for example, interfere with the healing process. Therefore, all possible efforts are made to keep an adequate blood supply in the healing area.

Because the patient's primary protective barrier is weakened when skin and mucous membrane break, the need for preventing microorganisms from entering the body becomes especially important. Careful handwashing before caring for the wound is probably the single most effective method for preventing infections. While it is not possible to sterilize the skin, practices of surgical asepsis are used when caring for an open wound. Precautions are also taken for persons with closed wounds because of the lowered resistance of the damaged tissue to infection.

Drainage, dead or damaged tissue cells, microorganisms, or imbedded fragments of bone, metal, glass, or other substances can act as foreign bodies and interfere with good tissue healing. Cleaning an injured area of this sort of debris is referred to as **débridement.** The physician ordinarily performs a débridement. However, the nurse is usually responsible if a wound irrigation is performed. When healing does not occur by wound care, it may be necessary to use skin grafts to close the wound. This is especially true when the skin covering a large area has been destroyed.

There are times when the body walls off a collection of pus or a foreign body and healing occurs around it. This is known as an **abscess.** Local treatment of an abscess varies. It may include a surgical procedure to open and drain the abscess. Local application of heat and immobilization of the part may also be used.

Care of the wound

The tissues of open and closed wounds are more susceptible to further injury than is normal tissue. Prevention of additional injury and the promotion of healing are two goals of wound care.

The Undressed Wound. Most closed wounds are left undressed. Some physicians also prefer leaving certain open wounds undressed if the wound has sealed itself and can be protected from injury and irritation. This is true even of wounds that have been surgically created and sutured. There may be occasions when a wound is left undressed for most of the day and then covered at bedtime. Many small cuts and abrasions are handled in this manner.

There are several reasons for leaving some wounds undressed. Friction and irritation of the dressing may destroy skin tissues. Organisms normally found on the skin can be rubbed into the wound. A dark, warm, moist area under the dressing is suitable for the growth of microorganisms. A dressing may interfere with good circulation to the part, causing a delay in healing. Exposure to air helps keep the area dry. For example, one approach to the care of extensive burns is the open or no-dressing method. As another example, the woman who has just delivered a baby almost always has some areas of broken tissue. Her care includes preventing contamination of the area. But the wound is ordinarily left undressed.

The Dressed Wound. The protective covering over a wound is called a dressing. Dressings serve several purposes. If used properly, they aid in preventing microorganisms from entering the wound. They help absorb drainage and can help to restrict movement that tends to interfere with healing. A dressing may be applied with pressure to reduce blood flow when bleeding is present. To assist in the healing process, dressings are applied in a manner that helps to approximate wound edges. For aesthetic reasons, a dressing serves to cover an area of disfigurement.

Some patients are taught to change their own dressings, or the nurse or physician changes the dressings. In some agencies, dressings may be changed in a treatment room or in an operating room. In others dressings are changed while the patient is in bed. Some agencies have dressing carts which are wheeled from one patient to another. However, to help prevent cross-infection, the preferred method is to have individual dressing trays which contain the equipment and supplies necessary for each patient. Commercially prepared, sterilized, and individually packaged supplies selected according to the patient's needs are used.

In some instances, patients do not wish to look at their wounds when they are dressed. They should neither be encouraged to do so nor chided about it. This is particularly true of patients whose wounds involve changes in their normal body functions or appearance, such as the removal of a breast or the amputation of an extremity.

After providing privacy, the patient is helped to assume a comfortable position for a dressing change. The position should also make it easy for the nurse to observe sound practices of surgical asepsis and to have a convenient work area. If the procedure is likely to produce considerable discomfort, a medication to relieve pain may be ordered and given before beginning the procedure.

The following are basic supplies needed for changing a dressing: a means for removing a soiled dressing without contaminating the wound or hands of the person removing it, such as sterile forceps or sterile gloves; materials for cleansing the wound and the area around it; dressings; and materials for securing the dressing. If the wound is to be irrigated or the skin needs special protection from drainage or adhesive, appropriate equipment and supplies should also be in readiness. A special solvent will be required to remove some spray-on plastic dressings.

Chart 18-1 describes how to change a dressing when there is drainage present. The procedure is easily adapted to meet the needs of patients having wounds without drainage.

Colostomies may have considerable fecal drainage before patients establish regularity. Ileostomies may have almost constant fecal drainage. Changing these dressings is similar to the procedure described in Chart 18-1. The skin around the stoma requires special care. It should be kept as dry and clean as possible to prevent odors and skin irritation. An ointment to protect the skin from irritation is applied and removed regularly as necessary, as described in Chart 18-1.

Securing the Dressing. This responsibility often requires considerable ingenuity and resourcefulness on the part of the nurse. It requires consideration for such factors as the size of the wound, its location, whether drainage is present, the nature of the drainage, the frequency with which the dressing needs changing, and the activities of the patient.

For securing a small dressing on a wound with little or no drainage, liquid adhesive may be used effectively. The edges of the outer piece of gauze that is cut to fit over the dressing are painted with liquid adhesive and then glued to the skin.

Strips of adhesive probably are used most frequently for securing dressings. Adhesive is dispensed in various widths. The length is cut according to need. Some adhesive is porous to allow for the escape of moisture and heat. Elasticized adhesive permits more movement of a body part without pull on adjacent tissues.

Adhesive often causes skin irritation, especially when dressings must be changed frequently. Therefore, it is good practice to apply a protective coating to the skin before using adhesive. A preparation used often is compound tincture of benzoin. Another suitable preparation is collodion, which is treated plant cellulose in ether or alcohol.

Chart 18-1 Dressing a draining wound
The purpose is to remove a soiled dressing, cleanse the wound, and apply a sterile dressing

Suggested Action	Reason for Action
Practices of surgical asepsis are used when caring for open wounds.	Organisms introduced into wound are likely to result in wound infection or increased problems if infection is already present.
Remove soiled dressings with sterile forceps or sterile-gloved hands.	This practice protects hands from heavy contamination from wound. Sterile equipment is used to help prevent possibility of introducing organisms into wound.
If dressing sticks to wound, moisten with solution, such as sterile water, normal saline, or hydrogen peroxide.	Removing dressing carefully will not disturb healing process or rubber drain.
Use caution when rubber drain is in place in wound so that it is not dislodged during wound care.	A drain helps keep wound open so that adequate drainage occurs, thus promoting healing.
Discard soiled dressings as well as materials for cleansing wound in waterproof bag for later disposal (preferably burning), being careful not to contaminate outside of bag.	Confining organisms within a waterproof bag and keeping outside of bag clean help prevent spreading organisms to others. Burning destroys organisms.
When considerable drainage is present, wash skin with soap or detergent and water around and away from wound, rinse, and dry well.	Thoroughly washing area removes excessive drainage effectively. Soap or detergent left on skin may irritate skin. Drying area helps prevent skin irritation.
If ointment is used to protect skin from drainage, remove it regularly, preferably daily, with appropriate solvent—soap or detergent and water or oil, for example. Use only sufficient friction to remove ointment.	Removing ointment allows for thorough cleansing. Minimum friction helps prevent skin irritation.
Cleanse wound carefully and then area around it with antiseptic solution of agency's choice.	Cleansing helps remove organisms, tissue debris, and drainage, thereby promoting healing.
When cleansing, move material (usually sterile cotton balls) over wound and then away from it, using one cotton ball for each stroke.	Moving away from wound and using one cotton ball for each stroke prevents bringing organisms from skin into wound.
Dry area with sterile material as necessary.	Protective ointments cannot be applied well to wet skin. Dressings become damp when applied to wet skin.
Apply ointment of agency's choice to skin when drainage is profuse and occurs over period of time.	Ointment protects skin from drainage that may cause irritation and destruction of skin tissues.
Cover wound with sterile dressings handled with sterile forceps or sterile gloves. Only outer surface of top of dressing is handled as clean rather than sterile.	Dressing handled by hands becomes contaminated and organisms may then enter wound.

Chart 18-1   continued

Suggested Action	Reason for Action
Fluffed and loosely packed dressings absorb more drainage and carry it up and away from wound and skin.	Capillary action causes liquid to rise on dressing fibers that act as small wicks. Loosely packed dressings promote air circulation, thus helping to prevent skin irritation by increasing evaporation of moisture and dissipation of heat.
Arrange dressing so that drainage flows into thickest part of dressing. Arrangement of dressing depends on patient's position in bed or whether he is up and about.	Gravity causes liquids to flow from a high to a lower level.
Change dressing often enough so that it does not become soaked with drainage.	Keeping skin clean and dry prevents irritation and destruction of skin tissue.
Handle contaminated instruments according to agency policy and in a manner that prevents them from touching other equipment and supplies.	Careless handling of contaminated equipment spreads organisms to others.

See text for suggestions for securing dressings.

Some patients are allergic to adhesive. The nurse should investigate any complaint or discomfort associated with adhesive tape. Symptoms include redness, swelling, and blister formation. Various kinds of non-allergic tapes are available for sensitive patients.

Because adhesive applied over hairy areas of skin can be painful to remove, shaving the area is often recommended. If the adhesive does not stick well to the skin, passing it over an alcohol flame or moistening it with a little alcohol or ether usually helps increase the stickiness.

When the dressing must be changed frequently, it is suggested that the nurse use straps for securing it. They do not require changing with each dressing and can be made or purchased. The adhesive end of the strap is placed on the skin well away from the wound. The end of the strap near the wound remains free since the adhesive side has been turned back upon itself. Gauze or cloth strips passed through eyelets are tied over the wound to secure the dressing. When the dressing is changed, the straps are untied and turned back to allow for wound care. The skin can be protected with compound tincture of benzoin or collodion before applying the straps to the patient. These straps are illustrated in Figure 18-1.

When a dressing is being secured, pressure on the wound should be exerted from the edges toward the center of the wound. This practice helps to approximate the wound edges and hence promotes healing. It should be remembered that circulation of air in the dressing is desirable, especially when there is drainage. For this reason the dressing should be secured in a manner that allows for maximum air circulation but that is snug enough to prevent the dressing from slipping about over the wound. Loose-fitting dressings cause friction as the patient moves which produces irritation on the wound and skin.

When drainage is profuse, adequate protection sometimes requires

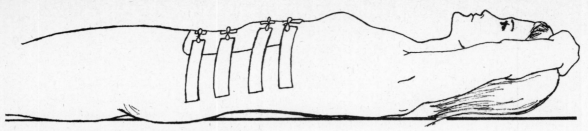

Fig. 18-1. A means for securing dressings that must be changed frequently.

judicious use of waterproof materials to prevent soiling linen and clothing. However, completely sealing a dressing with waterproofing is rarely advised. This practice traps moisture and heat which tend to cause irritation and a breakdown of the skin around the wound. Also, the warmth and moisture favor the growth of microorganisms.

When adhesive cannot be used safely and effectively, various types of binders and bandages may be used.

Use of bandages and binders

A **bandage** is a length of material applied in a manner to fit a part of the body. Usually, bandages are dispensed in rolls of various widths. A **binder** is a type of bandage. The term binder is generally used when the material fits a large body area, for example, the abdomen, chest, or breasts. Some texts use the terms synonymously, although in the strictest sense they do not have the same meaning.

Bandages and binders are used for a variety of purposes: to hold dressings and splints in place; to exert pressure over an area; to restrict or limit motion; to support a part of the body; and to protect an injured area. When the purpose is well served, a bandage or binder promotes healing, prevents further injury, and provides comfort and security.

Binders are usually made of muslin, flannel, or synthetics. Synthetic binders are often elasticized; some are self-adhering, that is, they stick to themselves rather than to the skin.

Usually, gauze is used for bandages. It is light and soft and can be adjusted readily to fit a body part comfortably. Because it is porous, it is cool and allows for circulation of air.

Muslin and flannel are also used for bandages. Strong and firm, they are useful when pressure and immobilization are desired. Flannel is more absorbent than muslin and molds easily to fit the contours of the body. Flannel also helps keep an area warm, which may be an advantage or a disadvantage, depending on specific circumstaces.

Muslin and flannel bandages are well suited for home use because they can be washed and reused.

Various types of elastic webbing can be purchased. They are particularly effective when bandaging is needed for firm support and immobilization and for exerting pressure. The webbing is strong and molds well because of its elasticity. It can be washed and used repeatedly.

One type of elastic webbing has a side with an adhesive surface so that it will stick to itself. This can be used like adhesive and has the

Measures to promote tissue healing

advantage of holding well to body contours. It does not withstand washing and therefore cannot be reclaimed for repeated use.

Stockinet is a stretchable tubular bandage, constructed so that a body part, such as a finger, a foot, or an arm, may be inserted into it. It is commonly used under casts to protect the skin. Stockinet is dispensed in various widths or diameters. It has advantages over the roller bandage in that it remains in place better, applies a uniform pressure, and is simple and quick to use.

Stockinet is especially useful for making caps for securing dressings on the head. The desired length is cut from a roll of an appropriate width, usually 6 inches. The stockinet is placed over the head and folded back on itself at the forehead for extra security. The opposite end is tied or pinned at the top of the head.

Stockinet seems to offer more security than other types of bandages on the head. It is also comfortable for the patient. In narrow widths, it is appropriate for finger bandages. An applicator is dispensed with the stockinet so that it can be slipped over the finger with ease.

Elasticized stockings are a special type of bandage for people who may need to have pressure applied to their legs. Examples include persons with varicose veins, those with circulatory disturbances, or women during pregnancy. Many patients routinely wear elasticized stockings following major surgery or when they are confined to bed for long periods of time. The stockings help to promote venous blood return and to avoid stagnation of blood in veins which may result in clot formation.

Several manufacturers make men's and women's hose which are capable of applying pressure to the leg from the foot to the midthigh. Some apply mild pressure while others are capable of applying pressure equivalent to an elastic bandage. They are more expensive than regular stockings, which may make them prohibitive for some patients. However, they wear well and many people who are on their feet or remain in one position for long periods of time, such as homemakers, nurses, and sales persons, find them very useful. The sustained pressure helps to prevent edema in the feet and lower legs. The stockings should be correctly fitted for the individual. Also, they should be applied as soon as the person awakens, before he gets out of bed.

Immobilized patients who wear elasticized stockings should have them removed and replaced twice a day. Their legs need to be inspected and bathed at least daily. The stockings are washed as necessary but at least twice weekly. Figure 18-2 illustrates a nurse teaching a patient how to apply an elasticized stocking.

The following measures promote safety and comfort when one is applying bandages and binders:

- Observe medical asepsis. The area to which bandages and binders are applied should be clean and dry. When an open wound is present, apply them over the sterile dressing. They are washed and sterilized between patients when reclaimed for repeated use.
- When possible, use porous rather than nonporous materials in order to allow air to circulate so that perspiration and heat can escape.
- Applying a small amount of talcum powder to the *unbroken* skin helps to keep it dry and decreases friction. Make certain that powder does not enter a wound if one is present.

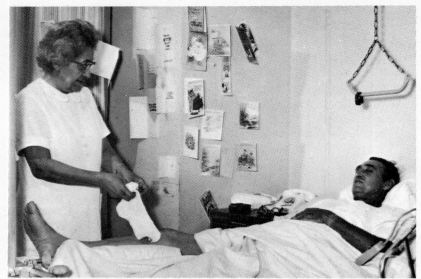

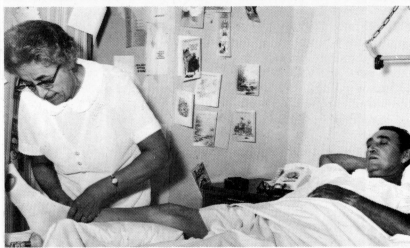

Fig. 18-2 The nurse teaches the patient how to hold the elastic stocking before putting it on, and then demonstrates how it is put onto the foot and leg. (Good Samaritan Hospital, Phoenix, Arizona)

- Do not allow two skin surfaces to touch each other under the bandage or binder. Use absorbent material, such as cotton wadding or gauze, between touching skin surfaces. For example, when fingers or toes are bandaged together, place padding between them first to prevent skin from rubbing against skin. Examples of other areas needing similar protection include the axillary area, the area under the breasts, and folds in the groin or abdomen.
- Pad bony prominences over which bandages and binders must be placed. Hollows in the body contour may be filled with padding which increases comfort and helps maintain equal pressure on body parts.
- Bandages and binders usually restrict some motion and often are intended to immobilize part of the body. It is important that the part involved first be placed at rest and comfortably in the position of normal functioning so that deformities will not result. For example, when bandaging the foot, support it so that the bandage will not force it into the footdrop position. Joints should be slightly flexed, rather than extended or hyperextended.
- Apply the bandage or binder with sufficient pressure to provide the

amount of immobilization or support desired, to make sure that it remains in place, and to secure a dressing if one is present. However, pressure should not be great enough to interfere with circulation. For example, weakened veins, especially in the lower extremities, can usually function more effectively when their walls are supported. Too much pressure can impair proper blood circulation.

- When bandaging an extremity, if possible, leave a small portion of the extremity, such as the fingers or toes, exposed so that any change in circulation can be noted. Signs of impaired circulation include coldness and numbness of the part, swelling, bluish coloring of the skin and nailbeds, or tingling pain. A simple test of circulation can be done by applying pressure on the nailbeds with your fingers. In normal circumstances, the area will blanch first and then return to its original color quickly when pressure on the nailbed is released. If the bandage is too tight, the blood neither leaves nor returns to the area quickly. Any one of the signs just described should be reported promptly so that steps may be taken to loosen the bandage. Prolonged poor circulation to an area can result in the death of tissue cells.
- A bandage that leaves a considerable portion of the end of an extremity uncovered is likely to produce swelling. Once swelling occurs, the tension on the lower border of the bandage increases, thus making the condition worse. Therefore, start bandaging an arm or a leg, for example, as near the ankle or wrist as possible, rather than beginning the bandage at midarm or midleg.
- Bandage an extremity *toward* the body to avoid congestion and interferences with circulation in the distal part of the extremity.
- Apply the bandage or binder securely enough so that it does not move about on the patient and cause friction with the skin.
- Do not apply a binder used on the chest so snugly that it interferes with breathing.
- Apply a bandage or binder over a wet dressing or a draining wound less tightly than usual. If the bandage or binder becomes wet, it is likely to shrink and become too tight for safety and comfort.
- Avoid an unnecessarily thick or extensive bandage. It will not be comfortable for the patient. Also, heavy and extensive bandaging makes the area unnecessarily warm.
- Place pins, clips, and knots used to secure the bandage or binder well away from a wound or a tender and inflamed area. Also, place them so that they do not cause unnecessary pressure on a part of the body. For example, a knot to secure a sling should be placed near the shoulder rather than over the cervical portion of the spine.
- Check bandages and binders at regular intervals, including the times when the patient is asleep. Note the circulation and see that the patient is in proper body alignment. If a bandage or binder has loosened or slipped out of place, reapply it whenever necessary.

Applying a Roller Bandage. A **roller bandage** is a continuous strip of material wound on itself to form a cylinder or roll. These rolls are prepared in various widths and lengths. The free end of the roll is the initial extremity while the terminal end is in the center of the roll. The rolled portion is called the body. The outer surface of the bandage is placed next to the patient's skin. When the bandage is begun, the initial

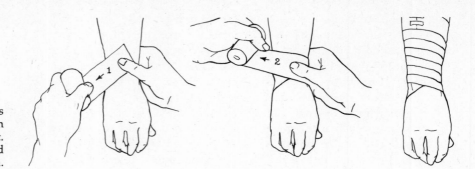

Fig. 18-3. (Left) Note that bandage is started obliquely at the wrist and then (center) anchored around the wrist. (Right) The spiral turn has been used on the forearm.

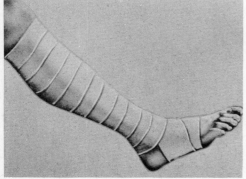

Fig. 18-4. Elastic roller bandage applied to the leg, using spiral turns. (Becton, Dickinson & Co., Rutherford, N. J.)

end is held in place with one hand while the other hand passes the roll around the part. Once the bandage is anchored, the body of the roll may be passed from hand to hand, care being taken that equal tension is exerted with each turn. It is easier to keep the tension equal by unwinding the bandage gradually and only as it is required. There are five basic turns used when applying roller bandages. They may be used separately or in any combination, depending on the purpose and the part being bandaged.

The **circular turn** encircles the part. The body of the bandage is returned to the exact point of starting on the first turn; the second turn completely overlaps the first; the third turn completely overlaps the second; and so on. The area covered is equal in width to the width of the bandage. This turn is used most frequently for anchoring the bandage when it is started and when it is ended.

An adaptation of the circular turn is often used for starting a spiral or figure-of-eight turn. The extremity of the bandage is crossed obliquely by the first turn, as illustrated in Figure 18-3.

For the **spiral turn,** each turn only partly overlaps the previous turn. The overlapping varies from one-half to three-fourths of the width of the bandage, depending on the purpose of the bandage. The turn is used most frequently when the part is cylindrical in shape. Examples include the fingers, forearm, leg, chest, and abdomen. The spiral turn is illustrated in Figures 18-3 and 18-4.

The **spiral-reverse turn** is a spiral turn in which reverses are made halfway through each turn. Spiral-reverse turns are particularly effective for bandaging a cone-shaped part, such as the thigh, leg, or forearm. Figure 18-5 illustrates this turn. The position of the nurse's thumb on the bandage shows the manner in which the reverse is made. This type of turn takes up the slack on the lower border of the bandage.

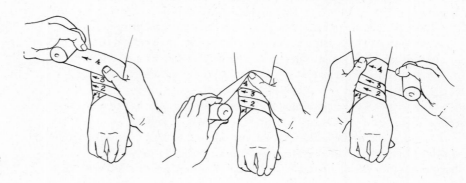

Fig. 18-5. Procedure for making the spiral-reverse turn.

Measures to promote tissue healing

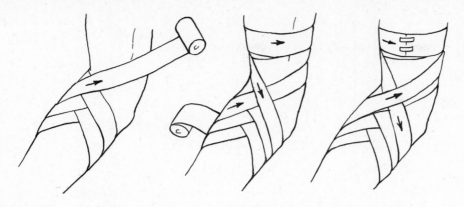

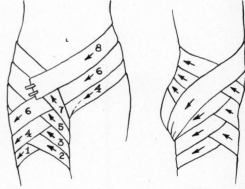

Fig. 18-6   Procedure for making the figure-of-eight turn.

The **figure-of-eight turn** consists of making oblique overlapping turns that ascend and descend alternately. Each turn crosses the one preceding it so that it resembles the figure eight. Figures 18-6 and 18-7 show how this turn is made. It is effective for use around joints, such as the knee, elbow, ankle, and wrist. It provides for a snug bandage and therefore is often used for immobilization.

The spica is an adaptation of the figure-of-eight turn. It consists of ascending and descending turns with all turns overlapping and crossing each other to form a sharp angle. It is particularly useful for bandaging the thumb, breast, shoulder, groin, and hip. Figure 18-8 illustrates its application.

The **recurrent turn** is used for bandaging rounded surfaces, such as the head or the stump of an amputated limb. After a few circular turns to anchor the bandage, the initial extremity of the bandage is placed in the center of the part being bandaged, well back from the tip to be covered. The body of the bandage is passed back and forth over the tip, first on one side and then on the other side of the center piece of bandage. Figure 18-9 illustrates the manner of applying a recurrent bandage to a stump. The last drawing in the Figure shows the use of the figure-of-eight turn to finish the bandage. Figure 18-10 shows an elastic bandage applied to a stump. Recurrent bandages are also used effectively for the head.

Whichever turn is being used, the tension on each turn should be equal. Unnecessary and uneven overlapping of turns should be avoided. All skin should be covered by the finished bandage to prevent pinching skin between turns. It should be completed well away from the wound or inflamed or tender area. The terminal end of the bandage may be secured with adhesive, clamps, by tying a bow, by sewing, or with safety pins. None of these methods of terminating the bandage should be done in a way that produces pressure on the patient's skin or over the wound.

Removing Roller Bandages. When the bandaging material is not to be reused, the bandage may be cut open with bandage scissors. Cutting should be done on the side opposite the injury or wound, from one end to the other, so that the bandage can be folded open for its entire length. If the material is to be reclaimed, it may be unwound by keeping the loose end together and passing it as a ball from one hand to the other while unwinding.

Applying Binders. A **T binder** looks like the letter T. A single T binder has a tail attached at right angles to a belt. A double T binder has two tails attached to the belt. T binders are particularly effective for

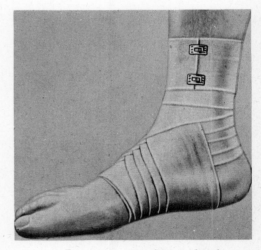

Fig. 18-7   The figure-of-eight turn used to apply elastic bandage to the ankle. (Becton, Dickinson & Co., Rutherford, N. J.)

Fig. 18-8   Procedure for making the spica bandage.

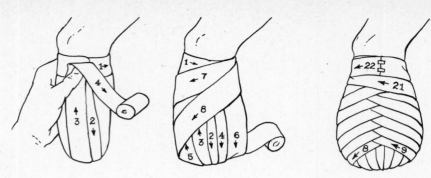

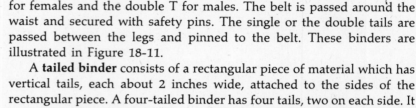

Fig. 18-9   Procedure for making a re-current bandage to cover a stump.

securing dressings on the perineum and in the groin. The single T is used for females and the double T for males. The belt is passed around the waist and secured with safety pins. The single or the double tails are passed between the legs and pinned to the belt. These binders are illustrated in Figure 18-11.

A **tailed binder** consists of a rectangular piece of material which has vertical tails, each about 2 inches wide, attached to the sides of the rectangular piece. A four-tailed binder has four tails, two on each side. It is useful for securing dressings on the nose and chin and is illustrated in Figure 18-12.

Many-tailed binders are called **scultetus binders.** They are used on the abdomen and chest. When a scultetus binder is applied to the abdomen, the patient lies on his back and on the center of the binder. The lower end of the binder is placed well down on the hips but not so low that it will interfere with the use of a bedpan or with walking. The tails are brought out to either side of the patient's body with the bottom tail in position to wrap around the lower part of the abdomen first. A tail from each side is brought up and placed obliquely over the abdomen until all tails are in place. The last tails are fastened with safety pins. Figure 18-13 illustrates the application of a scultetus binder to the abdomen.

A **straight binder** is a rectangular piece of material, usually about 6 to 8 inches wide and long enough to more than circle the body. It is generally used for the chest and abdomen. Straight binders must be applied so as to fit the contours of the body. This is usually done by making small tucks in the binder as necessary. In some instances, these tucks can be secured with safety pins. A straight binder for the chest often is provided with shoulder straps so that it will not slip down on the trunk.

A **sling** is a triangular binder. It is usually made of muslin in varying

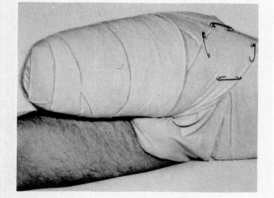

Fig. 18-10   Elastic bandage used to dress a stump. (Becton, Dickinson & Co., Rutherford, N. J.)

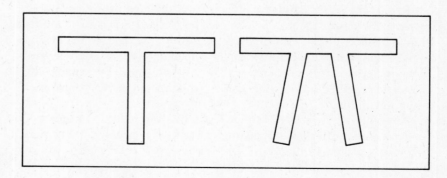

Fig. 18-11   (Left) The single T binder. (Right) The double T binder.

Measures to promote tissue healing

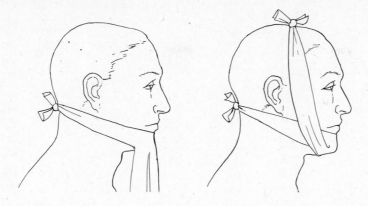

Fig. 18-12   Four-tailed binder.

sizes. For most adults, a 36- to 40-inch square cut in half diagonally to form two triangles is a common size. Figure 18-14 illustrates a triangular binder used as a sling (see p. 386).

To apply a sling, the open triangle is placed on the chest. One end of the base of the triangle is placed over the shoulder on the uninjured side and to the back of the neck. The apex or point of the triangle is placed under the arm on the affected side. The last end of the triangle is brought around the affected arm and over the shoulder on the same side. The ends are tied behind the neck with the knot at either side of the cervical spine. The material at the elbow is folded neatly and may be secured with a pin placed behind the sling so that it will be out of sight.

Triangular binders may also be made into mittens for covering foot and hand dressings. They are also useful for bandaging the head, shoulders, and hips. Occasionally, two triangular binders may be used if the area is large.

A **cravat binder** is made by folding a triangular binder over and over upon itself, starting at the apex, until the desired width is obtained. A cravat may be used as a small sling. It is also used on limbs and on the head. It is useful as a tourniquet and as a temporary measure to support a sprained joint. It is illustrated in Figure 18-15 (see p. 386).

Local applications of heat and cold

Before applying heat or cold to the body, the nurse will wish to be familiar with certain background facts in order to give safe care.

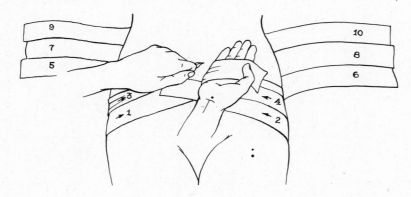

Fig. 18-13   Procedure for applying a many-tailed binder.

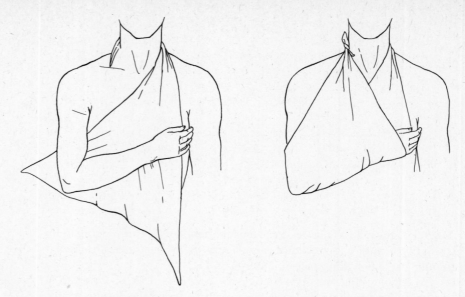

Fig. 18-14   Triangular binder used as a sling to support the arm.

- Nerve receptors for heat and cold lie in the skin. An important characteristic of heat and cold receptors is that they adjust readily if the stimulus is not extreme. For example, if the arm is placed in warm water, the sensation of warmth soon diminishes because of the adaptability of the heat receptors. The same phenomenon occurs if cool water is used. This is important to remember. Once the receptors adapt, the patient may become unaware of temperature extremes until tissue damage occurs. The patient usually is not familiar with this adaptability process and will often wish to increase the heat or cold beyond the point of safety.

- The temperature that the skin can tolerate varies with individuals. Some can tolerate warmer and colder applications more safely than can others. Certain areas of the skin are also more tolerant of temperature than are others. Those parts of the body where the skin is thinner, for example the chest and abdomen, generally are more

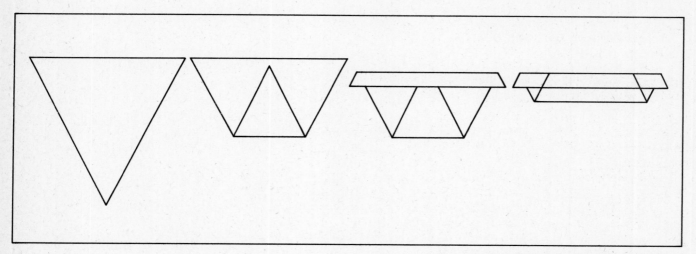

Fig. 18-15   Left to right, a cravat being made from a triangular binder.

Measures to promote tissue healing

sensitive to temperature than exposed areas where the skin is often thicker. Therefore, it is important to apply warm and cold applications well within the generally known safe limits of temperature. But, in addition, the skin should be observed so that persons who are more sensitive to temperature will not suffer tissue damage, even though applications have been applied within recommended temperature ranges.

- Heat and cold are transferred directly from one substance to another by conduction. A poor conductor is called an **insulator.** Water is a relatively good conductor of heat while air is a poorer conductor. Therefore, the skin will tolerate greater extremes of temperature if the heat or cold is dry rather than moist. For example, a moist hot dressing should be applied at a lower temperature than a cloth-covered hot-water bag in order to prevent burning the skin. The air between the bag and the dry cloth acts as an insulator.

- The body tolerates greater extremes in temperature when the duration of exposure is short. When duration is lengthy, the temperature range that the body can tolerate safely is narrower. The area involved is also important. In general, the larger the area to which heat or cold is applied, the less tolerant is the skin to the extreme in temperature.

- The condition of the patient is an important factor to consider when heat and cold are being applied to the body. Special care is indicated for patients who are debilitated and unconscious. The very young and the very old do not tolerate heat and cold well. Patients who have disturbances in circulation are more sensitive to heat and cold. Broken skin areas are also more subject to tissue damage and less tolerant of heat and cold.

- The immediate effect of cold applications is that blood vessels in the area constrict or become smaller. The prolonged use of cold causes vessels to dilate or become larger. The opposite occurs when heat is applied: the immediate effect is blood vessel dilation while prolonged use causes blood vessels to constrict. Therefore, applications should not be left in place for long periods of time. The recommended durations for various heat and cold applications are given when they are described later in this chapter.

- Cold is commonly used immediately following bruises, sprains, and strains in order to limit the accumulation of fluid in body tissue. If edema is already present, the application of cold will act to retard its relief since circulating blood in the area will be at a minimum and excess fluid will not be reabsorbed as efficiently. The application of cold will aid in controlling hemorrhage by constricting vessels. Cold has anesthetic value and can be used for this purpose in some surgical applications. Lower temperatures are also used for limiting inflammation and pus formation, inhibiting activity of microorganisms, and reducing body temperature.

- Heat applied for its local effects is used very often for the relief of pain, congestion, inflammation, and muscle spasms. Healing is often promoted by improved circulation to an injured area. Local heat also may be applied for comfort when patients feel chilly.

Applications of Cold. No one optimum temperature can be stated for cold applications. The selection of temperature depends on such factors as the duration of the application, the method of the application, the condition of the patient, the condition and sensitivity of the skin, and the area to be covered. For short periods of time and for small areas, colder temperatures can be tolerated without discomfort or tissue damage. For longer periods, it is usually considered dangerous to keep skin temperatures below 40°F. except when ice is used for anesthesia.

The temperature of water used for cold applications usually is described as tepid, cool, cold, or very cold. The temperature ranges stated frequently are as follows:

Tepid	80 to 93°F.
Cool	65 to 80°F.
Cold	50 to 65°F.
Very cold	Below 50°F.

Ice bags

The device used frequently for applying cold to an area is the rubber or plastic ice bag. Ice collars are smaller than most ice bags and are used for the neck and other small areas.

The ice bag or collar is filled with small pieces of ice, making it easier to mold to the contour of the body part. Also, chips reduce the amount of air which acts as an insulator. Water is run over cubes or chips to eliminate sharp edges. After the bag or collar is approximately one-half to two-thirds full, excess air is removed by twisting the top and then capping the bag or collar. Leaks are checked for at this time.

A covering is placed on the ice bag or collar to make it more comfortable for the patient and also to provide for absorption of the moisture which condenses on the outside of the bag. Some bags are made with a soft cover, making a second covering unnecessary.

Commercially prepared cold packs are available. They retain a constant degree of cold for several hours.

To be effective as a local application, the ice bag or collar should be applied for one-half to one hour and removed for approximately one hour. In this way, the tissues are able to react to the immediate effects of the cold. Signs of excessive cold include mottled and pale skin and numbness in the area being treated.

Cold compresses

Moist, cold, local applications are usually referred to as cold compresses. They might be used for an injured eye, headache, or tooth extraction. The texture and thickness of the material used will depend on the area to which the compress will be applied. For example, eye compresses could be prepared from surgical gauze compresses which have a small amount of cotton filling. A washcloth makes a good compress for the head or face.

The material used for the application is immersed in a clean basin, appropriate for the size of the compress, that contains pieces of ice and a small amount of water. The compress should be wrung thoroughly before it is applied in order to avoid dripping, which is uncomfortable for the patient and may also wet the bed and clothing. The compresses should be changed frequently. Usually, the patient can feel when they have become warm, and many patients like to apply their own compresses. The application should be continued for 15 to 20 minutes and repeated every two to three hours. The use of ice bags or certain commercial devices for keeping the compresses cold limits the frequency with which they must be changed.

Alcohol or cold sponge bath

There may be times when an alcohol or a cold sponge bath is recommended for reducing the patient's elevated temperature. It is more common in home situations than in health agencies. Alcohol added to tepid water is tolerated more easily than a cold bath by most patients. Alcohol vaporizes more quickly than water and therefore removes heat from the skin surfaces rapidly.

When an alcohol or cold sponge bath is given, it is important that it be continued until the initial reaction of chilliness, or shivering, is overcome and the body has adjusted to the temperature. Therefore, it is best if the procedure lasts for about 25 to 30 minutes. Each extremity should be bathed for a five-minute period at least, and then the entire back and buttocks for an additional five to ten minutes. The chest and abdomen are not bathed. The patient is draped and bed linens are protected as for a bed bath. It is handy to have two washcloths for this procedure. While using one, the other is cooling in the water.

During the procedure, moist, cool cloths are placed over large superficial blood vessels, as in the axillae and groin, as a further aid in lowering the temperature. Warmth placed at the feet helps to overcome a sensation of chilliness. To help provide comfort, an ice bag may be applied to the patient's head.

Hypothermia

Lowered body temperature is referred to as **hypothermia.** The cooling baths just described are intended to lower body temperature. However, mechanically operated blankets and pads through which a thermostatically controlled solution is circulated are used in many health agencies to produce hypothermia. The manufacturers' instructions and agency procedures should be observed since each type of equipment operates slightly differently. It is important that the patient's temperature be checked frequently. The cooling device is removed as the patient's temperature approaches the desired level. Ice packs placed in the axillae and groin may be used simultaneously. A drug may also be ordered which acts to depress the heat-regulating center in the brain, thereby helping to lower body temperature.

Applications of Heat. It is true of applying heat as well as cold that the optimum temperature for local applications cannot be stated arbitrarily. The condition and sensitivity of the skin, the size of the area being covered, the duration of the application, the method of applying heat, the condition of the patient, and the differences in heat tolerance need to be considered. When the temperature of the skin surpasses approximately 110°F., many individuals are likely to suffer burns.

The temperature of water used for applications is described usually as warm or neutral, hot, and very hot. The temperature ranges stated frequently are as follows:

Warm or neutral	93 to 98°F.
Hot	98 to 105°F.
Very hot	105 to 115°F.

PERMIT FOR USING ELECTRICAL APPLIANCES

I hereby agree that in using _A HEATING PAD_

and similar appliances in my room while a patient _Pine Memorial Hospital_, I do so at my own risk and hereby absolve the said hospital from any and all responsibility from burns, injuries or property damage which may result from or because of said appliance.

Signed _Helen Jones_

Date _JULY 16, 1974_ Hour _2:05 P_ .M. Witness _Jane Doe L.P.N._

Permit for Using Electrical Appliances

Fig. 18-16 An example of a form used by some health agencies that permits a patient to use a heating pad while freeing the agency of responsibility.

Measures to promote tissue healing

Electric heating pads

The electric heating pad is a popular means for applying dry heat locally. It is easy to use, provides constant and even heat, and is relatively safe when used properly. Careless handling can result in injury to the patient or the nurse, as well as damage to the pad.

Because of possible injury, many health agencies have a policy that prohibits the use of heating pads. If the patient insists on using one, the health agency requires him to sign a release to free the hospital of responsibility. An example of such a release is illustrated in Figure 18-16.

Since heating pads are commonly used in the home and in some agencies, the nurse should be familiar with their proper use. The heating element of an electric pad consists of a web of wires that converts electric current into heat. Crushing or creasing the wires may impair proper functioning, and portions of the pad will overheat. Burns or a fire may result. Pins should be avoided for securing the pad since there is danger of electric shock if a pin touches the wires. Pads with waterproof coverings are preferred, but they should not be operated in a wet or moist condition because of the danger of short-circuiting the heating element and consequently causing electric shock.

Heating pads for home use have the selector switch for controlling the heat within easy reach of the patient. After the heat has been applied and a certain amount of depression of nerve endings in the skin has taken place, the patient often increases the heat. Many persons have been burned in this manner. Health agencies which use heating pads usually have preset pads which cannot be set at temperatures that may burn the patient.

Heating pads should be covered with flannel or similar material. This helps to make the heat more comfortable for the patient. The pad can be used repeatedly when the cover is washed after each patient's use. However, it is important not to cover the pad too heavily, for heavy covering over an electric pad prevents adequate heat dissipation. The patient should not lie on a heating pad; heat will accumulate and may cause burns.

The devices described earlier which produce hypothermia may also be used to apply heat. To do so, the circulating fluid is heated and kept at an even temperature. Pads are useful on wet dressings when heat is applied.

Hot-water bags

Many health agencies do not allow the use of hot-water bags. Too often, they have been used carelessly and patients have been burned. However, they are commonly found in the home and the nurse should be familiar with their proper use.

It is considered essential to test the temperature of water accurately with a thermometer before pouring it into the bag. A safe temperature range for infants under two years of age is from 105 to 115°F.; for older children and adults, from 115 to 125°F.

To keep the bag easy to mold to body areas and as light as possible in weight, the nurse should fill it about two-thirds full. The air remaining in the bag must then be expelled. To do this, the nurse places the bag on a flat surface and permits the water to come to the opening; she then closes the bag. Or, she holds the bag up, twists the unfilled portion to remove the air, and then closes it. She holds the bag upside down to check for leaks, and applies a flannel cover to the bag before placing it on a body part. In order that the patient may feel warmth immediately, the cover may be warmed before it is placed on the bag.

Many patients seem to think that the water is not hot enough. Unless the patient receives a better explanation than that the temperature is correct, it is likely that the bag may be filled from the hot-water tap when the nurse is not around. If the patient cannot do it, a visitor or family member may oblige.

Miscellaneous methods of applying dry heat

A cradle with an electric light bulb enclosed in a metal frame is sometimes used to apply dry heat to extremities. It is a good way, for example, to help circulation in an extremity, to provide general warmth for the patient, and to help dry a cast. The bulb should be 25 watts and placed no closer to the patient than 2 to 3 feet.

Ultraviolet and infrared lamps can also be used to apply dry heat. Diathermy, which produces heat in tissues by the use of high-frequency currents, may be used. Generally, trained workers are responsible for using diathermy and ultraviolet and infrared lamps. But the nurse will wish to observe the patient's reactions to these types of heat applications.

Hip or sitz baths

As a means of applying tepid or hot water to the pelvic area, patients are often placed in tubs filled with sufficient water to reach the umbilicus. These baths are referred to as hip or sitz baths. Special tubs and chairs or basins are available which are designed so that the patient's buttocks fit into a rather deep seat which is filled with water of the desired temperature. The legs and feet remain out of the water. These appliances may be disposable and are practical for both home and agency use. A regular bathtub is not as satisfactory for a sitz bath because the heat is applied also to the legs. This alters the effect desired in the pelvic region.

If the purpose of the sitz bath is to apply heat, water at a temperature of 110 to 115°F. for 15 minutes will produce relaxation of the parts involved after a short initial period of contraction. Warm water is not used if considerable congestion is already present.

If the purpose of the sitz bath is to produce relaxation or to help promote healing in a wound by cleansing it of discharge and dead tissue, water at a temperature of 94 to 98°F. is used. The temperature of the water should be tested frequently to prevent too great a range from occurring.

Since a large body area is involved when a sitz bath is given, the patient should be observed closely for signs of weakness and faintness. The nature of the procedure also makes it necessary to protect the patient from exposure. Usually, a bath blanket is wrapped around his shoulders and draped over the tub. After the bath, the patient should be covered adequately and encouraged to remain out of drafts. It is preferable for him to rest until normal circulation has returned.

Sitz tubs and chairs are not adjustable to the comfort needs of patients, especially short patients. After the patient is in the tub or chair, he should be checked to see that there is no undue pressure against the thighs and legs. If the feet do not touch the floor, and the weight of the legs is resting on the edge of the chair or tub, the patient should be provided with a stool to support the feet and relieve pressure on vessels in the legs.

It may be necessary to place a towel in the water to support the patient's back in the lumbar region. Fifteen to 20 minutes can seem like a very long time if one's body is not comfortable and in good alignment.

Soaks

Placing part of the body in water or a medicated solution is referred to as a soak. If a soak is prescribed for a large wound, such as one which covers an entire arm or lower leg or even an area of the torso, a compromise with sterile technique may be necessary. The vessel into which the body area is placed is sterilized before use if possible. If this is not possible, the vessel should be cleaned scrupulously. Tap water may be used for soaks since it is generally accepted as free from pathogens.

During the treatment, which is usually 15 to 20 minutes per soak, the temperature should be kept as constant as possible. This may be done by discarding some of the fluid every five minutes or so and replacing it with solution at a higher temperature. But care must be taken to avoid burning the patient. When hot solution is added, the nurse stirs or otherwise agitates it into the cooler solution quickly to prevent discomfort or tissue damage. Unless otherwise ordered, a temperature range of 105 to 110°F. is used.

The vessel holding the solution should be placed so that the part to be immersed is comfortable and the patient is in good body alignment. For example, an arm basin placed on top of the bedside stand may cause the patient's shoulder to be thrown out of alignment. It may also cause pressure on the back of the patient's arm. Or, a hand basin may be so situated as to cause wrist fatigue. Whenever a soak basin is placed in position, the nurse should look for pressure areas and assist the patient to a comfortable position.

Local applications of heat and cold

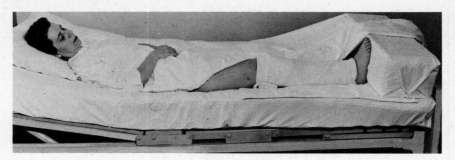

Fig. 18-17. In applying heat or cold to any body area, keep it in good alignment to prevent fatigue. Here the foot is kept free from the leg wrapping so that it may be supported in dorsiflexion. A small towel under the knee gives support but is placed to avoid popliteal pressure. The weight of a large pack often restricts motion and contributes to fatigue.

Hot moist packs and compresses

The application of warm moist cloths to a body area is referred to as a pack. Warm moist gauze dressings are called compresses. Packs usually are applied to a more extensive area than are compresses. Packs and compresses differ from soaks primarily in two ways: the duration of the application of packs and compresses is usually longer, and the initial application of heat is more intense. Packs and compresses usually are applied as hot as the patient can tolerate them comfortably.

Depending on the situation, a pack or compress may be applied using sterile technique. If so, all materials and the solution must be sterile, and the person applying the pack wears sterile gloves. Or, in the case of compresses, the dressings may be wrung out with sterile forceps.

If an area is to be kept warm, the frequency of the change of such applications will depend on the thickness of the material and the amount of protection used. A mechanical heating device can be used to maintain the temperature of the pack or compress. However, it must be remembered that to avoid tissue damage, a lower temperature for applying moist heat should be used than when dry heat is applied.

Because of the effect of the hot application on circulation, the patient is likely to feel chilly. Comfort measures should be taken during and following treatment to keep the patient warm and free from drafts, especially in the area which has been treated.

Figure 18-17 illustrates a patient with a leg pack supported in good alignment. Chart 18-2 describes applying a hot pack.

Irrigations

An irrigation is a flowing solution directed over an area. The purpose of the irrigation may be to cleanse the area and/or to apply local heat or antiseptic. Ear, eye, and vaginal irrigations are most commonly performed. Open wound irrigations are sometimes done to promote débridement.

The circumstances of the area determine the type of solution used. Water, normal saline, and antiseptic solutions are commonly used. Generally, if there are no breaks in the skin or mucous membrane, practices of medical asepsis are observed. If there is an open wound, sterile technique is used.

Eye Irrigation. An eye irrigation is usually done with normal saline for cleansing purposes. Mild antiseptic solutions may be prescribed if an infection is present.

Chart 18-2 Applying hot moist packs to a body area
The purpose is to apply hot moist heat to an area to produce changes in the blood vessels and the underlying tissues

Suggested Action	Reason for Action
Prepare material, preferably wool, of sufficient size to cover area well.	Materials with loosely woven fibers hold moisture well and trap air between fibers.
Prepare hot-water bag, heating pad, or other heating device if one is to be used over pack, according to agency policy	External heat helps to keep pack warm.
Place dry pack and waterproof cover under extremity or near area where pack is to be applied. Dry pack will cover moist one and waterproof material will be on outside. N.B. Some procedures recommend dry pack on outside and waterproof material next to wet pack: observe local policy.	Dry pack and waterproof cover will act as insulators and will prevent rapid heat and moisture loss from wet pack.
Lubricate skin in area of application with petrolatum if desired and if skin is not broken.	Petrolatum acts as insulator to delay transmission of intense heat from pack to skin, thus helping to avoid burning patient.
Immerse packs in hot water until they are saturated.	Allowing material to become saturated provides even heat by avoiding dry areas in pack.
Wring hot wet packs as dry as possible.	Saturated packs can burn patient with water.
Shake pack once or twice quickly.	Incorporating air into material acts as insulator to help keep pack warm and prevent patient from being burned with water.
Place pack on skin lightly, and after a few seconds, lift pack to inspect patient's skin for degree of redness.	Watching skin closely before wrapping outside pack around wet pack helps prevent burning of patient.
Wrap pack around area well and mold it to skin surface.	Air spaces between skin and pack will reduce the effect of application.
Cover moist pack with dry pack and waterproof material. Secure in place with safety pins or ties.	Insulation and covering help prevent heat and moisture loss.
Apply hot-water bag, heating device, or heating pad to area in a manner so weight is not increased over injured area. Leave in place for prescribed period of time.	External heat helps maintain pack temperature. Weight of heat supply over injured area can cause fatigue and discomfort.

Chart 18-3 Administering an eye irrigation
The purpose is to cleanse the eye

Suggested Action	Reason for Action
Prepare 2 to 8 ounces of physician's or agency's choice of solution at about body temperature, 100°F.	Amount of solution for cleansing depends on amount of material present to be removed.
Have patient sit or lie with his head tilted toward side of affected eye so that solution will flow from inner canthus of affected eye toward outer canthus near forehead.	Gravity will aid flow of solution away from unaffected eye and help prevent spread of material from eye to eye. Solution directed toward outer canthus aids in preventing spread of contamination to lacrimal sac and duct and nose.
Cleanse lids and lashes with normal saline or solution ordered for irrigation.	Materials lodged on lids and lashes may be washed into eye if not removed.
Place curved basin at cheek on side of affected eye to receive irrigating solution.	Gravity will direct flow of solution into basin.
Expose lower conjunctival sac and hold upper eyelid open.	To avoid possible injury to cornea, solution is directed onto lower conjunctival sac—not onto eyeball. Patient usually is unable to hold upper eyelid open during irrigation.
Direct flow of solution from inner canthus to outer canthus along lower conjunctival sac.	Solution directed toward outer canthus aids in preventing spread of contamination to lacrimal sac and duct and nose.
Use only sufficient force of solution to *gently* remove secretions from conjunctival sac.	Directing solutions with force may cause injury to tissues of eye.
Avoid touching any part of eye with irrigating tip.	Eye is easily injured. Touching eye is uncomfortable for patient.
Have patient close his eye periodically during proceudre.	Movement of eye when lids are closed helps move secretions from upper conjunctival sac to lower.
Continue irrigating lower conjunctival sac for duration of treatment.	Length of irrigation depends on cleansing effect desired.
After irrigating, have patient close his eye and wipe excess solution from lid and lashes.	Excess moisture on lids and lashes is uncomfortable for patient.

Several methods may be used for irrigating the eye. An eyedropper is satisfactory when small amounts of solution are used. For large amounts, a soft, rubber bulb syringe is appropriate. For home use, an eyecup, washed scrupulously after each use, usually is convenient. In an emergency, squeezing the solution from a soaked cotton ball offers a satisfactory method of irrigation. Chart 18-3 describes an eye irrigation.

Ear Irrigation. Irrigations of the external canal of the ear with normal saline generally are done for cleansing purposes. Antiseptic solutions are sometimes used for their local action. Irrigations may also be used for applying heat to the ear.

An irrigating container with tubing and an eartip may be used. The

Measures to promote tissue healing

container should be kept just high enough to allow a gentle flow of solution. An eartip fits easily into the external canal and has two extensions: one for the solution to enter the canal and the other for it to leave the canal and drain into a receiving basin. A soft, rubber bulb syringe is often used. It allows solution to enter and leave the ear simultaneously. It is not usually as comfortable for the patient since the flow of solution must be interrupted during the irrigation while the syringe is refilled. A metal or Pomeroy syringe is available in some agencies. This syringe requires careful use to prevent excess pressure when directing solutions into the ear. Chart 18-4 describes an ear irrigation.

Vaginal Irrigation. An irrigation of the vagina is usually referred to as a **douche**. An irrigation with normal saline is usually done for cleansing purposes. It may also be done to apply heat or an antiseptic to the area.

An irrigating container or bag connected with tubing to an irrigating nozzle is ordinarily used. Irrigating nozzles are curved to fit the normal contour of the vagina and are generally made of plastic. The nozzle should be inspected before use to prevent injury should it be damaged.

A large bulb fitted onto a nozzle is often used for home douching. The bulb is filled with solution and then squeezed to force solution into

Chart 18-4 Administering an ear irrigation
The purpose is to cleanse the external ear canal

Suggested Action	Reason for Action
Prepare about 500 ml. of physician's or agency's choice of solution at about body temperature, 100°F.	This amount of solution usually is sufficient for cleansing. Solutions warmer or cooler than body temperature feel uncomfortable, may injure tissue, and may cause nausea and dizziness.
Have patient sit up or lie with his head tilted toward side of affected ear. Have patient support basin under his ear to receive irrigating solution.	Gravity causes irrigating solution to flow from ear to basin.
Cleanse outer ear and meatus at entrance to ear canal as necessary with normal saline or irrigating solution.	Materials lodged on ear and at meatus may be washing into ear canal during irrigation.
Fill syringe with solution. If an irrigating can is used, allow air to escape from tubing.	Air forced into ear is noisy and therefore unpleasant for patient.
Straighten ear canal by pulling ear downward and backward for infants and upward and backward for adults.	Straightening ear canal aids in allowing solution to reach all areas of canal.
Direct steady slow stream of solution against roof of canal, using only sufficient force to remove secretions.	Solution directed at roof of canal helps prevent injury to tympanic membrane and prevents pushing material into canal.
Do not close off ear canal with irrigating nozzle.	Continuous in-and-out flow of solution helps prevent undue pressure in canal.
At completion of treatment have patient lie on affected side with a small dressing or cotton ball under the ear.	Gravity allows remaining solution in canal to escape from ear.

Chart 18-5 Administering a vaginal irrigation
The purpose is to cleanse the vagina

Suggested Action	Reason for Action
Prepare 1500 to 2000 ml. of physician's or agency's choice of solution at a temperature of 110 to 115°F.	This amount of solution usually is sufficient for cleansing. Vagina tolerates relatively high temperature but membranes around meatus do not.
Have patient void before beginning irrigation.	Full bladder interferes with distention of vagina with solution.
Place patient in dorsal recumbent position. Remove all but one pillow and lower head of bed. Place patient on bedpan so that hips are higher than vaginal meatus.*	Gravity will cause solution to flow into all portions of vagina. With elevated hips, solution will distend vaginal walls so that all areas are reached with solution.
Arrange irrigating container at a level just above patient's hips about 12 inches above meatus so that solution flows easily and gently.	Undue force could drive solution and contamination into uterus.
Cleanse vulva by separating labia and allowing solution to flow over area. If this does not seem sufficient, wash area with a soap or detergent and water solution.	Materials lodged around vaginal meatus can be introduced into vagina.
Permit some solution to run through tubing and out over end of nozzle to lubricate it.	Moist surface on nozzle causes less friction for easier and more comfortable insertion.
Gently rotate nozzle in vagina during irrigation.	Movement of nozzle aids in directing solution to all surfaces of vagina.
Place patient on absorbent pad after irrigation.	Remaining solution in vagina will drain to outside.

*Patients being taught how to give themselves a douche at home should be instructed to lie in a bathtub. Administering a douche while sitting on the toilet will not result in a thorough cleansing.

Chart 18-6 Administering an open wound irrigation
The purpose is to cleanse the wound

Suggested Action	Reason for Action
Practices of surgical asepsis are used when caring for an open wound.	Organisms introduced into wound are likely to result in wound infection or increased problems if infection is already present.
Prepare solution of physician's or agency's choice, usually 100 to 200 ml., at about 90 to 95°F.	Warmer solution may injure tissue. Colder solution may cause patient to feel chilly.
Remove soiled dressings as described in Chart 18-1, p. 376.	
Place patient in position so solution will flow from wound down to basin held below wound.	Gravity carries contaminated solution away from wound and into basin.
Irrigate wound generously but carefully, being sure to irrigate pockets in wound.	Solution will wash away organisms, tissue debris, and drainage. Irrigating with undue pressure may injure tissue.
Cleanse skin around wound as described in Chart 18-1, being careful not to touch wound.	Organisms normally present on skin should not be carried to wound where infection may develop.

Protect skin, dress wound, and secure dressing as described earlier in this chapter.

the vagina. This type of equipment is not generally recommended. There is a danger of using too much pressure which could cause solution to enter the uterus. Chart 18-5 describes a vaginal irrigation.

Wound Irrigation. Open wounds are occasionally irrigated for the cleansing effect of the flowing solution. Generally, tissue debris exists and its mechanical removal with solution will help hasten healing.

A large syringe without a needle or a bulb syringe may be used. Care should be taken that the solution flows directly into the wound and not over a contaminated area before entering the wound. Following irrigation, a sterile dressing is generally applied to the wound. Chart 18-6 describes a wound irrigation.

Teaching the patient to care for injured tissues

Patients with tissue injuries often are not hospitalized or may return home before wounds are healed. Therefore, they or family members need to learn to care for injured tissue.

The nature and the amount of teaching in relation to wound care will depend on individual circumstances. Nurses have observed that patients usually are concerned about odor from dressings, discomfort, and fear of soiling clothing when drainage is present. Other disturbing factors include fear that dressings will slip out of place and cause infection, concern for the reaction of friends and family to the appearance of dressings, and the cost of dressings.

It is too often taken for granted that patients who are to use heat or cold applications know how to do so without assistance. The nurse will wish to be sure these patients understand the dangers of using heat or cold to excess. Patients should also be taught signs that indicate heat or cold may be damaging tissue.

Patients who will use irrigations also need the nurse's help. They should understand the importance of using the correct solution at the proper temperature. The nurse should be sure that the patient understands the dangers of introducing solutions under too much pressure.

Conclusion

Tissue trauma is a common occurrence. The ability of the body to contain and heal the injury is remarkable. Nevertheless, the nurse plays an important role in using measures to promote healing and to teach patients how they can best help with the healing process.

References

Beaumont, Estelle, "Product Survey: Hypo/Hyperthermia Equipment," *Nursing '74*, 4:34–41, April 1974.

Laughlin, Victor C., "Doing It Better: Stopping the Constant Drip of Draining Wounds," *Nursing '74*, 4:26–27, December 1974.

Petrello, Judith M., "Temperature Maintenance of Hot Moist Compresses," *American Journal of Nursing*, 73:1050–1051, June 1973.

Powell, Mary, "An Environment for Wound Healing," *American Journal of Nursing*, 72:1862–1865, October 1972.

Rinear, Charles E. and Rinear, Eileen E., "Emergency Bandaging: A Wrap-Up of Better Techniques," *Nursing '75*, 5:29–35, January 1975.

Wallace, Gladys and Hayter, Jean, "Karaya for Chronic Skin Ulcers," *American Journal of Nursing*, 74:1094–1098, June 1974.

19 measures to promote respiratory functioning

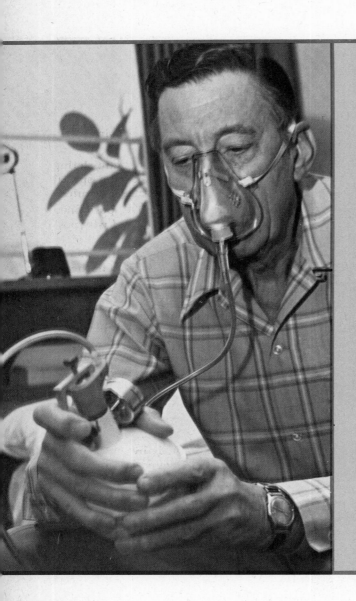

chapter outline

behavioral objectives

When mastery of content in this chapter is reached, the student will be able to

Define terms appearing in the glossary.

List three conditions for which patients may require oxygen therapy.

List five common symptoms of anoxia.

Describe why oxygen is humidified while it is being administered.

State safety precautions that are observed in the patient's room to help prevent accidents when oxygen is administered.

Describe how and why an oxygen tank is "cracked."

Describe how oxygen is administered by each of the following means: a nasal cannula, a nasal catheter, a face mask, and a tent.

Discuss special nursing care required for patients receiving oxygen by each of the four methods described in this chapter.

List two common reasons for using steam inhalations.

Describe the procedure for administering steam inhalations and the special nursing care the patient requires.

Describe how the patient is positioned for postural drainage and why postural drainage is used.

Explain why an inner cannula should always be in place when a tracheostomy is used.

Describe how to suction a tracheostomy.

Describe how humidity is added to the inspired air of the patient with a tracheostomy.

List three common reasons for using intermittent positive pressure breathing therapy.

Describe how and why percussion and vibration are used for patients with pulmonary diseases.

Describe three methods by which drugs can be administered by inhalation.

glossary

Aerosolization The suspending of medicated droplets in a gas for inhalation.

Anoxia An inadequate oxygen supply.

Atomization The breaking of a medicated solution into comparatively large particles for inhalation.

Intermittent Positive Pressure Breathing A mechanical means of providing gases or drugs under positive pressure for inhalation. Abbreviated I.P.P.B.

Nebulization The breaking of a medicated solution into small particles in order to produce mist or fog for inhalation.

Tracheostomy An artificial external opening into the trachea through which a tube for breathing is passed.

Ultrasonic Nebulization The use of high-frequency sound waves to break a medicated solution into minute particles for inhalation.

introduction

The act of respiration involves the exchange of gases in which oxygen from the air is delivered to the tissue cells and carbon dioxide is removed. Attention to the patient's respiratory functioning is as much a part of basic nursing care as any other measure. The increasing incidence of chronic lung diseases and newly developed methods of prevention and treatment have opened another vast area of preventive nursing care.

This chapter will describe various measures used to assist the respiratory function. These measures will almost always require a physician's order. Recording is done according to agency policy, and should include patients' reactions to these measures.

Oxygen therapy

Oxygen is essential for life, and the body has no reserve of it. **Anoxia** is defined as an inadequate oxygen supply. Regardless of its cause, this condition frequently requires oxygen therapy.

Oxygen therapy is given only as ordered by the physician. The order will specify the method of administration and the amount to be given. The nurse handles it as a medication and administers it with the same precautions and checking for accuracy as she would any drug she may give.

There are several conditions that often require oxygen therapy. When the lungs are diseased, oxygen is added to inhaled air so that the blood receives sufficient oxygen. An example is a lung infection such as pneumonia. Another example is chronic obstructive pulmonary disease (COPD). Certain heart conditions, such as congestive heart failure, impair the circulation of blood in the lungs. Increasing the intake of oxygen helps relieve anoxia in these instances. Strict bed rest is important in certain disease conditions, as for example, following a heart attack. Oxygen is then given to the patient so that he can breathe while using the least possible amount of energy.

Patients suffering from anoxia often feel as though they are suffocating and are unable to breathe. They are usually restless, worried, and frightened. Respirations are characteristically difficult and the skin becomes bluish in color. Faintness and dizziness are often present.

Respiratory therapists are available in many health agencies. They are responsible for starting and maintaining oxygen therapy. In those agencies not having respiratory therapists, it is important for the nurse to understand how oxygen is managed and used for therapy.

Oxygen therapy must sometimes be instituted with such speed that there is little time for explaining procedures to the patient. However, some concurrent instruction is generally possible. Once the patient is out of immediate danger, he should be told about the device being used and the essentials necessary to serve him effectively. It is a terrifying experience to be unable to breathe. The patient needs support and the comfort of feeling that all that is possible is being done for him.

Oxygen is delivered to the respiratory tract artificially under pressure. Therefore, excessive drying of mucous membranes lining the respiratory tract occurs unless the oxygen is humidified. Since oxygen is only slightly soluble in water, it can be passed through solution with little loss. Tap or distilled water is generally used for this purpose. The exact method of moisturizing oxygen depends on the agency's equipment. An illustration of one type of humidifier bottle appears in Figure 19-2, p. 404.

Oxygen is a tasteless, odorless, and colorless gas. It supports combustion and hence, must be used with great care. To help avoid fires, open flames and sparks must be kept away from the area where oxygen is being used. This precaution cannot be overemphasized since periodically tragic accidents occur. "No Smoking" signs should be placed in prominent places in the patient's room and the patient and his visitors taught the importance of the regulation.

When oxygen tents are used and when oxygen is brought to the patient's room in tanks, many agencies adhere to additional policies. Electric devices, such as razors, suction apparatus, hearing aids, radios, and television sets are removed or checked very carefully to be certain they are not emitting sparks. Care should be taken also in the management of linens and blankets, since many fabrics generate static electricity. Sparks from such sources as wool, silk, rayon, and nylon can be dangerous. Some agencies require that nurses working around oxygen wear cotton uniforms and undergarments to help avoid static electricity. Electric signal devices are generally not used because of the danger of sparks. It is better if the nurse gives the patient a mechanical device, such as an ordinary dinner bell, to call for assistance. The patient in an oxygen tent will need to have his bell in the tent with him. Oil and alcohol for backrubs are sometimes not used because of the fire danger they present. Candles for religious ceremonies cannot be used safely. Before starting oxygen therapy, the nurse should check the patient's room carefully to see that all safety measures have been taken and that agency policies are carefully observed.

In many hospitals, oxygen is piped into each patient unit and is immediately available from an outlet in the wall. The wall outlet can be prepared for use quickly. The oxygen is supplied from a central source through a pipeline, usually at 50 to 60 pounds per square inch of pressure. A specially designed flowmeter is attached to the wall outlet. The flowmeter opens the outlet and a valve makes regulation of the oxygen flow possible. Figure 19-1 illustrates a flowmeter.

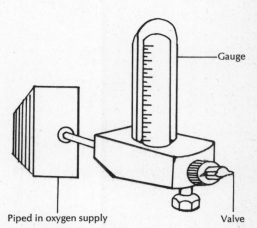

Fig. 19-1   A piped-in oxygen supply with flowmeter. The valve permits regulation of the oxygen flow at the rate indicated on the gauge. The lower connection attaches to the humidifier bottle. The oxygen is supplied from a central source piped into the patient's room.

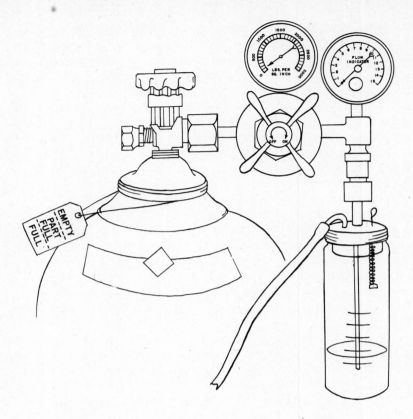

Fig. 19-2 Oxygen tank with regulator. The regulator is fastened to the tank valve and tightened with a wrench. The valve atop the tank admits oxygen to the regulator. When this valve is opened, the left-hand gauge will indicate the tank pressure. The regulator valve (below the tank gauge) than is turned; it releases the oxygen and then is adjusted for the correct rate (shown on the right-hand gauge). A humidifier attached to the apparatus is used when oxygen is administered by all methods except the tent.

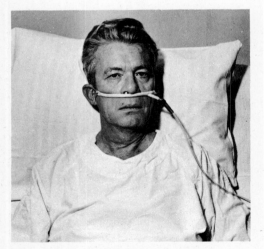

Fig. 19-3 Patient receiving oxygen via a nasal cannula.

When oxygen is not piped into a room, oxygen is compressed and dispensed in steel tanks. The tank is delivered with a protective cap to prevent accidental force against the tank outlet. When a standard, large-sized tank is full, its contents are under more than 2000 pounds of pressure per square inch. The force behind an accidently partially opened outlet could cause the tank to take off like a rocket with disastrous results. The tank should be transported carefully, preferably strapped onto a wheeled carrier. Once located, it should be stabilized by securing it in a properly fitting stand. No oil should be used near the gauge or the outlet because of the danger of the oil's igniting spontaneously.

Gases other than oxygen are used in many health agencies. For example, tanks may contain a mixture of carbon dioxide and oxygen which is sometimes used to stimulate respirations. Various gases used for anesthesia are dispensed in steel tanks. Therefore, the nurse should check to see that the tank is clearly labeled oxygen, just as she should check the label on a container before giving a medication. Administering the wrong gas is a serious error!

A regulator with a valve releases oxygen safely and at a desirable rate from the tank. There are two gauges on the regulator. The one nearest the tank shows the pressure, hence the amount of oxygen in the tank. The other indicates the number of liters per minute of oxygen being released to the patient. Figure 19-2 shows an oxygen tank with its regulator.

Because dust or other particles may lodge in the outlet of the tank and be forced into the regulator, the tank is "cracked" before the regulator is applied. The nurse uses two hands to "crack" a tank so that opening the tank can be well controlled. The wheel of the tank valve which releases the oxygen is turned slightly so that a small amount of oxygen may be released. This clears the outlet. The force with which the oxygen is released from this opening causes a loud hissing sound which usually startles anyone who is not aware of what it is. Hence, it is recommended that oxygen tanks be "cracked" away from the patient's bedside. If this is not possible, the patient should be prepared for the noise by proper explanation.

Use of the Nasal Cannula, Nasal Catheter, and Face Mask for Administering Oxygen. The simplest way to administer oxygen is via the nasal cannula. The cannula is a plastic device, usually disposable, with two protruding prongs for insertion into the patient's nostrils. It is held in place with an elastic strap around the patient's head. Figure 19-3 illustrates a cannula in place. This method is often used by patients receiving oxygen at home. Also, patients who are up and about often use a cannula and carry a small oxygen tank in their hands or strapped to their backs.

A nasal catheter is a very efficient means for administering oxygen. It is generally somewhat less comfortable than a cannula but capable of delivering oxygen at a relatively high concentration. It is illustrated in Figure 19-4.

Various types of face masks are available. A mask may cover only the nose. Or, it may be designed to cover both the nose and mouth. The latter type presents problems for eating, drinking, and talking. However, it is necessary when the patient breathes through his mouth. Masks are especially effective when very high concentrations of oxygen are needed. One is illustrated in Figure 19-5, p. 406.

Chart 19-1 describes the use of a nasal cannula, nasal catheter, and face mask. The chart assumes that the patient has been prepared, the room has been made safe, and the oxygen supply is in readiness.

Use of the Oxygen Tent for Administering Oxygen. An oxygen tent is a light, portable structure made of clear plastic and attached to a motor-driven unit. The motor circulates air in the tent. A thermostat in the unit keeps the tent at a comfortable temperature for the patient. The tent fits over the top part of the bed so that the patient's head and chest fit inside of it.

Patients are often frightened by the appearance of an oxygen tent. However, when the patient is prepared and knows its advantages, few object to its use. Many prefer it over other methods because it is cool, permits movement in bed, and prevents excessive dryness of mucous membranes. It is illustrated in Figure 19-6, p. 406.

The use of the oxygen tent is described in Chart 19-2. It is assumed the patient has been prepared, the room has been made safe, and the oxygen supply is in readiness (see p. 409).

Some patients at home keep oxygen handy for quick use as necessary. Figure 19-7 illustrates a patient giving himself oxygen with a mask from a small container of oxygen. He can refill the container as necessary and easily carry it with him (see p. 411).

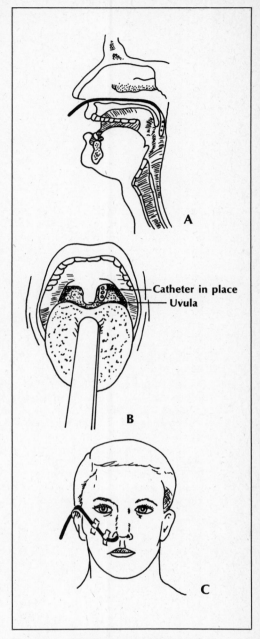

Fig. 19-4 (A) Diagram of the correct location of a nasal catheter in the nose and the oropharynx. (B) To make certain that the catheter is placed properly, it is necessary to ask the patient to open his mouth. The tip of the catheter should be located just below the uvula (C) The catheter should be taped close to the nares and on the cheek. It can then drape over the ear. This provides freedom of movement of the lips and reduces pull on the catheter.

Oxygen therapy 405

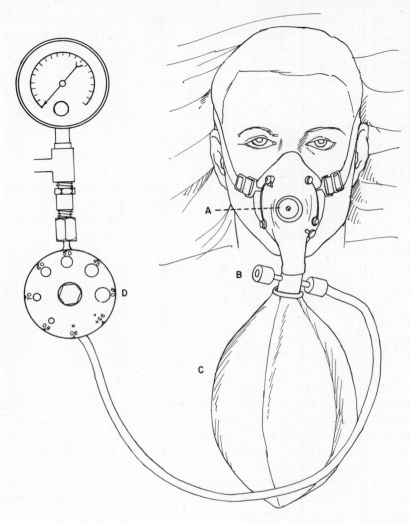

Fig. 19-5 There are many types of face masks. Some provide for an oxygen reservoir, a means for the expired carbon dioxide to be removed, and a means for mixing air with the oxygen, as the one in this sketch. (A) The flutter valve on the oronasal face mask, which provides an outlet for expired air. Pressure of the expired air forces the soft rubber disc away from the mask. (B) A safety valve that provides for an air inlet in the event of an emergency or increased depth of respirations. (C) The reservoir which contains the air and oxygen mixture inhaled by the patient. (D) The meter calibrated from 40 to 95 plus per cent, for adjusting concentration of oxygen to be delivered to bag.

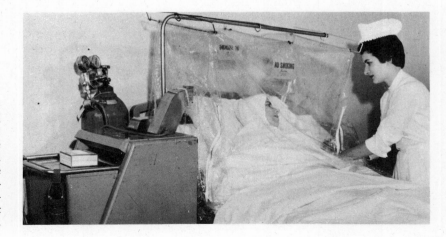

Fig. 19-6 Many nursing activities are carried out easily through the zippered openings provided in the oxygen tent. Because of the air circulation in the tent, protection for the patient's head may be necessary. Care should be taken also to avoid restricting the patient's activity by tucking the drawsheet which helps seal the bottom part of tent too tightly under the mattress.

Chart 19-1 Administering oxygen by means of the nasal cannula, nasal catheter, and face mask

The purpose is to administer a therapeutic concentration of oxygen to the patient

Suggested Action	Reason for Action
Observe practices of medical asepsis. Assist patient to comfortable position in bed, usually in a semi-Fowler's position.	Upper respiratory passages are not treated as sterile. A relaxed and comfortable patient is better able to assist with his oxygen therapy.
During course of therapy, check oxygen supply in tank or oxygen supply delivered to wall outlet and rate at which patient receives it at frequent intervals. Be familiar with agency procedure to obtain additional oxygen.	Keeping supply of oxygen continuous is important to maintain proper oxygen therapy for patient. Administering too little or too much oxygen may endanger patient's life.
During course of therapy, make certain that oxygen is properly humidified, procedure depending on agency's equipment.	Oxygen is drying to mucous membranes and hence, is humidified before administration.
During course of therapy, give patient special mouth care frequently.	Oxygen is drying to mucous membranes. Oral hygiene is needed to keep tissues moist and lubricated, and the mouth fresh and clean-tasting.

Use of Nasal Cannula

Suggested Action	Reason for Action
Attach cannula to oxygen supply and to humidifier and start oxygen at ordered rate, usually 2 to 4 liters per minute. Note that oxygen is being delivered properly by placing prongs of cannula in glass of water.	Starting oxygen and making certain that apparatus is functioning properly is less frightening, safer, and more comfortable for patient than starting oxygen after cannula is in place.
Place prongs of cannula in nostrils. Secure cannula with strap around patient's head, as illustrated in Figure 19-3, p. 404. Check regularly for position and tightness of cannula.	Oxygen is delivered from tips of prongs into nose efficiently when cannula is in good position on patient.
Place small gauze padding under cannula as indicated and move cannula slightly from time to time.	While still having cannula in place, these measures help prevent skin irritation and discomfort for patient.
Check flow of oxygen regularly to assure that oxygen is being given at rate ordered by physician.	Too little oxygen is not particularly helpful. High concentrations of oxygen tend to cause excessive drying of mucous membranes. Excessive or inadequate amounts of oxygen may be dangerous for patient.
Remove and clean cannula at least every eight hours, oftener if indicated.	A soiled cannula is uncomfortable and unpleasant for patient.
Instruct patient to breathe through his nose.	There is oxygen loss when patient breathes through his mouth.
Cleanse nostrils around cannula prongs as necessary.	Accumulated secretions at nostrils are uncomfortable for patient and will irritate skin and mucous membranes.

Chart 19-1 continued

Suggested Action	Reason for Action

Use of Nasal Catheter

Attach catheter to oxygen supply and to humidifier and start oxygen at ordered rate, usually 4 to 7 liters per minute. Note that oxygen is being delivered properly by placing end of catheter in glass of water.	Starting oxygen and seeing to it that apparatus is functioning properly is less frightening, safer, and more comfortable for patient than starting oxygen after catheter is in place.
Lubricate catheter well with water-soluble lubricant. Size 10 or 12 Fr. catheter about 16 inches long is usually used for adults.	Oily substances if aspirated into lungs can be harmful and many are irritating to nasal membranes. Lubricant reduces friction and thus minimizes irritation of catheter on nasal membranes.
Measure distance from nostril to earlobe as guide for distance to insert catheter. Hold tip of patient's nose up and insert catheter by moving it along floor of nose carefully until measured distance is reached.	Inserting catheter recommended distance along floor of nose usually places catheter in best position and with most comfort for patient.
Look for position of catheter by depressing tongue with tongue blade and adjust position as necessary. Correct position is illustrated in Figure 19-4, p. 405.	Catheter inserted too far will cause oxygen to enter gastro-intestinal tract and may cause patient to gag. Oxygen escapes when catheter is not inserted far enough.
Bring catheter across cheek to temple area, as illustrated in Figure 19-4. Or, bring it up and over bridge of nose and forehead. Secure to patient with adhesive. Tubing from oxygen supply to catheter may be secured to bed linen with clamp or pin.	Keeping catheter away from eyes is comfortable for patient. Securing catheter prevents it from slipping out of place.
Check flow of oxygen regularly and maintain at ordered rate.	Too little oxygen is not particularly helpful. High concentrations of oxygen may cause sore throat and excessive drying of mucous membranes. Excessive or inadequate amounts of oxygen may be dangerous for patient.
Remove and clean catheter at least every eight hours, oftener if indicated.	A soiled catheter is uncomfortable and unpleasant for patient.
Alternate nostrils when changing catheter if possible.	Alternating nostrils reduces irritation to mucous membranes.
Check patient's skin for irritation from adhesive. If patient is allergic to adhesive, fasten catheter by some other means, as gauze bandaging.	Irritation from adhesive is uncomfortable for patient.
Cleanse nostril around catheter as necessary.	Accumulated secretions at nostril are uncomfortable for patient and will irritate skin and mucous membranes.
Check regularly to see that catheter is not kinked.	Kinked catheter will decrease or halt flow of oxygen.

Chart 19-1   continued

Suggested Action	Reason for Action
Use of Face Mask	
Oxygen becomes humidified from patient's expirations into mask. Humidifier may be placed in room if indicated.	Humidified oxygen is less drying to mucous membranes.
Have oxygen flow at about 10 to 15 liters per minute to begin so that patient can feel oxygen and be less fearful of suffocating with mask.	Fear of mask and of suffocation is less likely when patient can feel oxygen entering mask.
Instruct patient to breathe normally and help him to relax while applying mask.	Well-prepared and relaxed patient can assist with his oxygen therapy.
Adjust mask in place to cover nose and mouth or only nose, depending on type of mask. Secure with strap around head, as illustrated in Figure 19-5, p. 406. Fill openings between mask and face with gauze or other suitable material as necessary for secure fit.	Well-fitting mask delivers oxygen in desired concentration by preventing oxygen leakage around mask.
Check flow of oxygen and maintain at ordered rate.	Too much or too little oxygen may be dangerous for patient. Too little oxygen is not particularly helpful. High concentrations of oxygen may cause excessive drying of mucous membranes.
Remove and clean mask at least every eight hours, oftener if indicated.	A soiled mask is uncomfortable and unpleasant for patient.
Wash and powder face regularly as indicated.	This helps prevent irritation of skin by mask.

Chart 19-2 Administering oxygen by means of a tent
The purpose is to administer a therapeutic concentration of oxygen to the patient

Suggested Action	Reason for Action
Assist patient to comfortable position in bed and in good body alignment. Head of bed may be elevated.	A relaxed and comfortable patient is better able to assist with his oxygen therapy. Patients in tent usually receive therapy over long period of time. Good body alignment helps prevent fatigue and musculoskeletal complications.
Bring tent to bedside, plug in motor, and start unit. Turn on oxygen flow. Check oxygen flow inlet in tent and exhaust outlet. Set temperature control at about 70°F.	Checking mechanical aspects of tent reduces possibility of causing further respiratory distress for patient in event of defects.

Chart 19-2 Continued

Suggested Action	Reason for Action
Close all openings of hood. Seal bottom opening by bringing sides together and folding over several times, or by tying, so that upper half of hood is flooded with oxygen at 15 liters per minute.	For immediate benefit for patient, air in tent should contain oxygen content of at least 30 to 40 per cent. Oxygen is heavier than air; therefore flood area which is to be over patient's head.
Flood tent for two to five minutes while hood is closed.	A therapeutic concentration is usually established in this length of time.
Move unit directly into position near head of bed before opening hood.	Having unit in place prevents oxygen loss when hood is placed over patient.
Open bottom of hood and arrange it over patient. Leaving some slack, tuck part at head of bed well under mattress as far as it will go.	Sufficient length of hood is necessary to raise and lower head of bed as desired.
Enclose part of hood which goes over patient's body in draw-sheet and arrange so that open spaces between hood and bedding are closed. Tuck ends under mattress to hold them well.	Oxygen, being heavier than air, will escape through open areas at edge of hood. Linen facilitates sealing openings and keeps edge of hood in place.
Test inside tent for drafts by placing your hand in various locations near patient's head. Protect patient's head and shoulders with shawl or other suitable garment.	Many tents have complete exchange of air in less than minute's time, thus causing drafts that are uncomfortable for patient unless he is well protected.
After tent is in place and secured, reduce flow of oxygen, usually to 10 to 12 liters per minute.	This rate of flow usually maintains 40 to 60 per cent concentration in tent.
Check temperature indicator frequently until temperature in tent is stabilized. Adjust to temperature most comfortable for patient.	Temperature of 68° to 70°F. usually is comfortable for most patients when they are protected from drafts in tent.
When giving most care, slip your hands into tent at zippered openings.	Special openings in tent for giving care help conserve oxygen concentration inside tent.
When giving bath, changing linen, and so on, tuck hood of tent under pillow so that patient's head remains in tent and least amount of oxygen escapes. Increase oxygen flow.	For extensive care, patient will receive good concentration of oxygen when tent is closed in best possible manner and when oxygen flow is increased.
Use normal tone of conversation when speaking to patient. Avoid conversation in his room that may disturb him.	An oxygen tent is not soundproof. Therefore patient can hear conversation in his room. Raising your voice unnecessarily is unpleasant for him.
Empty drainage near base or back of motor unit as often as recommended by manufacturer, usually at least once every 24 hours.	Moisture in air which has been withdrawn from tent condenses. There is also some condensation from refrigerator unit.

Steam inhalations

Steam inhalators are used to soothe inflamed and irritated mucous membranes and to loosen respiratory secretions. The inhaled air, carrying minute droplets of water, carries moist heat to the respiratory tract. This produces the same results as when moist heat is applied locally to other parts of the body, as described in Chapter 18.

Electrically heated steam inhalators are available for delivering warm moist heat in most agencies and they are also often used in the home. Drugs are sometimes added to the water of a steam inhalator. When vaporized in steam, the drugs are carried to the respiratory tract with inspirations. They act locally to help soothe irritated and inflamed mucous membranes. Compound tincture of benzoin is an example of a drug that may be added to steam inhalators. The steam is allowed to escape into the room. When windows and doors are closed, the room air becomes warm and moist.

When administering steam inhalations, the nurse must observe every precaution to avoid burns. Steam inhalators are very hot! Also, she must be sure electric inhalators are in good working order to prevent the danger of electrical shocks and burns.

When steam inhalation therapy is discontinued, the patient will usually feel damp and warm. He should be dried and his bed garments and linen changed as necessary. Also the patient should be protected from drafts and from chilliness with appropriate coverings.

Postural drainage

Postural drainage is the promotion of drainage from the respiratory tract by positioning the patient so that gravity helps promote drainage. The position places the patient's head and chest below the level of the hips. One position is illustrated in Figure 19-8. If the patient is unable to assume this position, he may lie on his abdomen over several pillows with his head lower than his hips. Postural drainage is often recommended for the patient with considerable heavy respiratory secretions when it is difficult for him to raise the material by coughing alone.

The tracheostomy

A **tracheostomy** is an artificial opening into the trachea. When a tube is inserted into the opening, the patient is able to breathe air, oxygen, or any other gas he may need through it. Tracheal and bronchial secretions may also be suctioned through the tracheostomy.

The care of a tracheostomy is a nursing responsibility. When the patient coughs, secretions are forced out of the tracheostomy. These secretions should be wiped away carefully around the opening so that the patient does not inspire them as he breathes. It is best to wipe away secretions with material that does not have lint. Inhaled lint may irritate the respiratory passages and may cause undue coughing.

The inner cannula should be removed, cleaned, and sterilized regularly so that it does not clog with mucus and other debris. As soon as

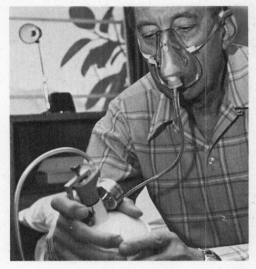

Fig. 19-7 Patient using face mask and oxygen from small portable container. Oxygen supply is quite limited but can be used temporarily when patient is in need. His right forefinger regulates amount of oxygen received.

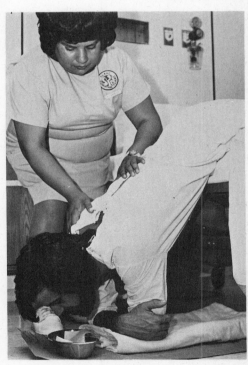

Fig. 19-8 A good position for postural drainage. Nurse remains ready to assist patient should the position tire or weaken him. Those unable to assume this position safely or comfortably may lie on their abdomens over pillows on the bed.

it is removed for cleaning, a second clean and sterile cannula is placed in the tracheosotomy (the outer cannula) immediately so that at no time is the patient without an inner cannula. When an inner cannula is not kept in place, the outer cannula may become clogged. This may endanger the patient's life and necessitate having the physician replace the entire piece of equipment in the surgical opening. Figure 19-9 illustrates the nurse removing the inner cannula.

The inner cannula, while in place, is suctioned frequently and kept open and free of mucus. Figures 19-10, 19-11, and 19-12 illustrate a nurse suctioning the tracheostomy tube.

Dry air irritates respiratory tract membranes quickly. Therefore, the air inspired by a patient with a tracheostomy is often humidified. A moist gauze bib may be placed over the opening. Or, an air humidifier may be attached, as illustrated in Figure 19-13. Oxygen therapy may also be administered in the same manner as moisturized air is delivered to the patient.

Other methods for assisting respiratory functioning

Certain drugs are administered by inhalation. Most of these drugs are used to improve respiratory functioning. Much of the absorption occurs on the surfaces of lung tissue. Because of the large surface area in the lungs, absorption after inhalation generally is rapid.

Before drugs can be inhaled, they must be vaporized to permit their entry into the body with each inspiration. Drugs may be added to a vehicle, such as water, and placed in steam for inhalation, as described earlier in this chapter. Still another method is to use a nebulizer which

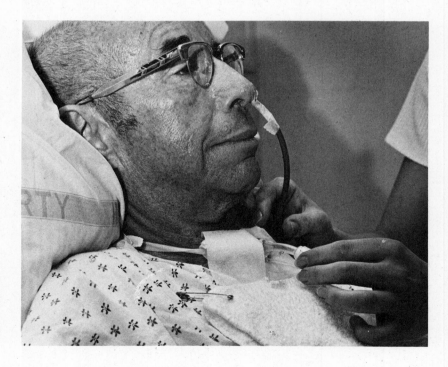

Fig. 19-9 The nurse removes the inner cannula only for regular cleaning and sterilizing, or for discarding when the cannula is disposable. She replaces it immediately after removal with another cannula. The inner cannula remains in place during routine suctioning.

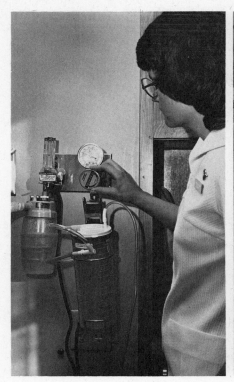
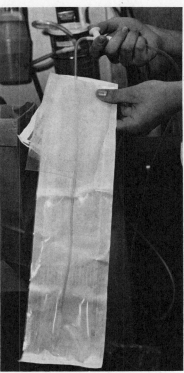

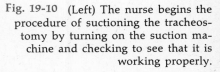

Fig. 19-10 (Left) The nurse begins the procedure of suctioning the tracheostomy by turning on the suction machine and checking to see that it is working properly.

Fig. 19-11 (Right) The catheter for suctioning the tracheostomy is sterile when dispensed in its plastic bag. The top is turned down only sufficiently to connect the catheter with the suction machine. The nurse checks to see that there is suction by placing her thumb over the valve, as shown. When her thumb is off the valve, there will be no suction in the catheter.

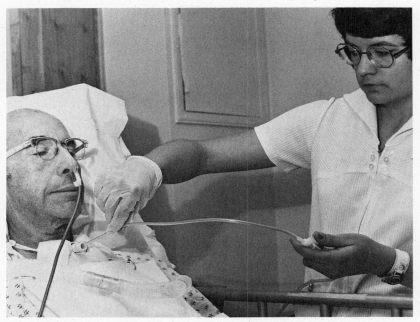

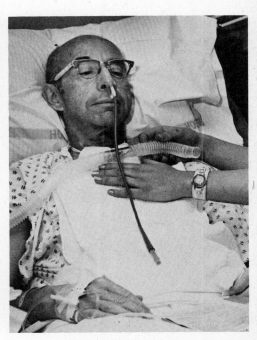

Fig. 19-12 After donning a sterile glove, the nurse handles the sterile catheter as she suctions. The catheter is inserted through the inner cannula and into the respiratory passage. The nurse regulates the amount of suction with her thumb, as shown. The catheter should be inserted carefully and slowly without forcing it so as not to injure mucous membranes in the respiratory passage. Suctioning should not be continuous for more than 10 or 15 seconds. Suctioning removes oxygen as well as secretions. Hence, longer periods of continuous suctioning will result in too severe oxygen deprivation for the patient.

Fig. 19-13 The large plastic tubing fastened over the tracheostomy opening supplies moisturized air for the patient. The tube in the patient's nostril is a gastric gavage tube, used for giving this patient nourishment and oral medications.

separates a drug in solution into minute particles for inhalation. Drugs administered by nebulization are frequently used to relieve bronchial spasms. The condition often occurs with asthma. **Atomization** usually refers to the production of rather large droplets. **Nebulization** is the production of a mist or fog. The smallest particles are produced by high-frequency waves. The procedure is called **ultrasonic nebulization.** Suspending the droplets in a gas is called **aerosolization.** In lay language, aerosolization is frequently referred to as "cold steam."

The finer the particles, the farther they will travel into the respiratory tract. If the inhalation is intended to produce effects in the nasal passage as well as in the remainder of the respiratory tract, the patient closes his mouth while he breathes and inhales the substance through his nose. Otherwise, the mist is inhaled through the mouth.

There are several ways in which a spray may be produced. The hand nebulizer uses a bulb attachment. When the bulb is compressed by hand, air is forced through the container holding the drug in solution. The increased pressure in the unit then forces solution into a specially constructed strictured device. The force with which the solution is made to move through this stricture and to leave the container is sufficient to break the large droplets of fluid into a fine mist. Commercially prepared aerosol containers with medications are also available. It is the type being used by the patient in Figure 19-14.

Nebulization can also be accomplished by using the force of an oxygen stream or compressed air to be passed through the drug in solution in a nebulizer. This method is valuable for patients who require 10 to 15 minutes of a drug several times a day when a hand nebulizer would prove to be quite fatiguing. A machine used to administer intermittent positive pressure breathing may also be used to nebulize a drug, as will be explained next.

A common means for administering oxygenated air and a nebulized drug is by **intermittent positive pressure breathing,** usually abbreviated I.P.P.B. This method uses a machine that provides a specific amount of air and medication under increased pressure for the respiratory tract. I.P.P.B. forces deeper inspiration by positive pressure inhalation and permits the patient to exhale normally. The amount of pressure varies according to the patient's tolerance and needs. Usually, I.P.P.B. therapy is ordered to be used two to four times daily for 15 to 20 minutes each time.

There are many models of I.P.P.B. machines on the market. The one illustrated in Figure 19-15 is portable and especially useful for the patient at home. Figure 19-16 illustrates the patient using his machine.

In many health agencies, respiratory technicians are responsible for administering I.P.P.B. therapy. The nurse will wish to be familiar with the machine used in the agency where she gives care in order to understand the exact nature of the therapy her patients receive.

Common reasons for using intermittent positive pressure breathing include aiding respiratory ventilation; administering aerosol therapy; and helping patients to expectorate respiratory secretions.

Figure 19-17 illustrates the container in which drugs in solution are placed for nebulization. Drugs commonly used are antibiotics, expectorants, and those that help to dilate the bronchiol tubes.

Many patients with chronic pulmonary diseases have difficulty raising mucus from the respiratory tract. Postural drainage may be

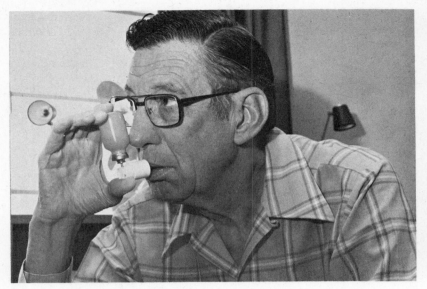

Fig. 19-14 The patient uses a nebulizer which can be purchased in most drug stores with a physician's prescription. He is about to place the mouthpiece into his mouth. Then, by pressing his fingers and thumb together on the nebulizer, his drug in solution will be nebulized and forced into his respiratory passage.

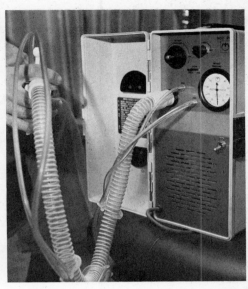

Fig. 19-15 A portable intermittent positive pressure breathing machine. The patient controls the amount of pressure he can tolerate and needs with a dial on the face of the machine.

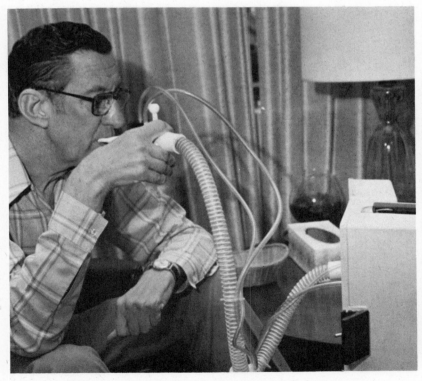

Fig. 19-16 The patient holds the mouthpiece securely between his lips as he gives himself intermittent positive pressure breathing therapy. The pressure forces deep inspirations but allows the patient to exhale normally.

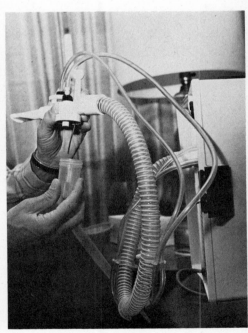

Fig. 19-17 Drug in solution can be placed in the small container near the mouthpiece. The pressure created by the machine produces nebulization while the patient gives himself therapy.

Assisting respiratory functioning   415

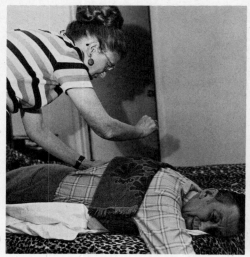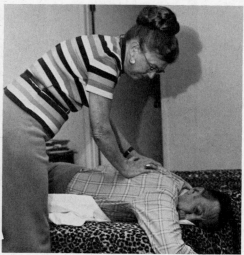

Fig. 19-18 (Left) The patient's wife strikes areas over the lungs with her closed hands for percussion and (right) rubs the areas, using firm and strong circular movements with her opened hands, for vibration. The patient is placed in various positions—on his sides, back, and abdomen—so that all areas over both lungs can be percussed and vibrated. The treatment assists the patient to raise respiratory secretions that have accumulated in his lower respiratory passages.

ordered for these patients. Or, if postural drainage does not seem effective, percussion and vibration over the area of the lungs may be ordered. Percussion and vibration help to break up the mucus and raise it so that the patient can more readily expectorate it. Figure 19-18 illustrates the wife of a patient administering percussion and vibration. I.P.P.B. therapy is usually used immediately before having percussion and vibration.

Still another way to assist proper respiratory functioning is to teach the patient how to cough and breathe deeply. These procedures are most often used when caring for the postoperative patient and will be discussed in Chapter 21.

Conclusion

Adequate respiratory functioning is essential for life. Persons who have difficult breathing are generally anxious and fearful. The nurse can play an important role in helping to relieve psychological distress which is often as important to improving respiratory functioning as specific physical measures.

References

Brannin, Patricia Kay, "Oxygen Therapy and Measures of Bronchial Hygiene," *The Nursing Clinics of North America*, 9:111–121, March 1974.

Chrisman, Marilyn, "Dyspnea," *American Journal of Nursing*, 74:643–646, April 1974.

Deal, Jacquelyn, "Breathing," *Nursing Care*, 7:21, October 1974.

———, "When Breathing Becomes Work," *Nursing Care*, 6:11–15, November 1973.

———, "When Breathing Becomes Work. Part 2." *Nursing Care*, 6:12–16, December 1973.

Davis, Anne L., "Chronic Respiratory Problems in the Older Patient: Battling for Breath: Chronic Obstructive Pulmonary Disease," *The Journal of Practical Nursing*, 23:18–21, 32, October 1973.

Foss, Georgia, "Postural Drainage," *American Journal of Nursing*, 73:666–669, April 1973.

O'Dell, Ardis J., "Doing It Better: The Administration of Airway Humidification," *Nursing '74*, 4:66–67, April 1974.

Roberts, Joyce E., "Suctioning the Newborn," *American Journal of Nursing*, 73:63–65, January 1973.

Sweetwood, Hannelore, "Bedside Assessment of Respirations," *Nursing '73*, 3:50–51, September 1973.

Tinker, John H. and Wehner, Robert, "The Nurse and the Ventilator," *American Journal of Nursing*, 74:1276–1278, July 1974.

Tyler, Martha L., "Artificial Airways: Suctioning, Tubes & Cuffs, Weaning & Extubation," *Nursing '73*, 3:21–38, February 1973.

Weber, Betty, "Eating with a Trach," *American Journal of Nursing*, 74:1439, August 1974.

"When Your Patient Is On Respiratory Therapy," *Nursing Update*, 6:1, 3–13, January 1975.

20

the nurse as an assistant

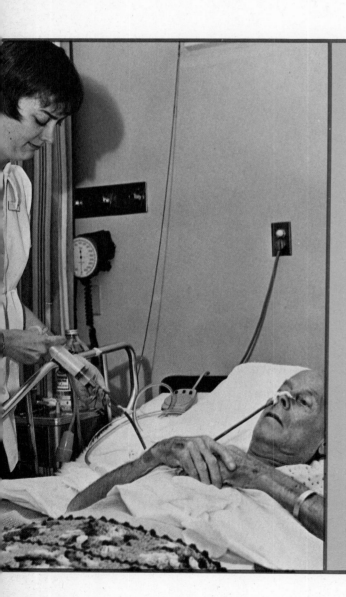

behavioral objectives

When mastery of content in this chapter is reached, the student will be able to

Define terms appearing in the glossary.

Discuss ten primary responsibilities of the assisting nurse.

State the common indications, basic equipment and supplies required, and usual duties of the assisting nurse for each of the six procedures described in this chapter.

glossary

Blood Transfusion The intravenous infusion of whole blood.

Crossmatch A laboratory examination which determines whether blood specimens are compatible.

Donor The person giving blood.

Empyema The presence of pus in the pleural cavity.

Gastric Analysis The laboratory examination of stomach contents.

Gastric and Duodenal Suction The use of suction for the continuous removal of contents from the stomach and the first part of the small intestine (duodenum).

Lumbar Puncture The insertion of a needle into the subarachnoid space. Synonym for spinal tap.

Paracentesis The withdrawal of fluid from a body cavity; a term usually used to refer to the removal of fluid from the abdominal cavity. Commonly known as an abdominal tap.

Queckenstedt's Test A test that arrests blood flow in the neck or abdomen by applying pressure to the area; the test is used to help determine whether there is an obstruction in the subarachnoid spaces.

Recipient The person receiving blood.

Spinal Tap The insertion of a needle into the subarachnoid space. Synonym for lumbar puncture.

Thoracentesis The withdrawal of fluid from the pleural cavity. Commonly known as a chest tap.

Typing of Blood A laboratory examination which determines a person's blood type.

There are various procedures used for diagnosis and treatment that require the assistance of a nurse. These procedures may be done by a physician or by other specially trained personnel. This chapter discusses the role of the nurse who acts as an assistant to the operator carrying out the procedure.

Responsibilities of the assisting nurse

The primary responsibilities of the assisting nurse fall into several broad categories, each of which will be briefly described below.

Understanding the Procedure. When the nurse assists, she must first know the nature of the procedure. Answers to such questions as the following will help to provide the necessary information:

- What is the procedure and how is it defined?
- What are the purposes, or indications, for which the procedure is commonly used?
- What part of the body will be entered?
- What practices of medical and surgical asepsis will be required?
- How shall the patient be positioned in order that the procedure may be carried out efficiently and safely and with comfort for the patient?
- Will a specimen be obtained?
- What symptoms will the patient have that indicate the purpose for carrying out the procedure is being reached?
- What symptoms indicate that the patient is not responding well to the procedure and what measures can be used to prevent complications?

Understanding the Patient, His Illness, and His Plan of Care. Answers to questions such as these will help the nurse to understand the patient, his illness, and his plan of care:

- What is the patient's diagnosis?
- What is the probable cause of the patient's illness?
- How is the patient's illness interfering with normal body functions?
- What is the patient's physical and mental condition?
- How well is the patient responding to his present prescribed plan of care?
- How does the procedure to be carried out fit into the patient's plan of care?

Preparing the Patient. Ordinarily, the physician assumes responsibility for explaining the procedure to the patient. The nurse assists by helping the patient as necessary so that he understands the procedure. No exact rules can be stated as to how best to prepare each patient for each procedure. In general, the nurse is guided by the physician's wishes, the patient's condition, and individual circumstances. She is further guided by suggestions offered in Chapter 3 concerning developing a good relationship with the patient in order to meet his individual needs.

The physical preparation of the patient varies, depending on the procedure. However, the following measures ordinarily apply for any procedure:

- Have the patient void before the procedure. Usually the patient feels somewhat anxious, which may stimulate the urge to void, even though he has been well prepared. Also, most patients feel more comfortable and relaxed after voiding. It is usually inconvenient and sometimes almost impossible to offer a bedpan or urinal during the procedure.
- Plan to have the patient wear a garment that will protect him from unnecessary exposure while still allowing the operator convenience in carrying out the procedure.
- If the skin is to be entered, check the condition of the patient's skin at the site of entry. If the area is not clean, wash it with soap or detergent and water. At the time of the procedure, an antiseptic will be used at the site of entry. However, every effort should be made to have the skin as clean as possible before using an antiseptic. This helps to minimize the danger of introducing microorganisms into the body and causing an infection.
- If any special preparation is required for the procedure, check to see that it has been done correctly. For example, prior to a gastric analysis, the patient usually is not allowed food or fluids for a period of time. If proper preparations have not been carried out, report this promptly. It usually becomes necessary to cancel the procedure in such instances.
- If there is considerable hair at the site of entry, check with the physician or supervising nurse to see whether shaving the area is indicated. This suggestion applies particularly for a paracentesis, a thoracentesis, and a lumbar puncture.
- Be prepared to transport the patient to the room where the procedure will be carried out if it is not to be done at the patient's bedside. The nurse will wish to explain the reason for the move so that the patient understands that it is for his comfort and safety.

Observing Agency Policy. The nurse will wish to be familiar with any agency policy relating to the procedure with which she will assist. For example, if legal consent by the patient, his guardian, or a family member is required, she will check to see that a consent form has been executed properly. Similarly, she will wish to be familiar with agency policy indicating who may carry out the procedure and when and where it is to be done.

Preparing Supplies and Equipment. In most instances, the assisting nurse is responsible for having the proper supplies and equipment ready for the procedure. Such equipment and supplies will depend on the procedure and will vary among agencies. Some agencies have pre-packaged trays with most, if not all, of the necessary items in readiness. Other agencies may require the nurse to assemble the appropriate equipment and supplies. While assembling and preparing materials, the nurse observes practices of medical and surgical asepsis as indicated. Proper draping materials and extra covering for the patient's comfort as indicated, are also necessary.

The basic equipment and supplies necessary for common procedures requiring an assisting nurse are given in Chart 20-1.

Preparing the Working Unit. Whether the procedure is carried out in a special room or at the patient's bedside, the nurse is responsible for seeing that privacy is provided, that the room is comfortable in terms of temperature and ventilation, and that there is a good source of light. The equipment and supplies should be placed so that they are convenient for the operator and for observing sound practices of asepsis.

Assisting During the Procedure. The assisting nurse is responsible for placing the patient in the appropriate position. The patient should be made as comfortable as possible but in a position that makes it convenient for the operator to work safely and easily. The patient is then draped, exposing only the area involved.

In some instances, the nurse prepares the skin at the site of entry. Cleansing with soap or detergent and water has already been mentioned. In addition, the skin is cleansed, usually with cotton balls or gauze swabs, with an antiseptic of the agency's choice. Sufficient pressure is used so that friction will help the cleaning process. The nurse begins by cleaning the site of entry; she then moves outward from the site of entry.

The operator may hand certain pieces of equipment to the nurse for connection to containers for specimens, suction, drainage, and so on. She may also hold drugs and injectable anesthetics. The nurse will check drugs and anesthetics by reading the label carefully as described in Chapter 17. In addition, she will hold the container so that the operator can also read the label. These practices help to avoid errors and misunderstandings. More specific guides for the assisting nurse are given in Chart 20-1.

After Care of the Patient. After the procedure is completed, the nurse helps the patient to his bed and to a comfortable position. She should observe the patient for symptoms, desirable and undesirable, that will indicate the effects of the procedure. These may occur soon afterward, but in some cases delayed reactions may occur as late as 24 to 48 hours or longer after the procedure has been completed.

Recording the Procedure. Local policy determines the exact manner in which the nurse records. The following information is usually included: the date and time; the name of the procedure; the name and amount of the drug injected, if one has been given; the nature and amount of drainage when present; the nature of the specimens collected; the name of the person who carried out the procedure; and the name of the nurse who assisted. In addition, the patient's reactions are recorded, including those which occurred during and immediately after the procedure and any delayed reactions.

Caring for Equipment and Supplies. Local policy will indicate whether the assisting nurse is responsible for caring for equipment and supplies used during the procedure. When she is responsible, she will observe suggestions discussed in Chapter 4, being very careful to take precautions to avoid the spread of microorganisms.

Common procedures with which the nurse ordinarily assists

Chart 20-1 describes common procedures with which the nurse ordinarily assists: lumbar puncture; thoracentesis; paracentesis; gastric analysis; and gastric and duodenal suction. The blood transfusion, described below, is carried out by adapting the procedure for an intravenous infusion which was described in Chapter 17.

Chart 20-1 Common procedures with which the nurse ordinarily assists

Procedure and Definition	Common Indications	Basic Equipment and Supplies	Guides for the Nurse Who Will Assist
Lumbar Puncture or **Spinal Tap** Insertion of needle into subarachnoid space.	Obtain specimen. Measure pressure of cerebrospinal fluid, normal being 100 to 200 mm. of water. Relieve undue pressure. Inject dye for x-ray visualization. Inject drug.	20- to 22-gauge lumbar puncture needle, 3 to 5 inches long. 22- to 25-gauge needle and 2 ml. syringe for injecting local anesthesia, usually procaine hydrochloride. Fenestrated drape; opening of drape is placed over area of back where spinal canal will be entered. Manometer for measuring pressure. Drug and syringe for injecting it, if ordered. Test tubes for specimens. Antiseptic and cotton balls to cleanse skin at site of entry. Sterile gloves. Gauze and adhesive for dressing at site of entry when needle is withdrawn.	Observe practices of surgical asepsis. Position patient as shown in Figure 20-1 on page 427. Cleanse skin at and around site of entry. Anchor drape to patient with adhesive to prevent its slipping from place. Area of drape around working area is kept sterile. Check label on anesthesia container and hold container so operator can also read label to avoid errors. Explain to patient importance of remaining motionless. Moving about makes it difficult to insert needle and needle may break. Help patient to remain in position as necessary. Note pressure readings on manometer as requested. Apply pressure with your hand on patient's abdomen or on jugular vein in neck as requested. Normally, pressure will rise and fall quickly as pressure is applied to patient and then released. This is called **Queckenstedt's test.** Check label on drug or dye container and hold container so operator can also read label to avoid errors. Handle and label specimens. Note patient's color and pulse and respiratory rates during procedure and if unusual, report to operator in a manner that will not alarm patient. Apply gauze dressing at site of entry and secure with adhesive after procedure is completed. Place patient flat in bed after procedure to help avoid headache; report if patient develops headache, which may last from a few hours to a few days. Report unusual signs occurring after procedure, such as twitching, slow pulse rate, or nausea and vomiting.
Thoracentesis Withdrawal of fluid from pleural cavity. Commonly known as chest tap.	Remove fluid for study and to ease respirations. If fluid contains pus, condition is called **empyema.** Obtain specimens.	Blunt thoracentesis needle, usually 15-gauge, 2 to 3 inches long. 50 ml. syringe with three-way stopcock and container to receive drainage. Or, tubing to connect needle with drainage bottle that has a partial vacuum obtained with pump and two-way stopcock.	Observe practices of surgical asepsis. Assist patient to sitting position, as described and illustrated in Figure 20-2 on page 427. If patient cannot sit up, have him lie on his affected side. Cleanse skin at and around site of entry. Anchor drape to patient with adhesive to prevent its slipping from place. Area of drape around working area is kept sterile.

Chart 20-1 continued

Procedure and Definition	Common Indications	Basic Equipment and Supplies	Guides for the Nurse Who Will Assist
		22- to 25-gauge needle and 2 ml. syringe for injecting anesthesia, usually procaine hydrochloride. Fenestrated drape; opening of drape is placed over area of back where pleural cavity will be entered. Sterile gloves. Gauze and adhesive for dressing at site of entry when needle is withdrawn.	Check label on container of anesthesia and hold container so operator can also read label to help avoid errors. If syringe method is used to remove drainage, hold container to receive drainage from syringe. If vacuum-bottle method is used, connect tubing to bottle and operate pump to create partial vacuum. Handle and label specimens. During procedure, observe for sign of faintness, nausea, and vomiting. Note patient's color and pulse and respiratory rates and report anything unusual to operator in a manner that will not alarm patient. Apply gauze dressing at site of entry and secure with adhesive after procedure is completed. If respirations were difficult before procedure, note whether thoracentesis has eased respirations.
Paracentesis Withdrawal of fluid from any body cavity, but term most commonly used to refer to withdrawal of fluid from abdominal cavity. Commonly known as abdominal tap.	Obtain specimen. Remove fluid to relieve pressure caused by accumulation of fluid in abdominal cavity.	Trocar and cannula, a 4 to 5 inch long instrument with bore of about 1/8 inch; cannula is removable from trocar; trocar is cylindrical part through which fluid will drain. 22- to 25-gauge needle and 2 ml. syringe for injecting anesthesia, usually procaine hydrochloride. Scalpel to make incision at site of entry; suture material, small clamp or forceps, and scissors for closing incision. Tubing to connect trocar to drainage container. Fenestrated drape; opening of drape is placed over area of abdomen where abdominal cavity will be entered. Antiseptic and cotton balls to cleanse skin at site of entry. Catheter to thread trocar when it is in place, if ordered. Specimen containers. Sterile gloves.	Observe practices of surgical asepsis. Be sure patient voids before procedure to help prevent striking distended bladder with trocar. Report if patient cannot void; catheterization may be ordered. Assist patient to sitting position, preferably in chair at bedside, as illustrated in Figure 20-3 on page 428. Cleanse skin at and around site of entry. Anchor drape to patient with adhesive to prevent its slipping from place. Area of drape around working area is kept sterile. Check label on container of anesthesia and hold container so operator can also read label to help avoid errors. If fluid drains too rapidly, elevate container on stool to slow down rate, as requested. Handle and label specimens. During procedure, observe for signs of faintness and weakness. Note patient's color and pulse and respiratory rates and report anything unusual to operator in a manner that will not alarm patient. Respirations can be expected to ease as pressure of fluid on diaphragm is relieved. An incision is sutured. Place dressing over site of entry and secure it. Leakage from wound is common.

Purpose	Equipment	Suggestions
		Assist patient to comfortable position in bed. Apply abdominal binder for patient's comfort.
Gastric Analysis Laboratory examination of gastric content. Obtain specimens.	Rubber or plastic tube, as ordered, 12 to 24 inches longer than distance from patient's mouth to his stomach. Clamp for tube. Syringe, usually 50 ml. Water soluble lubricant; dish of chipped ice. Glass of water. Specimen containers. Test meals if ordered. Towel.	Observe practices of medical asepsis. Patient ordinarily should have been fasting, as ordered, prior to procedure. Have tube well chilled in dish of ice, if it is rubber, to make it easier to insert. Lubricate end of tube for easier insertion. Assist patient to comfortable sitting or lying position. Observe agency policy concerning who is allowed to insert a gastric tube. If it is the nurse's responsibility, have patient breathe through his mouth and swallow as tube passes through area in back of mouth to help prevent gagging. Offering sips of water, if allowed, helps tube insertion. Place end of tube in water; if air bubbles occur, tube is incorrectly placed in lung tissue. Also, misplaced tube may cause difficult breathing and coughing. Handle and label specimens. Tube may be left in place, clamped, and additional specimens taken after test meals. Receive tube in towel as it is removed.
Gastric and Duodenal Suction Continuous removal of contents from stomach and duodenum by use of suction. Keep stomach and duodenum at rest and empty, as for example, following surgery on stomach. Relieve distention. Prevent severe vomiting.	Rubber or plastic tube as ordered. Some have metal tip while others have inflatable bag, to help keep tube in place. Syringe and specified solution to inflate bag. Water-soluble lubricant and dish of chipped ice. Glass of water. Container for drainage. Source of suction; either an electric pump or wall suction apparatus is generally used. Adhesive and clamp for securing tube. For irrigating tube, 50 ml. bulb or regular syringe and irrigating solution (normal saline or water).	Observe practices of medical asepsis. Assist patient to comfortable lying position. If possible, place patient on right side if tube is to enter small intestine so that tube can more easily drop through pyloric valve at end of stomach. While inserting tube, follow guides given earlier for gastric analysis. It may be necessary to continue introducing tube every 20 to 30 minutes after it has reached stomach until desired length has entered upper intestinal tract. Attach tube to bottle to receive drainage. Attach bottle via a second tube to suction apparatus. Chill and lubricate tube as described for gastric analysis. Assist with inserting tube as necessary. Secure tube to patient with adhesive and to bed, as necessary, with clamp to allow patient to move without danger of tube slipping out of place. Fluids by mouth are limited to prevent washing out chemicals from gastrointestinal tube. Hence, give special mouth care frequently to prevent drying of mucous membranes and to relieve thirst. Care for nose to prevent accumulation of secretions.

Chart 20-1 continued

Procedure and Definition	Common Indications	Basic Equipment and Supplies	Guides for the Nurse Who Will Assist
			Irrigate tube as ordered with syringe and 30 to 60 ml. of normal saline or water. Tube is not clogged when irrigating solution returns as soon as suction is started again. Record solution as intake.
			Check drainage regularly to note that system is functioning. Note character and amount of drainage, and record according to agency policy.
			Figures 20-4 through 20-6 on pages 428 and 429 illustrate gastric suction and the irrigation of the gastric tube.

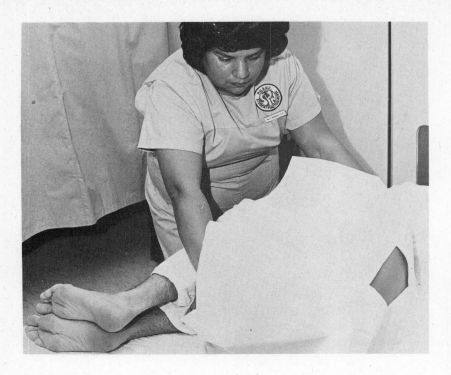

Fig. 20-1 The patient is in position for a lumbar puncture. Note that his back is sharply arched as the nurse holds him at his knees and at his shoulders. The sterile drape has been secured in place with adhesive strips.

Policies vary markedly among health agencies concerning who may start a blood transfusion. In many agencies, only a physician or specially trained personnel are allowed to give a transfusion. Hence, it is described in this chapter since in those instances, the nurse acts as an assistant. In agencies where the nurse is expected to assume responsibility for starting a transfusion, the procedure for administering an intravenous infusion described in Chapter 17 is followed.

A **blood transfusion** is the intravenous infusion of whole blood. It is usually given when the patient's total blood volume has been decreased, as for example, following a hemorrhage. Certain parts of whole blood are sometimes given when a selective need exists. For example, a patient may need red blood cells but not the plasma. In other situations, only plasma is required. Plasma is particularly useful in emergencies in order to replace fluids quickly since plasma presents no compatibility problems. Hence, time need not be lost with crossmatching and possibly seeking suitable donors.

The person giving the blood is referred to as the **donor.** The person receiving the blood is called the **recipient.** Blood may be given either by the direct or the indirect method. In the indirect method, which is the most common method, the blood is used after it has been collected from a donor. In the direct method, the blood is infused as it is being collected. This method is rarely used except in certain emergency situations.

Before blood is to be given to a patient, it must be determined that the blood of the donor and that of the recipient are compatible. Blood is categorized into four major groups: O, A, B, and AB. In addition to the four groups, there are many other factors which differentiate one blood from another, Rh factor being one example. The laboratory examination to determine a person's blood type is called **typing.** The process of

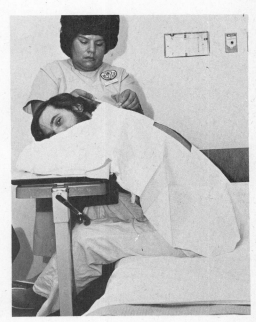

Fig. 20-2 The patient rests over his bedside table in readiness for a thoracentesis. The nurse is securing the sterile drape with adhesive strips so that it cannot slip out of place and over the working area.

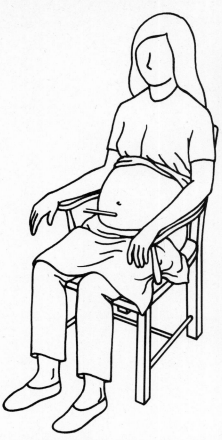

Fig. 20-3   The patient is in proper position for an abdominal paracentesis.

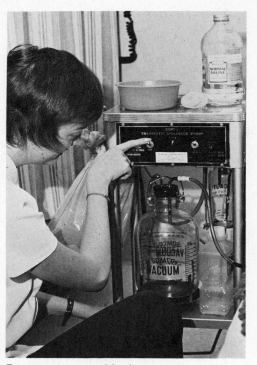

Fig. 20-4   A portable drainage pump commonly used for gastric suction. The calibrated bottle on the lower shelf receives drainage from the patient. Some health agencies provide suction from a wall outlet in the patient's room, making portable equipment as shown here unnecessary.

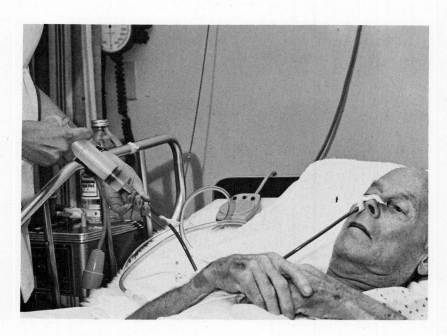

Fig. 20-5   The nurse is irrigating by injecting normal saline solution into the tube that drains the patient's stomach. She uses approximately 30 to 60 ml. of normal saline for each irrigation.

determining compatibility between blood specimens is known as **cross-matching.**

Blood is dispensed in bottles or in plastic containers by a blood bank or a laboratory and is ready for use. The container is the one used for obtaining the blood from the donor and contains a solution to prevent clotting.

Blood is normally not warmed before administration in order to prevent cell damage. Exceptions to this are occasionally made in emergency situations when large amounts of blood are transfused rapidly. To reduce the adjustment of the patient's body to a large volume of cold blood, special heat exchange coils are used to warm the blood. Hot water is not recommended.

For most transfusions, the equipment necessary is similar to that used for an intravenous infusion. The drip chamber in a transfusion set contains a filter. A slightly larger needle, usually an 18 gauge, is used because of the viscosity of the blood. Or, a catheter may be used as described in Chapter 17 and illustrated in Figure 17-34 on page 356. If the patient is very sensitive to the pain of a large needle as it pierces the skin, a small amount of local anesthesia or a volatile anesthetic spray may be used, if ordered by the physician. Occasionally, when small amounts of blood are being given, as for children, a syringe is used to introduce the blood.

Gentle inversion of the blood container will resuspend the red cells before the transfusion. Normal saline solution with a connection between it and the blood container is frequently used to start the transfusion. This type of equipment is illustrated in Figure 17-46 on page 364. A glucose solution should not be used because the solution is likely to destroy red blood cells and cause clotting in the intravenous tubing. Also drugs are not to be added to blood being transfused.

In the management of blood for transfusion, every safety precaution should be taken. The nurse should check and double check the labels, the numbers, the Rh factor, and compatibility. After identifying infor-

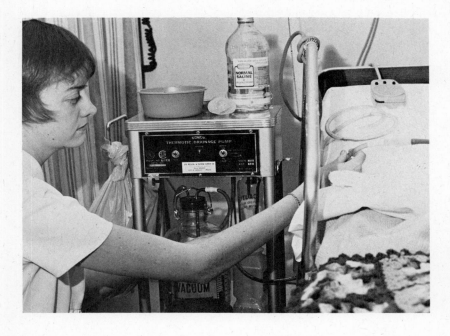

Fig. 20-6 After irrigating the tube, the nurse checks to see that there is a return of the irrigating solution through the tube at the glass connector. When the solution returns, she knows that the suction is working properly and that the patient's stomach is being emptied of its contents.

Procedures with which the nurse assists   429

mation on the patient's record is checked, identification of the patient should be reaffirmed at the bedside.

The nurse should be prepared to recognize signs and symptoms of untoward effects of a transfusion. She should remain with the patient for at least the first 15 minutes after a transfusion has been started and check the patient frequently while the blood infuses. The most serious and quickest complication is the reaction when incompatible bloods have been mixed. Incompatibility reactions generally occur after the first 100 to 200 ml. of blood have infused. A feeling of chilliness, any sign of general discomfort, or a change in the patient's appearance or expression should be noted carefully. Additional symptoms may include headache, difficulty in breathing, pain in the lumbar region, rapid pulse and respiratory rates, and a fall in blood pressure.

Reactions which may be due to some contaminate in the blood usually occur late in the course of the transfusion or after it has been completed. The patient generally has an elevated temperature, flushing of the skin, and general malaise. The following are additional signs that may indicate trouble: moist coughing and expectoration of blood-tinged mucus; feeling itchy, especially in the areas where the skin is warm; and hives.

Whenever untoward symptoms occur, the nurse stops the transfusion and reports her findings immediately. Reactions to blood transfusions can be very serious.

It is the nurse's responsibility to see that the blood is regulated at a flow as ordered. The nurse should check the rate of flow carefully and regularly while blood is being infused.

A blood transfusion is discontinued in the same manner as is an intravenous infusion. This was described in Chapter 17.

Some patients do not need all of the constituents of whole blood. For example, one may need red blood cells but not the plasma and its constituents. Packed red blood cells may be given to such a patient. In other situations, only plasma is required. Human serum or plasma is particularly useful in emergencies for immediate restoration of fluids, since serum presents no compatibility problem, and time need not be lost matching bloods and seeking donors. Fractions, such as serum albumin and gamma globulin, have been separated out of plasma and used for the treatment and prevention of certain diseases.

Conclusion

The primary responsibilities of the nurse acting as an assistant for procedures discussed in this chapter have been described. Possibly none is more important than that of observing the patient. Persons carrying out these procedures are often with the patient for short periods of time. Therefore, the assisting nurse's observations are important in order for the physician to plan the patient's medical regimen.

References

Beaumont, Estelle and Wiley, Loy, eds., "Helping Patients Cope With Painful Procedures," *Nursing '74*, 4:16, March 1974.

Child, Judy, et al, "Blood Transfusion," *American Journal of Nursing*, 72:1602–1605, September 1972.

Isler, Charlotte, "Blood: The Age of Components," *RN*, 36:31–42, June 1973.

Kelly, Sister Patricia, "Speaking Out: Diagnostic Tests: What Should We Tell the Patient?" *Nursing '74*, 4:15–16, December 1974.

Luciano, Kathy and Shumsky, Claire J., "Pediatric Procedures: The Explanation Should Always Come First," *Nursing '75*, 5:49–52, January 1975.

Marzluf, Sister Mary John, "Transfusion Recipients: New Battleground in a 5000-Year-Old Cold War," *Nursing Care-Bedside Nurse*, 6:12–15, April 1973.

21 preoperative and postoperative nursing care

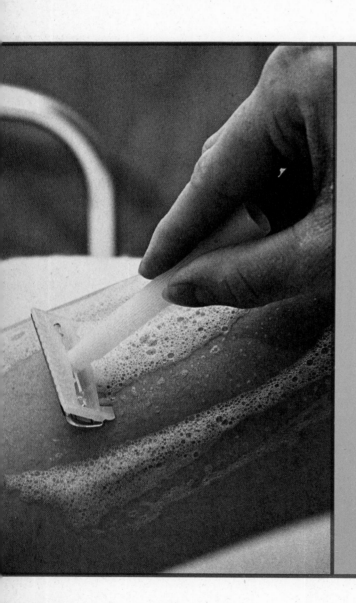

behavioral objectives

When mastery of content in this chapter is reached, the student will be able to

Define terms appearing in the glossary.

Design a plan of care for a surgical patient that will help to meet his psychological needs.

Design a teaching program that will help prepare a patient for the best possible respiratory functioning postoperatively.

Describe how the patient's skin in the area where surgery is to be done is prepared preoperatively and indicate why the preparation is done.

List at least 16 items of importance in the physical preparation of a preoperative patient and indicate the reason for each.

Discuss the nurse's role when she receives a patient from the recovery room.

State two primary goals of postoperative care.

List ten postoperative discomforts and complications for which the nurse should be alert; indicate care that will help to prevent them and common symptoms that will tell the nurse they may be developing.

List three postoperative complications that generally require emergency care and indicate how each is usually handled.

Discuss ways in which the nurse can assist the family of a surgical patient.

Explain why the key to the success of a surgical experience may very well depend on the patient's preoperative care.

glossary

Early Ambulation Assisting the patient to get out of bed and to walk as soon after a surgical procedure as it is possible.

glossary cont.

Embolus A dislodged blood clot that travels in the bloodstream.

Evisceration The separation of a wound with exposure of body organs.

Shock The reaction of the body to inadequate circulation or circulatory collapse.

Singultus Hiccups.

Thrombophlebitis Inflammation of a vein, usually in the leg, generally associated with the presence of a blood clot.

Thrombus A blood clot adhering to the wall of a blood vessel.

Trendelenberg Position The position of the patient in bed with the feet elevated and the head lowered.

introduction

This chapter discusses the preoperative and postoperative care of the surgical patient. The discussion will not include care of patients with specific disorders requiring surgery which is described in clinical nursing texts. Rather, it will include care that, in general, applies to all surgical patients, regardless of diagnosis and type of surgery.

Preoperative care prepares the way for postoperative care. For example, teaching the patient how to assist with respiratory functioning during the postoperative period is done before the patient has surgery. Experienced health practitioners have found that the well-prepared and well-informed patient has fewer postoperative discomforts and complications than the uninformed and ill-prepared patient. Therefore, good preoperative care is an important part of the total care of the surgical patient. It is often the key to the success of a surgical experience for the patient.

Psychological care of the surgical patient

In most instances, the patient is told about the surgery he needs by his physician before admission to the hospital. Occasionally, the patient may know for days, even weeks, that surgery is planned. In other instances, he may be admitted for study and then learn that surgery is advised. In emergency situations, when time is of the essence, the patient may know only minutes, or an hour or two beforehand that surgery is necessary. In any of these situations, the nurse has an important role in helping with the psychological preparation of the patient.

Chapter 3 pointed out that helping patients with psychological problems begins with knowing oneself. Put yourself in the patient's position. Try to understand how you would feel in a similar situation. Consider what action you would like a nurse to take in order to offer you support and comfort. It is the rare patient who faces surgery without worries. Most patients have fears of the unknown, of being unconscious, and of being helpless to control events. For patients, there is no such thing as minor surgery.

Psychological preparation will vary greatly among patients. For example, the patient's age, diagnosis, cultural and educational background, family responsibilities, sex, and occupation are typical factors that will guide the nurse when preparing the patient for surgery. In addition, the nurse is guided by the physician's role in the patient's preparation. For example, the physician may prefer to discuss the patient's diagnosis with him during the postoperative period when a diagnosis has been established with certainty. Or he may have given the patient rather specific information concerning the surgery. To repeat everything the patient already knows can be annoying.

Some patients may feel they understand the surgery from information they have gathered from friends. Unfortunately, this type of information is very often misleading and inaccurate.

Psychological preparation includes observing and listening to the patient. It is usually of no help simply to tell him that everything will be all right and that he should not worry. The helpful nurse will be available to the patient and give him an opportunity to discuss his problems and express his feelings.

Usually, it would be very frightening for the patient if the nurse were to suggest that he visit with his minister, priest, or rabbi before surgery. However, by observing and listening, she can often determine whether the patient wishes to see his clergyman. She can then take steps to arrange a visit if this has not already been done.

While there is no standard formula for preparation for surgery, experience has shown that the following concerns are most frequently expressed by the patient:

* What is the surgical procedure and why is it being done?
* Will I lose control of my body functions while I am unconscious?
* How long will I be in the operating and recovery rooms?
* When can I see my family after surgery?
* Will I have pain when I wake up?
* Will I be sick from the anesthesia?
* Will I have tubes in me when I wake up?
* Will I need a blood transfusion?
* What can I eat and drink after surgery?
* What kind of incision will I have? How long will it take to heal? Will I be disfigured? Can I lead a normal life?
* How long will it take before I can return to work and normal activity? For example, the breadwinner may be worried about time lost at work. A mother may be concerned about the care of her children. A student will want to know when he can return to school.

Some patients may pose still other questions. On the other hand, not every patient will be interested in answers to every question just listed. But the questions may help to guide the nurse in being alert to areas where the patient may have concerns.

Even though the patient may not have asked, it is usually helpful to tell him why bed siderails are likely to be used, why infusions or gastric suction may be necessary, why an indwelling catheter will be in place, how he will be prepared for walking, and so on. He may need to know the nature and advantages of recovery room care. The nurse is helping the patient psychologically when she prepares him before surgery for things to expect during the postoperative period.

Psychological care continues during the postoperative period in a manner similar to the preoperative care just described. The nurse

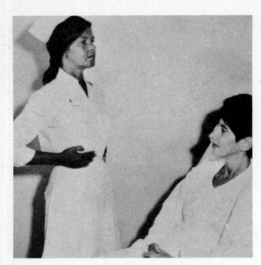

Fig. 21-1 The nurse demonstrates to the patient deep breathing exercises. She is showing her how to take a deep inspiration so that she can feel the pull between the ribs.

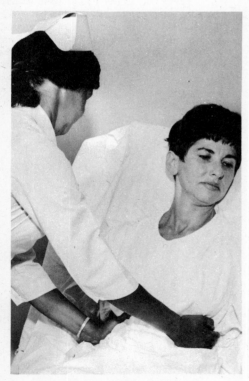

Fig. 21-2 The nurse is showing the patient how she can support the lower chest when doing deep breathing or coughing exercises.

continues to explain what is happening to the extent to which the patient is interested or able to understand. She watches for signs that suggest the patient may be covering fears. For example, he may ask, "How am I doing?", when he really means "Do you think I'll make it?". Such questions can alert the nurse to feelings and worries which patients may not be able to express more specifically.

To summarize, the nurse will wish to know her patient well before she begins preparing him for surgery. She should know what he already knows and what additional information he may need. The nurse can then purposefully consider just what her patient's needs may be and proceed with individualized pre- and postoperative care accordingly.

Preparing the patient for optimum postoperative respiratory functioning

Postoperative patients tend to take shallow breaths. They often try not to move about anymore than is necessary. They do not want to cough for fear of pain and of breaking open their wounds. If patients are allowed to continue in this manner, respiratory problems are likely to arise. Secretions will accumulate in the respiratory tract, parts of the lung will not be used and may collapse and fill with fluid, and lung infections may occur.

An important part of preoperative care is teaching the patient how to cough and deep breathe and explaining to him the importance of moving about postoperatively. It has been found that patients are much more cooperative and willing to cough, move about, and deep breathe when explanations and the opportunity to practice are given before surgery.

Positioning the patient is important for proper breathing. The patient should practice lying, sitting, and standing positions that allow for free movement of the diaphragm and expansion of the chest wall. Good body alignment, as described in Chapters 5 and 12, promotes best use of the respiratory process, whether the patient is lying down, sitting, or standing.

There are some variations in what is considered to be the best method for teaching the patient how to breathe deeply. Most experienced persons recommend that the patient be instructed to inhale slowly and evenly to the greatest chest expansion possible for him. Next, he should hold his breath for at least three seconds. Longer periods do not seem more beneficial than the three second hold. He then exhales normally. The patient's condition is a guide to how often deep breathing should be done. For some persons, two to three times every three or four hours postoperatively is satisfactory. For patients in danger of respiratory complications, it may need to be done as often as every hour or two.

Blow bottles are sometimes used to assist the patient to learn how to deep breathe. Water is placed in a bottle and the patient is given an ordinary drinking tube or a rubber or plastic tube. He is then instructed to blow bubbles vigorously in the bottle after taking deep inspirations. Some agencies run tubing between two bottles and have the patient force water from one bottle to the other by blowing into a second piece of tubing. The first bottle is capped but has openings to receive the two pieces of tubing; the second bottle is uncapped so that air can escape as water enters.

Inhaling and exhaling in an ordinary paper bag may be used. Carbon dioxide accumulates in the bag and stimulates deeper respirations. Occasionally, a mixture of carbon dioxide and oxygen may be ordered for inhalation to stimulate respirations.

The person with known lung pathology needs to learn more specific exercises. Persons with chronic pulmonary diseases in particular profit by developing respiratory muscles through exercises. Texts dealing with respiratory diseases describe these exercises in detail. Intermittent positive pressure breathing, described in Chapter 19, is also used for some patients. The preoperative patient should be taught how the I.P.P.B. machine functions if he is not familiar with it.

The cough mechanism causes an explosive movement of air from the lower to the upper respiratory tract. To be effective, a cough should have enough muscle contraction to force air to be expelled and to propel a liquid or a solid on its way out of the respiratory tract. The cough is a cleansing mechanism of the body. It is an effective way to assist in keeping the airway clear of secretions and other debris.

When teaching the patient how to cough, the nurse places him in a sitting position, and asks him to inhale deeply and then cough forcefully. The area of the incision is supported when the patient is deep breathing and coughing. Support may be offered with the nurse's hands, a pillow, or a folded blanket. This offers both comfort and support to the incision. Figures 21-1, 21-2, and 21-3 illustrate a nurse teaching the patient how to deep breathe and cough.

A good way to promote respiratory functioning is to have the patient change positions in bed frequently during the postoperative period. This should be done every three to four hours during the immediate postoperative period. At first, the patient may need assistance in changing his position. As soon as he can change position for himself, he is encouraged to do so frequently.

Being out of bed and walking as soon after surgery as possible is called **early ambulation.** It is usually a morale booster and most patients will report early ambulation with pride and joy. In addition to helping respiratory functioning, early ambulation helps prevent other postoperative discomforts and complications, as Chart 21-3 describes. Explaining the importance of early ambulation and how the patient will be prepared for it will usually result in the patient's desire to cooperate in this important aspect of postoperative care.

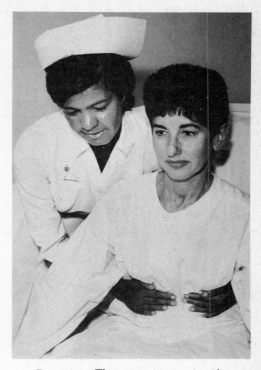

Fig. 21-3 The nurse is assuring the patient that if she has discomfort that there are means for helping her to do deep breathing and coughing exercises. For example, the nurse will go behind the patient and support her while she does deep breathing and coughing exercises.

Preoperative care of the patient

Most health agencies have a check list to guide the nurse as she carries out the physical preparation of the preoperative patient. An example of one is illustrated in Figure 21-4. After the nurse enters appropriate notations on this form, it is placed in the patient's record which accompanies him to surgery. Note that the nurse checks to see that an operative permit for surgery has been signed. An example of such a permit is illustrated in Figure 21-5 on page 439.

Chart 21-1 describes the basic physical preparation of the preoperative patient. It includes items found on most agency check lists plus additional preparation the patient ordinarily requires (see p. 441).

The skin at and around the site of the surgery is prepared preoperatively, as Chart 21-1 indicates. The purpose is to have the operative area free of hair and scrupulously clean. Hair shafts often harbor organisms. The skin cannot be sterilized, but proper skin preparation helps to reduce the chances of introducing organisms into the operative site.

The area of skin prepared is ordinarily much larger than the immediate area around the incision. This precaution further reduces the changes of infection. When the physician has not indicated the exact area to be prepared, Figure 21-7 may be used as a guide (see p. 440).

In some instances, the surgeon may order that sterile dressings be applied to the shaved area after the skin has been swabbed with an antiseptic. This is likely to be the case when orthopedic surgery is done.

Chart 21-2 and Figures 21-8 through 21-16 describe and illustrate shaving the operative site and applying sterile dressings to the part (see pp. 445 to 448).

When items in Chart 21-1 have not been carried out, the nurse will

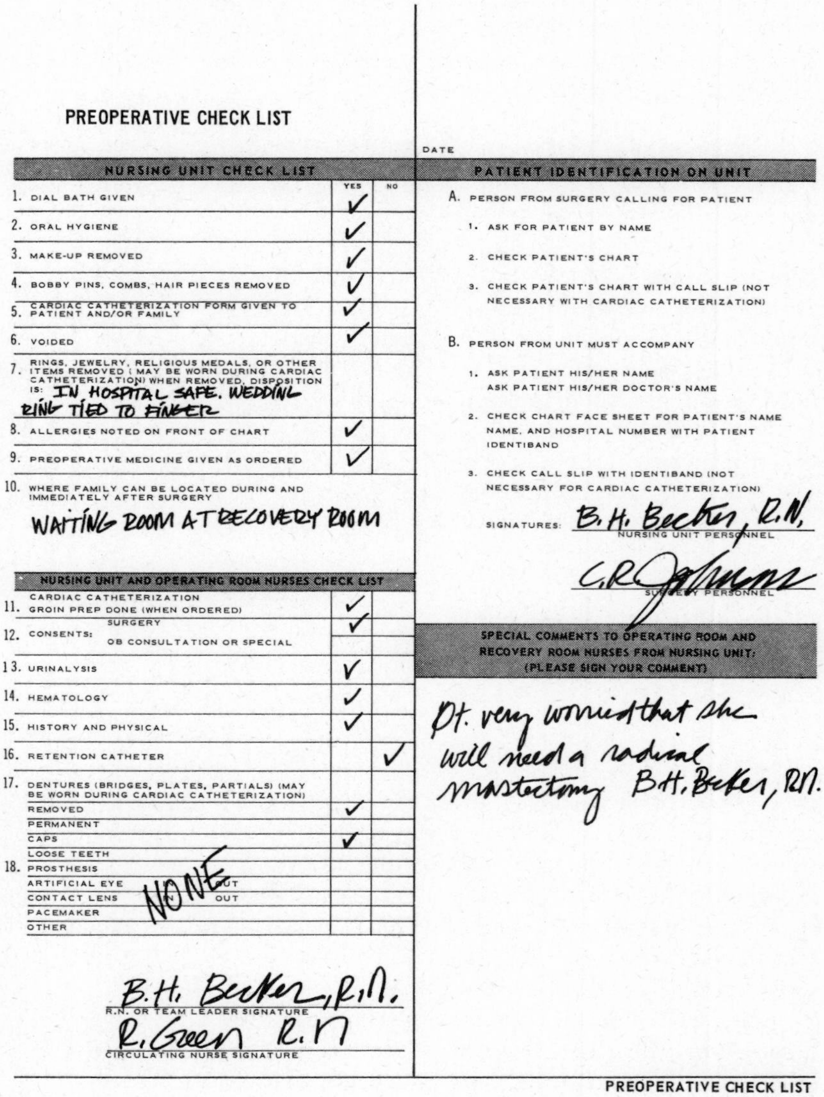
PREOPERATIVE CHECK LIST

DATE

NURSING UNIT CHECK LIST (YES / NO)

1. DIAL BATH GIVEN ✓
2. ORAL HYGIENE ✓
3. MAKE-UP REMOVED ✓
4. BOBBY PINS, COMBS, HAIR PIECES REMOVED ✓
5. CARDIAC CATHETERIZATION FORM GIVEN TO PATIENT AND/OR FAMILY ✓
6. VOIDED ✓
7. RINGS, JEWELRY, RELIGIOUS MEDALS, OR OTHER ITEMS REMOVED (MAY BE WORN DURING CARDIAC CATHETERIZATION) WHEN REMOVED, DISPOSITION IS: IN HOSPITAL SAFE. WEDDING RING TIED TO FINGER
8. ALLERGIES NOTED ON FRONT OF CHART ✓
9. PREOPERATIVE MEDICINE GIVEN AS ORDERED ✓
10. WHERE FAMILY CAN BE LOCATED DURING AND IMMEDIATELY AFTER SURGERY
WAITING ROOM AT RECOVERY ROOM

NURSING UNIT AND OPERATING ROOM NURSES CHECK LIST

11. CARDIAC CATHETERIZATION GROIN PREP DONE (WHEN ORDERED) ✓
12. CONSENTS: SURGERY ✓ / OB CONSULTATION OR SPECIAL
13. URINALYSIS ✓
14. HEMATOLOGY ✓
15. HISTORY AND PHYSICAL ✓
16. RETENTION CATHETER — NO ✓
17. DENTURES (BRIDGES, PLATES, PARTIALS) (MAY BE WORN DURING CARDIAC CATHETERIZATION)
REMOVED ✓
PERMANENT
CAPS ✓
LOOSE TEETH
18. PROSTHESIS
ARTIFICIAL EYE — IN / OUT
CONTACT LENS — IN / OUT
PACEMAKER
OTHER
NONE

B.H. Becker, R.N.
R.N. OR TEAM LEADER SIGNATURE
R. Green R.N.
CIRCULATING NURSE SIGNATURE

PATIENT IDENTIFICATION ON UNIT

A. PERSON FROM SURGERY CALLING FOR PATIENT
1. ASK FOR PATIENT BY NAME
2. CHECK PATIENT'S CHART
3. CHECK PATIENT'S CHART WITH CALL SLIP (NOT NECESSARY WITH CARDIAC CATHETERIZATION)

B. PERSON FROM UNIT MUST ACCOMPANY
1. ASK PATIENT HIS/HER NAME
ASK PATIENT HIS/HER DOCTOR'S NAME
2. CHECK CHART FACE SHEET FOR PATIENT'S NAME NAME, AND HOSPITAL NUMBER WITH PATIENT IDENTIBAND
3. CHECK CALL SLIP WITH IDENTIBAND (NOT NECESSARY FOR CARDIAC CATHETERIZATION)

SIGNATURES: B.H. Becker, R.N.
NURSING UNIT PERSONNEL
C.R. Johnson
SURGERY PERSONNEL

SPECIAL COMMENTS TO OPERATING ROOM AND RECOVERY ROOM NURSES FROM NURSING UNIT: (PLEASE SIGN YOUR COMMENT)

Pt. very worried that she will need a radical mastectomy. B.H. Becker, RN.

PREOPERATIVE CHECK LIST

Fig. 21-4 An example of a preoperative check list. The nurse responsible for the patient's care signs it when she has completed the form. Note that the persons who will transport the patient to the operating room are required to sign the form. Also, note that an operating room nurse signs this form when she receives the patient for surgery. These checks and double checks help to avoid errors and to assure that the patient has been properly readied for surgery.

1. I authorize and direct _JOHN BROWN_ _____ M.D.,
my surgeon and/or associates or assistants of his choice, to perform the following operation upon me
EXPLORATORY LAPAROTOMY AND APPENDECTOMY

_____

and/or to do any other therapeutic procedure that (his) (their) judgment may dictate to be advisable for the
patient's well-being. The nature of the operation has been explained to me and no warranty or guarantee has
been made as to the result or cure.

    2. I hereby authorize and direct the above-named surgeon and/or his associates or assistants to pro-
vide such additional services for me as he or they may deem reasonable and necessary, including, but not
limited to, the administration and maintenance of the anesthesia, and the performance of services involving pathology and radiology, and I hereby consent thereto.

    3. I understand that the above-named surgeon and his associates or assistants will be occupied solely
with performing such operation, and the persons in attendance at such operation for the purpose of administering anesthesia, and the person or persons performing services involving pathology and radiology, are not
the agents, servants or employees of the above named hospital nor of any surgeon, but are independent
contractors.

    4. Permission for observation of operation for visiting M.D.'s, nurses, medical students, interns and residents
is hereby granted at the discretion of the physician in charge, subject to current rules and regulations of the hospital.

    5. I hereby authorize the hospital pathologist to use his discretion in the disposal of any severed tissue

or member, except _____

Susan White   _Jane Doe, L.P.N._   _2:30 P.M. 7/18/74_
(PATIENT)   (WITNESS)   (TIME & DATE)

(If patient is a minor or unable to sign, complete the following:)

Patient is a minor _____, or is unable to sign, because_____

_____

_____

_____   _____   _____
(FATHER/MOTHER)   (WITNESS)   (TIME & DATE)

_____   _____   _____
(OTHER PERSON & RELATIONSHIP)   (WITNESS)   (TIME & DATE)

CONSENT TO OPERATION

Fig. 21-5 An example of a consent
form which is signed by the patient to
grant permission for surgery, anesthesia, and rendering of other medical
services. It also grants permission for
select persons to observe the operation
under certain circumstances.

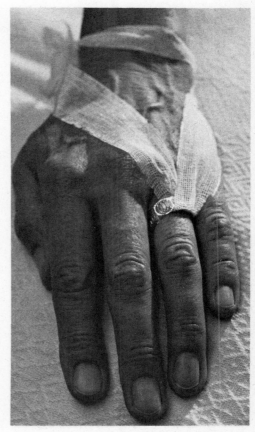

Fig. 21-6 Occasionally a patient may
not wish to remove a ring before going
to surgery. This illustrates how a ring
can be secured so that it will not slip
off the patient's finger.

need to discuss this with the supervising nurse or the physician. Appropriate steps can then be taken as the situation indicates. For example,
surgery may need to be delayed if a cleansing enema was inadvertently
not given.

    As the nurse prepares the patient, she will wish to explain the various
items with him so that he understands what is being done and why. It
is particularly important that he know, for instance, why he is not to have
fluids and food before surgery so that he does not eat or drink in the
nurse's absence.

    Judgment is required in emergency situations. The preoperative
preparation of the patient is adapted to meet the patient's needs in the
best possible manner while still conserving time.

Receiving the patient from the recovery room   439

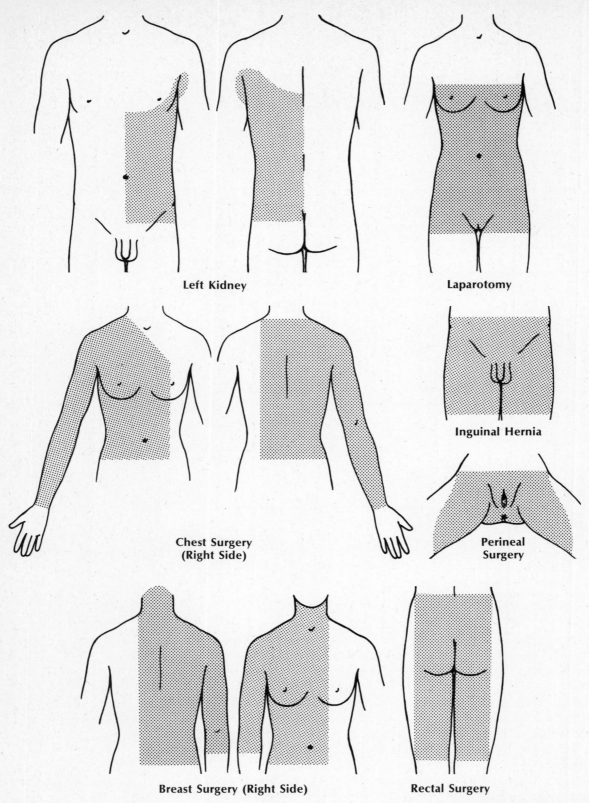

Left Kidney

Laparotomy

Chest Surgery (Right Side)

Inguinal Hernia

Perineal Surgery

Breast Surgery (Right Side)

Rectal Surgery

Fig. 21-7 These sketches illustrate the areas that are ordinarily shaved preoperatively for various types of surgery. Follow the physician's order or local policy which may differ slightly at times from the areas designated here.

Chart 21-1 Physical preparation of the preoperative patient

The purpose is to prepare the patient for surgery in a manner that will help
prevent complications and reduce surgical risks

Item	Reason for Preparation	Comments
	During Preoperative Period	
Complete physical examination, including laboratory studies, such as blood analysis, urinalysis, chest x-ray, and so on	Knowledge of patient's condition is important in order to help prevent complications and reduce surgical risk.	Physical examination is usually done in physician's office prior to admission. Laboratory studies may be done or completed in hospital. Blood analysis includes typing and cross-matching when blood transfusion is anticipated. Study of clotting time is done so that steps can be taken as necessary to help prevent postoperative hemorrhage. Study of electrolyte and blood gas status indicates whether electrolyte therapy is indicated.
		Laboratory findings suggesting patient has an infection may mean delaying surgery. Report any unusual symptoms promptly.
Rest and nutritional status	Having patient in best possible physical condition helps prevent complications and helps reduce surgical risk.	Patient may need assistance to improve physical condition before surgery, such as blood transfusion, intravenous fluids and chemicals, nutritious diet, adequate fluid intake, extra rest, and so on.
	Day/Evening Before Surgery	
Consent for surgery	Legal implications are serious when surgery is performed without proper consent. See Chapters 2 and 7 for further discussion.	Consent forms are usually executed at time of admission. Check to see that this has been done.
Vital signs	Abnormal signs may indicate presence of infection or of other conditions that may increase surgical risk.	Report abnormal vital signs promptly since surgery may have to be canceled if they are not within normal range.
Skin preparation	Having area free of hair and scrupulously clean reduces chances of introducing organisms into operative field.	See pp. 445 to 448 concerning how to prepare skin.
Cleansing enema	Full colon may act as obstruction for surgeon. While anesthetized, patient may have involuntary bowel movement when colon has not been emptied preoperatively.	Type and number of enemas will vary, depending on type of surgery to be performed. Chapter 14 described administration of enemas. Note results of enema carefully; if patient expells little or no fecal material, report this observation.

Chart 21-1 continued

Item	Reason for Preparation	Comments
Personal hygiene	Cleanliness helps prevent infections. Patient usually feels more relaxed and comfortable when personal hygiene needs have been met.	Bath or shower usually is given evening before surgery since there is often insufficient time to give bath or shower on morning of surgery. Early AM bath or shower may disturb patient's rest. Many agencies require using soap containing antiseptic for preoperative bath or shower. Be sure to include special mouth care as indicated.
Bedtime medication	Medication, usually a sedative, is given to assure good night's rest before surgery and to help relieve fears and worries.	Preparation for good night's rest should also include nursing measures discussed in Chapter 13.
Light evening meal and nothing by mouth after midnight	Fluids and food are withheld so that gastro-intestinal tract is at rest and empty. Having tract empty at time of surgery helps decrease postoperative nausea and vomiting. Vomiting while anesthetized may result in patient's aspirating material into lungs and serious complications.	Nothing by mouth is often abbreviated NPO, from Latin, *non per os*. In some instances, evening meal may also be withheld. Or, if surgery is scheduled for late in day, NPO may be ordered for after 6 AM.
	Day of Surgery	
Vital signs	Abnormal vital signs may indicate presence of infection or other conditions that may increase surgical risk and complications.	Report abnormal vital signs promptly since surgery may have to be canceled if they are not within normal range.
Nothing by mouth	Fluids and food continue to be withheld for reasons given above.	
Care of valuables, such as jewelry, watch, or money	Lost or damaged valuables may result in serious legal problems. Observe agency policy for proper labeling and safekeeping.	If patient objects to removing ring, secure it as illustrated in Figure 21-6.
Prostheses, such as artificial limbs, partial or complete removable dentures, artificial eye, wig, false eyelashes, and contact lenses	Prostheses may be lost or accidentally damaged during surgery. Dentures may become dislodged and cause choking during surgery. Contact lenses may damage eyes.	Store prostheses properly and safely according to agency policy.

Cosmetics, such as lipstick, nail polish, and rouge	Health practitioners in operating and recovery rooms will observe skin, lips, and nails for signs of cyanosis. Cosmetics interfere with these observations.	Patient or nurse removes patient's cosmetics before surgery.
Hair	Long hair can be bothersome for health practitioners in operating and recovery rooms. Hairpins and clips may accidently damage scalp.	Remove hairpins and clips. If patient does not object, braid long hair. Rubber bands may also be used to secure hair in place.
Personal hygiene	Cleanliness helps prevent infections. Patient usually feels more relaxed and comfortable when personal hygiene needs have been met.	Partial bath may be given as indicated. Special mouth care is included as indicated.
Wearing apparel	Hospital garments are used for convenience and to prevent possible damage to personal garments. Cap and stockings may be used for extra protection for patient.	Observe agency policy concerning use of protective cap and stockings.
Bowel and bladder	Full bowel and bladder may act as obstruction for surgeon. While anesthetized, patient may have involuntary bowel movement or urination when colon and bladder are not empty.	Occasionally, enema may be ordered given on day of surgery. Give it early enough so that patient has sufficient time to expel it well. Note results carefully. Report immediately if patient is unable to void. He may need to be catheterized. In most instances, an indwelling catheter if it is to be used, is inserted in operating room.
Preoperative medication	A sedative, usually a narcotic, is given to help relieve fear and to have patient in relaxed state for administration of anesthesia. A drug, such as atropine sulfate, is usually given also to dry secretions in mouth and respiratory tract, thus minimizing danger of aspirating mucus.	Explain to patient that he may feel thirsty after receiving medication, such as atropine sulfate.
Complete patient's record, check patient's identity, and assist with transferring patient to surgery	Health practitioners in operating and recovery rooms will need patient's completed record, including preoperative check list and all laboratory reports. Confusing patients because of poor identification is a serious error.	Completed record is placed on bed or stretcher but out of patient's view since entries on record may disturb him if he chooses to read them. A drowsy patient in a strange environment cannot be depended upon for self-identification. Use proper restraints or bed siderails so that patient will not fall out of bed or off stretcher.
Check patient's identity carefully, using identification bracelet and hospital number, with operating personnel receiving patient	Confusing patients because of poor identification is a serious error.	A drowsy patient in a strange environment cannot be depended upon for self-identification.

Receiving the patient from
the recovery room

Most health agencies now have recovery rooms. Ordinarily, patients are moved to the recovery room immediately after surgery is completed. They remain there until they are conscious and their condition stabilizes. Nurses working in recovery rooms have special training and advanced courses in the immediate care of the postoperative patient. Their role will not be described here.

While the patient is in the operating and recovery rooms, the nurse prepares an open bed, as described in Chapter 6. Or, she fan-folds the top linen to the far side of the bed. In this case, the top linen is not tucked under the mattress at the foot of the bed until the patient is comfortably positioned in bed. Extra protection may be placed at the top of the drawsheet to protect bottom linens from soilage. In addition, equipment and supplies that are likely to be needed are in readiness. They will include such items as blood pressure equipment, extra tissue wipes, several gauze dressings, an emesis basin, and a padded tongue blade or an airway. An airway is illustrated in Figure 21-17. A tongue blade is padded by wrapping it in gauze and then securing the gauze well with adhesive. Intravenous infusion solutions, a standard for holding them, suction and oxygen equipment, an endotracheal tube, and tracheostomy equipment should be available when judgment indicates they may be necessary. An endotracheal tube is a tube that is passed into the trachea through the upper respiratory passages. Like an airway, it is an artificial means to help the patient breathe. It can be suctioned like a tracheostomy and can be used to supply the patient with air or oxygen.

When the patient arrives from the recovery room, the nurse should be prepared to

- Assist with moving him from the stretcher to his bed, as described in Chapter 12.
- Place him on his side when possible so that secretions from his nose and mouth can drain more readily. Or, if he must be on his back, turn his head to one side. If he had spinal anesthesia, he should be kept flat in bed for as long as ordered, usually eight to twelve hours, although some anesthesiologists suggest a much shorter time. This position helps prevent headaches commonly associated with spinal anesthesia.
- Check his pulse and respiratory rates and his blood pressure and report any unusual findings promptly.
- Check his dressings and report immediately if there is fresh blood present.
- Check his postoperative orders and carry out any that need immediate attention. Examples include attaching a gastric suction tube, attaching an indwelling catheter to a drainage system, adding infusion solutions, starting oxygen therapy, and so on.
- Check his state of consciousness. Simple methods, such as calling him by name and touching him are used. Slapping him and moving him about unnecessarily to arouse him should be avoided.

As soon as immediate care has been given and before leaving the bedside, bed siderails are put in place and the patient's signal device is placed conveniently for him.

Additional typical postoperative orders include the following:

Chart 21-2 Shaving the skin of the preoperative patient
and applying sterile dressings to the area

The purpose is to prepare the skin so that it will be as free of microorganisms as
possible to help minimize organisms entering the wound and causing infection

Suggested Action	Reason for Action	Figure to Illustrate
Assemble equipment. Expose area and drape patient appropriately.	Having equipment in readiness saves time. A comfortable patient is more relaxed.	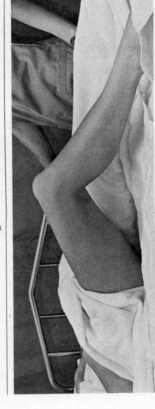 Fig. 21-8 The operative area is the knee, but the entire leg will be prepared. Note that the nurse has draped the patient, exposed the leg for shaving, and protected the bed linen under the leg.
Apply soap solution to small areas of skin and work up lather.	Soap emulsifies normal fatty substances on skin and loosens dirt so that water can penetrate and soften hair.	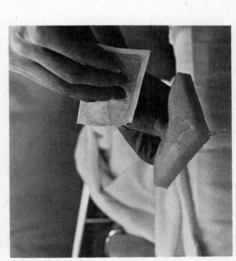 Fig. 21-9 The nurse pours pre-packaged liquid soap onto a sponge.

Chart 21-2 continued

Suggested Action	Reason for Action	Figure to Illustrate
Shave with one hand while stretching skin with other hand. Hold razor at about a 30° angle and take long, gentle strokes in direction of hair growth.	Stretching skin eliminates pits and wrinkles so that nurse can see area and accomplish a close shave. Gentle, long strokes with razor at about a 30° angle helps prevent knicking and cutting skin. Shaving in direction of hair growth helps minimize skin irritation.	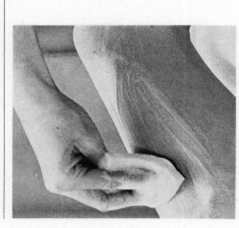 Fig. 21-10 The nurse works up a good lather over one area of the leg where she will begin the shave. 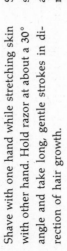 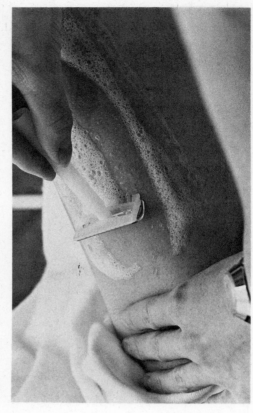 Fig. 21-11 Note that the nurse holds the patient's skin taut with one hand while shaving with the other.

To check to see whether hair has been removed, stoop so that eyes are at level of shaven area; repeat with shaving until all hair is removed.

Looking at area with eyes at level of skin helps nurse to see whether or not all hair has been removed.

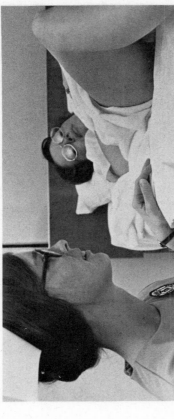

Fig. 21-12 After completing the shave, the nurse stoops so that her eyes are at the level of the patient's leg. She then inspects the leg carefully in order to be sure that all hair has been removed.

When all hair has been removed, don sterile gloves, rinse skin well with sterile water and sterile gauze, and dry with sterile gauze. Change gauze with each stroke while rinsing and frequently while drying.

Rinsing off soap helps prevent skin irritation. Drying area well prevents dilution of antiseptic. Using sterile water and gloves and using sterile gauze for only one stroke helps reduce number of organisms on skin in operative area.

Cleanse area with antiseptic of agency's choice, using firm but gentle strokes and in same manner in which soap was rinsed from skin. Allow antiseptic to dry on skin.

Cleansing area with antiseptic and in manner as described for rinsing helps reduce number of organisms on skin in operative area, thereby minimizing danger of organisms entering operative site.

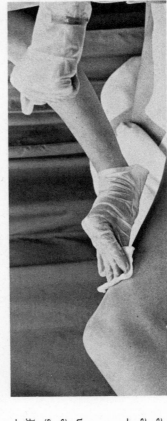

Fig. 21-13 The nurse has donned sterile gloves and now rinses soap from the skin with sterile gauze and sterile water.

Chart 21-2 continued

Suggested Action	Reason for Action	Figure to Illustrate

Cover area with sterile gauze dressings; wrap with sterile towels.

Covering and wrapping area with sterile dressings and sterile towels help protect operative area from contamination.

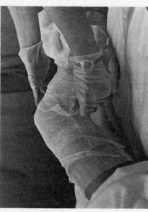

Fig. 21-14 Sterile dressings are applied to the entire leg.

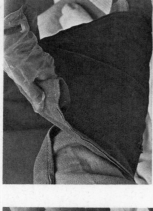

Fig. 21-15 Sterile towels are then used to cover the dressings on the patient's leg.

Secure dressings snugly but not so tightly that they cause discomfort or endanger proper circulation in area.

Well-secured dressings will stay in place to prevent contaminating operative site. Dressings applied too snugly are uncomfortable and could endanger circulation to the part.

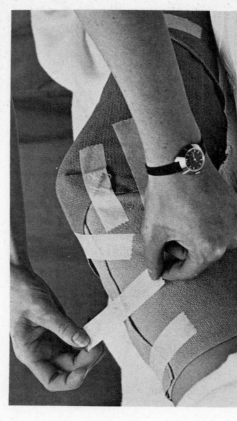

Fig. 21-16 The nurse completes the procedure by securing the sterile dressings well to prevent them from slipping out of place. Note how she has used strips of tape along the long axis of the leg to hold the two sterile towels together.

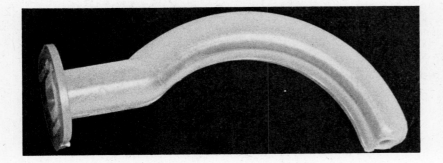

Fig. 21-17 A plastic disposable airway. It is inserted through the mouth and shaped to follow the contour of the mouth and upper respiratory tract. When in place properly, the airway holds the tongue so that it cannot drop back and into the throat. It can be suctioned easily should secretions accumulate.

- Frequency with which vital signs are to be checked, as for example, every 15 minutes for an hour, every half-hour for the next two hours, every hour for four hours, and then, if stable, routinely according to agency procedure.
- Laboratory examinations to be done immediately or during the first day, as for example, urinalysis, blood examinations, or x-rays.
- Type of food and fluids the patient may have, as for example, ice chips and sips of water as desired and tolerated, followed by clear fluids as desired and tolerated, and then a soft diet.
- Medications to be given. Ordinarily, orders are written for drugs to be used as necessary to control pain and sleeplessness. Other medications may include antibiotics and any other drugs to meet specific patient needs.
- Frequency with which patient is turned and frequency with which he is to cough and deep breathe. Usually, these orders specify every one to four hours for 24 to 48 hours.
- Frequency with which patient is to have intermittent positive pressure breathing therapy when this therapy is considered necessary.
- Recording the patient's intake and output.
- When patient is to dangle and ambulate.

Postoperative care of the patient

The primary goals of postoperative care are to prevent discomforts and complications and to help rehabilitate the patient. Chart 21-3 is offered as a guide for the care of the postoperative patient.

As you study Chart 21-3, you will note that measures to prevent postoperative discomforts and complications often include early ambulation. You are encouraged to review Chapter 12 which discussed how to prepare patients for walking and for being out of bed. It included descriptions also of how to assist the patient to get out of bed and to walk. Very often, the sooner a patient is able to ambulate, the fewer postoperative discomforts and complications he is likely to experience.

Note also that Chart 21-3 lists infection several times as a postoperative complication. The surgical patient has an open wound and he has suffered tissue trauma. His general resistance is often lowered. Therefore, the care of the postoperative patient includes every effort to decrease the likelihood of infection. Observing practices of medical and surgical asepsis as indicated is essential. In addition, helping the patient to regain his strength and general resistance to infection is important. Examples of measures to help do so include seeing that the patient has

Chart 21-3 Postoperative discomforts and complications, preventive measures, and nursing care

Item	Discomfort/Complication/Symptoms	Preventive Measures and Nursing Care
Circulatory problems	**Hemorrhage** Excessive blood on dressings; drop in blood pressure; rapid, thready pulse; pale or cyanotic and cold, clammy skin; rapid and labored respirations, as if gasping for breath; low body temperature; restlessness and anxiety, then listlessness, and finally unconsciousness.	Hemorrhage and shock are considered emergency situations; can be fatal. Check vital signs frequently and report adverse changes immediately. Check dressings frequently for sign of hemorrhage. Unless circulation is restored, damage to vital organs, such as brain and kidneys, may result.
	Shock Body's reaction to inadequate circulation or circulatory collapse, usually resulting from hemorrhage.	Patient in shock is usually placed in **Trendelenberg position,** that is, with head lowered and feet elevated. This position is *not* used for patients who have had spinal anesthesia or brain surgery. Some agencies require a physician's order before patients can be placed in this position.
		For hemorrhage and shock, be prepared to administer ordered emergency drugs, intravenous infusion, blood transfusion, and/or oxygen therapy. Place extra covering on patient for warmth.
	Thrombophlebitis Inflammation of vein, usually in leg, generally associated with blood clot. Pain, redness, and swelling are common symptoms.	Preventive measures include early ambulation, use of elastic stockings, as described in Chapter 18, and avoiding massage of legs. When thrombophlebitis is present, affected leg is elevated, patient is kept at rest in bed, hot packs often are used, and drug therapy usually is ordered. Presence of embolus can be fatal when it travels and lodges in vital organs, such as lung, heart, or brain.
	Thrombus Blood clot adhering to wall of blood vessel.	
	Embolus Dislodged blood clot that travels in circulatory system.	
Respiratory problems	Blocked respiratory passageways result in cyanosis and noisy, shallow, and difficult respirations or no respirations.	Blocked respiratory passageway is considered an emergency situation; can be quickly fatal. Check respirations frequently and report adverse changes immediately. Open patient's mouth by pressing down on chin and up at angle of jaw under ear; pull tongue out with gauze if tongue has fallen back into throat; hold mouth open with padded tongue blade. Or an airway may be used; one is illustrated in Figure 21-17. Use suction as indicated to remove secretions and debris that may be blocking passageway. Endotracheal tube or tracheostomy may be needed when other measures do not open respiratory tract.

	Poor respiratory functioning and lung infection are observed by rapid, shallow, and possibly labored respirations, elevated pulse rate, elevated temperature, flushed skin, and general malaise.	Observe measures to promote optimum respiratory functioning described in this chapter in order to help prevent poor respiratory functioning and infection. Clinical texts describe care of patient with lung infection.
	Singultus Hiccups.	Having patient breathe into paper bag usually helps hiccups. Physician may order whiffs of carbon dioxide and oxygen mixture.
Wound care	Infection in wound will display typical signs of local and possibly general systemic infection. **Evisceration** Wound separation with body organs exposed.	Check vital signs and wound regularly and report any signs of infection or wound separation promptly. Care for wound as described in Chapter 18. Evisceration is considered an emergency situation. Patient is likely to say that "something gave way." Report immediately and cover exposed organs with sterile gauze moistened with sterile normal saline.
Pain, restlessness, and sleeplessness	Patient may complain of pain at site of surgery and/or pain over larger body area. Wakefulness is common, especially when pain is present.	Medications to relieve pain and sleeplessness are ordinarily ordered, to be used as nurse considers necessary. Check dressings to see that they are secure but not causing unnecessary discomfort. Observe measures described in Chapter 13.
Urinary tract problems	Retention. Retention with overflow. Infection in urinary tract.	Early ambulation and adequate fluid intake help prevent these problems. Observe measures described in Chapter 16.
Upper gastrointestinal tract problems	Nausea and vomiting. Thirst. Anorexia.	Keep patient on side or with head turned to side so that he will not aspirate vomitus. Use suction as necessary to prevent blocking of respiratory passageways. Offer fluids as ordered; intravenous infusions which help prevent marked thirst and nausea and vomiting often are used during postoperative period. Observe measures described in Chapter 11 to help prevent and relieve these problems.
Lower gastrointestinal tract problems	Constipation. Distention.	Symptoms usually result from inactive gastrointestinal tract due to medications, anesthesia, handling of intestinal organs during surgery, patient's inactivity, and change in fluid and food intake. Early ambulation helps to prevent these problems. Observe measures discussed in Chapter 14.
Musculoskeletal problems	General muscle weakness. Contractures.	Early ambulation helps prevent general muscle weakness. Observe measures discussed in Chapter 12 to help prevent these problems.
Nutritional state	Malnutrition.	Intravenous infusions, certain drugs, and a nourishing diet may be ordered to help prevent results of inadequate food and fluid intake. Observe measures discussed in Chapter 11.
Problems related to skin and mucous membranes	Decubitus ulcer. Infection of mucous membranes in mouth. Discomfort and symptoms of poor personal hygiene.	Observe measures to promote personal hygiene and for the prevention and care of decubitus ulcers as described in Chapter 10.

appropriate physical activity, adequate fluid intake, a nourishing diet, and a sufficient amount of rest and sleep.

To maintain good respiratory functioning, suctioning may be necessary, as Chart 21-3 indicates. It is used when the patient is not able to raise secretions for himself. A rubber or plastic catheter is attached to a suction machine. Or, some hospitals have wall suction outlets which can be used. When mechanical removal of secretions is necessary, damage to the delicate respiratory membranes, excessive removal of essential oxygen, and the introduction of microorganisms are hazards. The catheter is inserted into the patient's respiratory tract. When an airway or endotracheal tube is in place, the catheter may be passed through it for suctioning. The procedure is similar to suctioning a tracheostomy, which was described in Chapter 19.

Assisting the family of the surgical patient

Family members are also fearful and worried about the patient. They too need the nurse's help and support. Many of their questions may be similar to those of the patient. Agency visiting policies may need to be explained. For example, can they visit the patient immediately before he goes to the operating room? If they may, the nurse explains that the patient will be drowsy. Also, she explains to them when the patient is likely to have tubes in place, oxygen therapy, or an infusion, for example. Once prepared, they will not necessarily assume that the patient's condition has worsened.

Family members appreciate knowing where they can wait and how long the patient is expected to be in the operating and recovery rooms. It is better not to state specific times. Delays sometimes occur, causing relatives unnecessary worry. Also, the nurse will wish to tell them where meals and snacks are available while they wait and where they can make telephone calls.

Most relatives are eager to be cooperative and helpful. The nurse who considers their feelings will almost always find a most helpful ally as she cares for the surgical patient.

Conclusion

Adequate preoperative preparation of the surgical patient readies him for his postoperative care. Most patients want to do whatever they can to make the surgical experience as easy as possible. Good psychological care can often help a fearful patient face surgery with calmness and confidence.

References

Beaumont, Estelle and Wiley, Loy, eds., "Innovations in Nursing: "Little Things" That Reduce Complications of Surgery," Nursing '74, 4:49–50, July 1974.

Blackwell, Ardith K. and Blackwell, William, "Relieving Gas Pain," *American Journal of Nursing*, 75: 66–67, January 1975.

Codd, John and Grohar, Mary Ellen, "Postoperative Pulmonary Complications," *The Nursing Clinics of North America*, 10:5–15, March 1975.

Glenn, Frank, "The Elderly As Surgical Patients," *RN*, 37:60, 61, 62, 64, 67, 68, 70, June 1974.

Lewis, Kathryn M., "Teaching: Teamwork: A Key to Better Preop Teaching," *RN*, 37:61–63, May 1974.

Luciano, Kathy, "The Who, When, Where, What & How of Preparing Children for Surgery," *Nursing '74*, 4:64–65, November 1974.

Metheny, Norma A., "Water and Electrolyte Balance in the Postoperative Patient," *The Nursing Clinics of North America*, 10:49–57, March 1975.

Obis, Paul, "Consultation: Remedies for Hiccups," *Nursing '74*, 4:88, September 1974.

Parsons, Mickey Camp and Stephens, Gwen J., "Postoperative Complications: Assessment and Intervention," *American Journal of Nursing*, 74:240–244, February 1974.

Smith, Betty J., "After Anesthesia," *Nursing '74*, 4:28–32, December 1974.

Tharp, Gerald D., "Shock: The Overall Mechanisms," *American Journal of Nursing*, 74:2208–2211, December 1974.

Wiley, Loy, "Diseases Today: Shock: Different Kinds . . . Different Problems," *Nursing '74*, 4:43–52, May 1973.

———, "Diseases Today: Staying Ahead of Shock," *Nursing '74*, 4:19–27, April 1974.

Winslow, Elizabeth Hahn and Fuhs, Margaret Frances, "Preoperative Assessment for Postoperative Evaluation," *American Journal of Nursing*, 73:1372–1374, August 1973.

22 communicable disease control

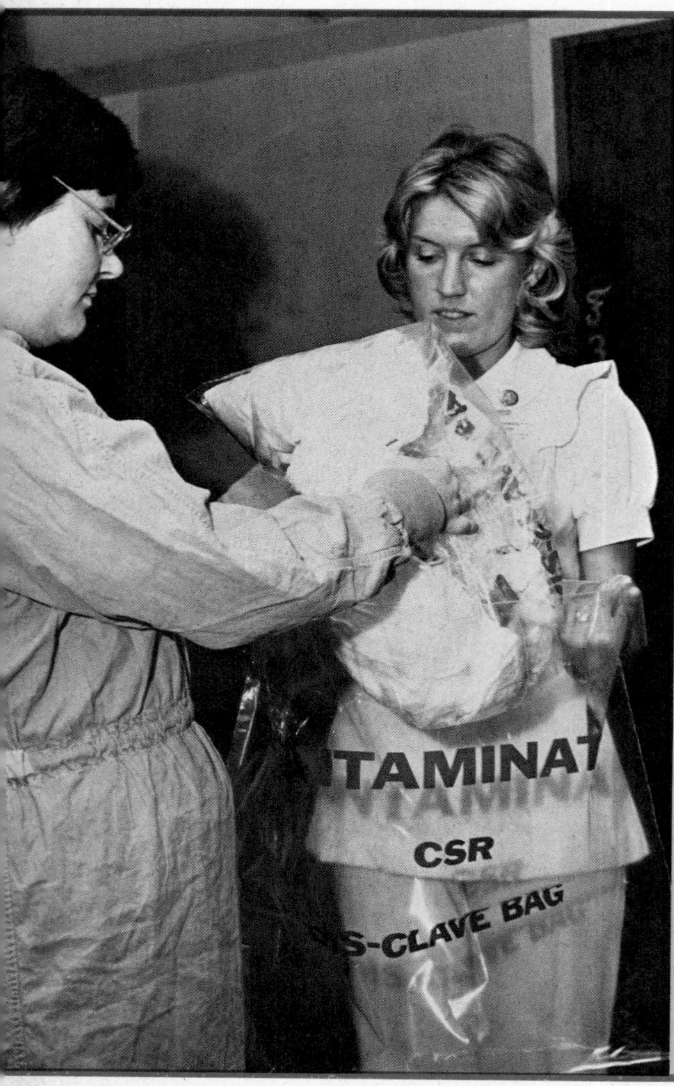

chapter outline

behavioral objectives

When mastery of content in this chapter is reached, the student will be able to

Define terms appearing in the glossary.

List two reasons why there has been dramatic progress in recent years in the control of the various communicable diseases.

Describe how a gown and mask are donned and removed and state the purposes of using them.

Describe how to dispose of excretions and secretions safely.

Describe how these supplies and equipment are handled after being used while caring for a patient with a communicable disease: thermometer, bed linens, blankets, and china and silverware.

List five desirable features of the physical environment of the patient when isolation technique is being observed.

Discuss why frequent and careful hand-washing is a vital part of any type of isolation technique.

List seven types of isolation technique, the purpose and basic requirements of each, and two examples of illnesses requiring the use of each type of technique.

Explain why it is desirable that the room of a patient on protective isolation should be under slight positive pressure while for other types of isolation, it is desirable that there be slight negative pressure in the patient's room.

Describe how to transport a patient with a communicable disease from one department of a health agency to another.

Design a plan that would help meet the psychological needs of a patient when communicable disease techniques are being used.

Blood Isolation Practices to prevent cross-infection by pathogens from the blood of the infected person.

Communicable Disease Technique Practices to limit the spread of microorganisms. Synonym for isolation technique.

Concurrent Disinfection Practices which are observed in the daily care of the patient to limit the spread of microorganisms.

Contagious Disease A disease that is easily spread from person to person.

Direct Contact The physical transfer of microorganisms between a susceptible host and an infected person.

Discharge Precautions Practices to limit cross-infection by pathogens from wounds where the likelihood is slight but possible.

Double-Bag Technique The placing of contaminated items in a bag which in turn is placed within another bag, the outside of which is kept clean for safe handling.

Droplet Spread The contact of a susceptible host with material released from the nose and mouth of an infected person as he coughs, sneezes, and talks.

Enteric Precautions Practices to limit the spread of organisms through direct or indirect contact with infected feces.

Indirect Contact The contact of a susceptible host with contaminated inanimate objects.

Infectious Disease A disease which is caused by a pathogen but which is not always contagious.

Isolation Technique Practices to limit the spread of microorganisms. Synonym for communicable disease technique.

Protective Isolation Practices to prevent contact between potential pathogens and a highly susceptible person. Synonym for reverse isolation.

Respiratory Isolation Practices to limit the spread of organisms by means of droplets that are coughed, sneezed, or breathed into the environment.

Reverse Isolation Practices to prevent contact between potential pathogens and a highly susceptible person. Synonym for protective isolation.

Strict Isolation Practices to limit the spread of highly communicable diseases that are transmitted by contact and airborne routes.

Terminal Disinfection Practices to remove pathogens from the patient's environment and belongings after his illness is no longer communicable.

Vector An insect or animal carrying pathogenic organisms.

Wound and Skin Precautions Practices to limit cross-infection by pathogens from wounds and the skin.

introduction

While all phases of medicine have undergone radical changes in recent years, one of the most dramatic and encouraging is the control of many communicable diseases. There are several reasons for the marked reduction in communicable diseases. The foremost possibly is the discovery of immunizing agents. Helping individuals to build up a resistance to many of the common communicable diseases has become a routine aspect of most preventive care in this country. One example is the use of immunizing agents to help prevent poliomyelitis.

A word of caution is issued lest success result in a careless attitude regarding routine immunizations. Some health practitioners are expressing concern that a false sense of security may result in neglect of immunizations and in an increased incidence of preventable communicable diseases in the future.

Also important in communicable disease control is the discovery of drugs that are effective against the organisms. While many people still become ill with some of the communicable diseases, drug therapy often helps bring the infection under control rapidly. In addition, the use of drugs often reduces the period of communicability. Many of the drugs make it possible for patients with pneumonia, streptococcic sore throat, and tuberculosis, for example, to require special precautions for much shorter periods of time than previously was true.

While the incidence of some communicable diseases has decreased, the prevalence of others remains or has increased. Special techniques used to help prevent the spread of communicable diseases are described in the remainder of this chapter.

Definition of terms

Chapter 4 described terms and practices with which the nurse should be familiar before proceeding with the study of this chapter. Also, knowledge of the spread of organisms, as illustrated in Figure 4-1 on page 45 is important to an understanding of much of the information presented in this chapter.

Communicable disease or **isolation technique** refers to practices that limit the spread of communicable microorganisms. It is made up of two parts: separating infected persons and their pathogens from the uninfected, and rendering contaminated items safe for reuse or disposing of them safely.

A **contagious disease** is one that spreads with relative ease from the sick to the well. The common cold is an example of a contagious disease. An **infectious disease** is caused by a pathogen, but it is not always contagious. Examples include nephritis and pancreatitis, which are infectious diseases of the kidney and pancreas. The terms "contagious" and "infectious" are often used interchangeably. However, they are not synonymous.

Microorganisms are transmitted by four main routes: contact, vehicle, airborne, and vector-borne.

The contact route is composed of three subgroups. **Direct contact** involves the physical transfer between a susceptible host and an infected person. For example, a nurse may acquire a communicable disease as she helps meet the patient's personal hygiene needs. Another example is a venereal disease, such as gonorrhea, which is spread by direct contact between a susceptible host and an infected person. **Indirect contact** involves contact of a susceptible host with contaminated inanimate objects, such as bed linen, clothing, and dressings. **Droplet spread** involves contact by a susceptible host with organisms spread by the patient when he coughs, sneezes, and talks. This is usually considered contact, since these droplets do not travel very far.

The vehicle route applies to diseases transmitted through contaminated food, water, and blood. Airborne transmission occurs when diseases are spread by dust, lint, and droplets that remain suspended in the air for long periods of time. Organisms carried in this manner are

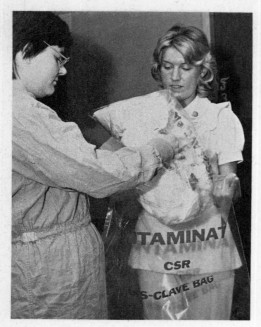

Fig. 22-1 The nurse wearing a gown drops a bag of contaminated items used in the care of a patient requiring isolation into a second bag, the outside of which is kept clean. Note that the nurse holding the second bag has folded back a cuff on her bag which helps prevent contamination of the outside of the second bag as she receives contaminated items. These plastic bags are clearly marked so that personnel handling them are made aware of their contents.

inhaled or deposited on the susceptible host. Vector-borne diseases are those carried by insects and animals. Malaria, for example, is spread by a **vector**—the mosquito.

Concurrent disinfection is the term used to refer to ongoing practices which are observed in the daily care of the patient. The purpose is to limit the spread of pathogenic organisms. Concurrent disinfection includes caring for items used by the patient, his body secretions and excretions, and other contaminated equipment and supplies used in patient care. Specific practices are determined on the basis of knowledge of the causative organism. All practices concerning the care of equipment and supplies observed routinely as a part of medical asepsis are considered concurrent disinfections, since they are intended to control the spread of pathogens.

Terminal disinfection refers to practices used to remove pathogens from the patient's immediate environment and belongings once his illness is no longer communicable. Equipment and supplies in contact with the patient should be thoroughly cleaned with a germicidal solution or other means of disinfection, as discussed in Chapter 4. Specific measures depend on the causative organism. In some instances, measures are prescribed by the sanitary codes of the community.

The **double-bag technique** is frequently used when caring for patients with a communicable disease. It consists of placing contaminated items, such as dressings or linens, in a bag which in turn is placed inside another bag. The outside of the second bag is kept clean for safe handling. The bag is then marked so that personnel are aware of the fact that the contents are contaminated items for disposal or for whatever special care they require to prepare them for reuse. Figure 22-1 illustrates the double-bag technique.

Personal contact precautions

Figure 22-2 illustrates how barriers prevent common vehicles from carrying pathogens from the patient to the general environment. Frequently used barriers are presented in this section and in the following two sections of this chapter.

Handwashing. The technique for handwashing was described in Chapter 4. It is generally believed that inadequately cleaned hands transmit more microorganisms than any other vehicle. Therefore, *handwashing is the single most important means of preventing the spread of microorganisms.* The hands should be washed before and after contact with each patient or with his secretions and excretions. This should be done even on those occasions when gloves are worn.

Gown Technique. In situations when gowns are necessary, individual gown technique is recommended. This means that gowns are worn only once and then discarded for disinfection and reuse. Disposable gowns are destroyed in an appropriate manner. Multiple gown technique means that the same gown is used several times by one or more persons. This technique was practiced extensively in the past and requires careful removal and donning of the gown to avoid contamination. Since contamination does often occur, the Center for Disease Control recommends that this technique be abandoned.

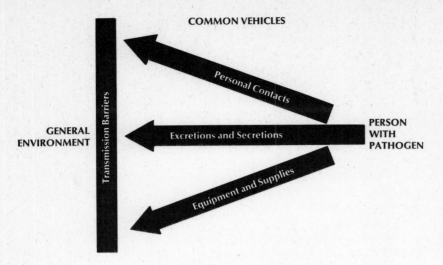

COMMON VEHICLES

GENERAL
ENVIRONMENT

Transmission Barriers

Personal Contacts

Excretions and Secretions

Equipment and Supplies

PERSON
WITH
PATHOGEN

Fig. 22-2 The transmission barriers are communicable disease or isolation techniques. Note that the transmission barriers prevent common vehicles from carrying pathogens from the infected person to the general environment. When possible, the room of the patient requiring isolation should be kept under slight negative pressure. Then, when a door or window is opened, air currents that could carry organisms from the patient will move *toward* the patient rather than away from him and into the general environment.

Gowns that are used for isolation technique are made of washable or disposable material. Most are made to be worn over the outer garments of the wearer. They are designed with the opening in the back and a tie around the waist to help keep the gown secure and closed. Some have stockinet at the wrists. Others have buttons. They may have buttons or tie strings at the neck. These minor variations do not affect the use or the value of the gown. All have the same purpose of protecting the clothing of those who come in contact with the patient from contamination.

Supplies of gowns should be available outside the immediate patient environment, so the wearer can put one on before entering the patient's area. There is no special way in which a clean gown must be put on. However, it should be closed well in the back, so that all parts of the wearer's clothing are covered.

When the wearer is ready to leave the unit, the gown is unfastened and removed by turning it inside out. The wearer takes off the gown and rolls it up so that the contaminated part is inside. Then the gown is discarded in a special hamper provided for it. The wearer now washes her hands thoroughly, making certain that special precautions are taken to prevent contaminating the faucets at the sink.

Masks. A variety of practices is observed in the use of the mask. It serves as a barrier in caring for a patient who has a communicable disease which can be transmitted via the respiratory tract. In some instances, all personnel and visitors to the patient wear masks. In others, personnel, visitors, and also the patient wear masks. Or it may be that only the patient wears the mask.

The mask is intended to filter inspired and expired air in order to trap organisms in its meshes. The purpose of the mask should be understood by the wearer. For example, if a patient has active pulmonary tuberculosis, it is recommended that he wear the mask to provide a barrier for the pathogens he may exhale. In situations where the patient is unable to cooperate by wearing the mask, persons coming in contact with him may need to wear masks. In nurseries for the newborn, the infants are protected from air expired by the workers. Hence, generally personnel wear masks.

When masks are worn by persons coming in contact with the patient, they should be stored with the gowns outside the patient area and put on before persons enter the room. They should cover both the nose and mouth and be worn only once. Masks are of no value and are a danger to the wearer when they are lowered around the neck.

Moisture makes masks ineffective. Therefore, they should be removed and appropriately discarded as frequently as necessary to keep them dry. The actual length of time a mask can be worn safely, which is partly determined by the type of mask, is a debatable question. Newer high-efficiency, disposable masks are more effective than reusable cotton gauze masks and are preferred for preventing airborne and droplet spread infections.

Gloves. Gloves may be worn in some situations during certain phases of patient care. They may be used as a barrier when the nurse handles wound dressings or when she carries out treatments if drainage is present. Sterile gloves may also be worn to protect a particularly susceptible patient from the introduction of organisms when the nurse cares for an open wound. Gloves are worn only once and then discarded appropriately. They should be changed after direct handling of potentially contaminated drainage and before completing the patient's care. Both reusable and disposable gloves are available.

Hair and Shoe Covers. Hair and shoe covers are not used generally except in some protective precautions. When hair covers are worn, they should cover all hair on the head. Shoe covers should protect the shoes as well as the open ends of trouser legs.

Excretion and secretion precautions

Organisms can escape from the host through body secretions and excretions. Urine, feces, and respiratory, oral, vaginal, and wound drainage may require special precautions.

Urine and feces may need to be treated before disposal into the sewage system. This precaution is unnecessary in those communities in which the sewage system is adequate for the destruction of organisms.

The disadvantages of the usual health agency bedpan flusher were discussed in Chapter 4. The safest practice is to empty the bedpan, rinse it thoroughly with cold water, wash it with soap or detergent and water if necessary, and sterilize it with steam under pressure before reuse by another patient.

Tissue wipes and other items may be contaminated by wound, mouth, nose, or vaginal drainage. The usual technique is to place the contaminated materials in a waterproof bag and then double-bag it. The entire bag is then discarded by incineration or other methods of the agency's choice.

Specimens of body secretions or excretions may need to be collected for laboratory analysis. As with dressings and other items, it is important for the protection of laboratory personnel that the outside of the container not be contaminated with the pathogens.

Equipment and supplies precautions

Equipment and supplies contaminated by pathogens can become vehicles for infection transmission if effective barriers are not developed. Common equipment used in providing patient care, such as the sphygmomanometer, stethoscope, and other physical examination equipment, should be left in the patient's room whenever possible for his exclusive use until the illness has subsided. Disinfection of the equipment should be done in the manner appropriate to the causative organisms and situation. A thermometer should also be left at the patient's bedside in a container of disinfectant. Cleaning the thermometer before placing it in the disinfectant and appropriate changing of the disinfectant solution are important. Needles and syringes must be handled carefully, especially if contaminated by the hepatitis virus. Nondisposable syringes and needles should be rinsed thoroughly in cold water and disinfected before they are prepared for sterilization and reuse. The extensive availability of disposable equipment in today's world makes the safe handling of contaminated supplies much easier.

Contaminated linens and personal laundry should be removed from the patient's immediate environment using the double-bag technique. Vigorous movements when changing bed linen should be avoided to prevent air movement and the spread of microorganisms.

Modern hospital laundering processes make it possible for almost all linens of patients with communicable diseases to be handled in the usual manner. There are some exceptions, as when linens are contaminated with organisms that are spore-forming, such as the bacilli of tetanus, gas gangrene, and anthrax. For such causative organisms, the linens should be sterilized by steam under pressure before they are handled by laundry personnel.

For items of clothing that are not washed easily in a machine, airing in sunlight for six to eight hours is effective against many organisms. This would be suitable for such items as blankets, decorative bed jackets, and so on. Also, a gas sterilizer, discussed in Chapter 4, may be used.

Most health agencies use dishwashers that leave dishes free of pathogens. When such equipment is not available, it then becomes necessary to take special precautions for the patient with a communicable disease. This is especially true when the disease is spread by secretions from the mouth. In some agencies, after dishes are rinsed they are boiled. Other agencies use disposable dishes, so that only silverware needs boiling. The technique of placing soiled dishes in a container of water and boiling them before they are washed is a questionable practice. The heat of the water often coagulates the food particles remaining on the dishes. If organisms are contained within these solids, they may survive the washing process. Therefore, dishes and silverware should be rinsed well before being washed and subjected to heat. Many mechanical dishwashers used in restaurants and hospitals provide for rinsing dishes before they are washed. Rubber gloves should be worn if dishes are rinsed by hand.

Leftover food should be wrapped and discarded along with other wastes from the patient's room. Liquids should be poured down the drain or the toilet if a satisfactory sewage system is available; if not, they may be disinfected before discarding.

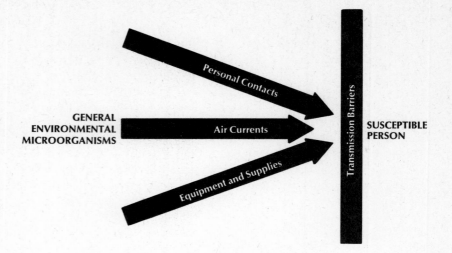

Fig. 22-3 This diagram illustrates protective or reverse isolation. Note that the susceptible person is protected from common vehicles that could carry microorganisms from the general environment by transmission barriers. When possible, the room of the patient requiring protective isolation should be kept under slight positive pressure. Then, when a door or window is opened, air currents that could carry microorganisms will move *away* from the patient's environment rather than into it.

Types of isolation and precautions

Isolation techniques vary among health agencies. Nurses working in one situation may be observing practices that are not followed in others. Therefore, it is important to know the procedures and policies of the agency where the nurse is giving care.

The patient needs to be in a physical environment in which it is feasible to carry out whatever precautions are necessary. Handwashing facilities in the immediate area are vital. Adjoining bathing and toilet facilities are desirable. Adequate space separating the person harboring the pathogen and others helps to decrease the possibility of transmission. A separate room with a door that can be kept closed is essential in circumstances where the causative organisms are airborne. To prevent cross-infection or recirculation of air between the isolation room and other areas, slight negative pressure in the room in relation to adjoining areas is desirable. Exhaust fans can be used for this purpose. The exception to this is when protective or reverse isolation is used, as Figure 22-3 explains. Facilities to discard excretions, drainage, and other contaminated substances safely are important.

The Center for Disease Control of the U. S. Public Health Service has categorized isolation and precaution techniques into seven groups: **strict, respiratory, enteric, wound** and **skin, discharge, blood,** and **protective.** A patient's particular pathogens and means of transmission determine which category of precautions is appropriate to use. The techniques are described in the publication, *Isolation Techniques for Use in Hospitals.* Chart 22-1 summarizes them.

462   Communicable disease control

Chart 22-1 Methods of communicable disease techniques

Technique	Purpose	Specifications	Examples of Diseases Requiring Technique
Strict Isolation	To prevent transmission of highly communicable diseases spread by contact and airborne routes.	Private room necessary; door must be kept closed. Gown must be worn by all persons entering room. Mask must be worn by all persons entering room. Hands must be washed on entering and leaving room. Gloves must be worn by all persons entering room. Articles must be discarded, or double-bagged before being sent to other departments for disinfection/sterilization.	Extensive burns infected with staphylococcal or streptococcal organisms. Staphylococcal or streptococcal pneumonia. Diphtheria. Smallpox. Rabies.
Respiratory Isolation	To prevent transmission of organisms by droplets coughed, sneezed, or breathed into environment and by freshly contaminated articles.	Private room necessary; door must be kept closed. Gown not necessary. Mask must be worn by all persons entering room if susceptible to disease. Hands must be washed on entering and leaving room. Gloves not necessary. Articles contaminated with secretions must be disinfected/sterilized. Persons susceptible to specific disease should be excluded from patient area; if contact is necessary, susceptibles must wear masks.	Chickenpox. Mumps. Meningococcal meningitis. Pertussis (whooping cough). Pulmonary tuberculosis with positive or suspect sputum. Rubeola (measles). Rubella (German measles).
Protective or Reverse Isolation (See Figure 22-3)	To prevent contact between potentially pathogenic organisms and uninfected person who has seriously impaired resistance. Patient is being protected from contamination.	Private room necessary; door must be kept closed. Gown must be worn by all persons entering room. Mask must be worn by all persons entering room. Hands must be washed on entering and leaving room. Gloves must be worn by all persons having direct contact with patient. Articles must be sterile or disinfected. Cap and shoe covers are worn in some cases. See Figure 22-3 for additional comments.	Agranulocytosis A disease characterized by great reduction in leucocytes, thus decreasing body's ability to fight infection. Certain patients with leukemia. Certain patients with extreme and severe dermitis, such as bullous.
Enteric Precautions	To prevent transmission of organisms through direct or indirect contact with infected feces.	Private room necessary for children only. Gown must be worn by all persons having direct contact with patient. Mask not necessary. Hands must be washed on entering and leaving room. Gloves must be worn by all persons having direct contact with patient or with articles contaminated with fecal material.	Cholera. Hepatitis. Typhoid fever.

Chart 22-1 continued

Technique	Purpose	Specifications	Examples of Diseases Requiring Technique
		Articles must be disinfected or discarded. Special precautions necessary for articles contaminated with urine and feces.	
Wound and Skin Precautions	To prevent transmission of organisms by contact with wounds and heavily contaminated articles.	Private room desirable. Gown must be worn by all persons having direct contact with patient. Mask not necessary except during dressing change. Hands must be washed on entering and leaving room. Gloves must be worn by all persons having direct contact with infected area. Special precautions necessary for instruments, dressings, and linen.	Impetigo. Staphylococcal skin and wound infections. Streptococcal skin infection. Wound infection, extensive. Burns, extensive, but not infected with staphylococcal or streptococcal organisms.
Discharge Precautions	To prevent transmission of organisms by contact with wounds, secretion, excretions, and heavily contaminated articles when likelihood of cross-infection is slight but possible.	Care of patient is as for other patients except for wound care. Hands must be washed before and after care. Gloves must be worn if there is direct contact with wound or soiled dressings. Forceps may be used instead, as indicated. Use sterile equipment for wound care and double-bag soiled dressings, linens, equipment, and so on before removing them from room.	Infected burns and wounds and burns (minor). Conjunctivitis. Gonorrhea and syphilis. Scarlet fever. Staphylococcal food poisoning.
Blood Precautions	To prevent transmission of organisms by contact with blood or items contaminated with blood.	Use disposable needle and syringe when possible. If needle and syringe are to be reused, sterilization with steam under pressure is recommended. Personnel should be careful not to prick and break their own skin with needles contaminated with blood from patient.	Hepatitis. Malaria.

Miscellaneous procedures recommended when caring for patients with communicable diseases

There are a few additional procedures that help prevent spreading pathogens when caring for patients with communicable diseases.

The Nurse's Watch. When a gown is worn, the nurse must be prepared to use her watch without contaminating it. To do so she lays her watch on a clean paper towel in a place where she can use it conveniently. She does not touch the watch until she has washed her hands after completing care. Figure 22-4 illustrates proper handling of a watch.

Transporting Patients. Patients for whom isolation techniques are being used are transported from their rooms to other health agency facilities only for essential purposes. For example, a patient requiring x-rays may need to be transported to the agency's x-ray department. The department receiving the patient should be familiarized with techniques being observed. The outer covering on the patient is kept clean. Also, whenever possible, the patient is taught how to assist with appropriate precautions that will help prevent the spread of pathogens.

Books and Magazines. The question often arises concerning how to deal with books and magazines handled by patients with communicable diseases. According to reports of experienced practitioners, they play little if any part in disease transmission. Therefore, extra care is rarely needed. In those few instances when they are likely to become heavily contaminated with secretions, it is best to have the patient use reading materials that can be destroyed without distressing him.

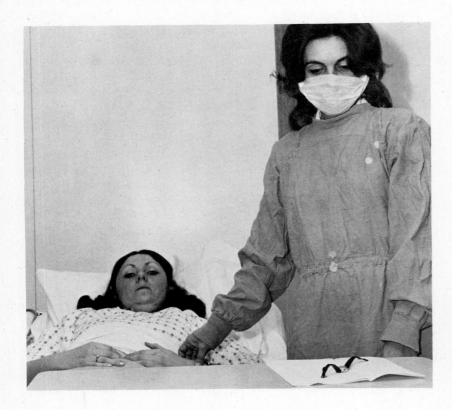

Fig. 22-4 The nurse has placed her watch on a clean piece of paper on the overbed table so that she can read it easily as she counts the patient's pulse rate. When she has finished caring for the patient, the nurse removes her gown and washes her hands before she picks up her watch.

Signing Documents. Just as with reading materials, it will rarely be necessary to use special precautions when the patient is required to sign an agreement or document. An exception may be the patient with smallpox. The paper to be signed is placed on a clean paper towel on a table where the patient can write. The area of the document on which the patient's hand will rest is covered with a second paper towel. The nurse's hands remain clean during this procedure so that she can pick up the document after it is signed and take it to the proper place.

Psychological implications when using communicable disease techniques

Regardless of the specific technique that is used and whether the patient is at home or in a health care facility, one need in his care does not change: attention to the psychological effects of the necessary restrictions. The implications are considerable whether the patient is strictly separated from others or whether he merely needs to observe simpler precautions. He may feel he is an undesirable person to others. He often feels frightened, "unclean," guilty, and rejected. Loneliness is often a problem, since the patient is usually without normal companionship and contacts with others. Because the person responds as a total being, his emotional state can influence his recovery.

Studies have shown that the extensive separation of persons from others can be very traumatic. The goal now is to minimize the extent of the precautions and the length of time they must exist as much as can safely be done. The problem of striking a balance is sometimes a delicate one. The skill and ingenuity of the nurse are often taxed in caring for the patient with a communicable disease.

Teaching and supportive measures are among the biggest contributions the nurse can make to this aspect of the patient's illness. The patient and his family need to have an accurate understanding of the situation and of how to carry out the necessary precautions. Particular emphasis needs to be placed on the idea that it is the organism which is unwanted, not the patient.

If the patient is being cared for at home, family members may need much help in understanding why the patient's behavior may change and in how to cope with it. The patient who resents and ignores the precautions needs help in being accepted as a person and in expressing his feelings.

A well-informed nurse who understands how to protect herself and others and a well-informed patient and family who are cooperating in his care are the best combination of communicable disease precautions.

Conclusion

Isolation techniques are based on knowledge of the causative pathogen, its reservoir, exit mode, transmission vehicles, entry portals, and susceptibility of new hosts. Barriers to prevent transmission of pathogens are among the most realistic means of preventing the spread of microorganisms. The nurse must use her knowledge judiciously in order to provide safe patient care when dealing with infections and communicable diseases.

References

Castle, Mary, "Isolation: Precise Procedures for Better Protection," *Nursing 75*, 5:50–57, May 1975.

Garner, Julia S. and Kaiser, Allen B., "How Often Is Isolation Needed?" *American Journal of Nursing*, 72:733–737, April 1972.

Hardy, Charlene S., "Infection Control: What Can One Nurse Do?" *Nursing '73*, 3:18–21, August 1973.

Isolation Techniques for Use in Hospitals, U. S. Department of Health, Education, and Welfare, Public Health Service, U. S. Government Printing Office, Washington, D.C., 1970, 87 p.

"Symposium on Infection and the Nurse," *The Nursing Clinics of North America*, 5:85–177, March 1970.

23
caring for the patient
when death appears
imminent

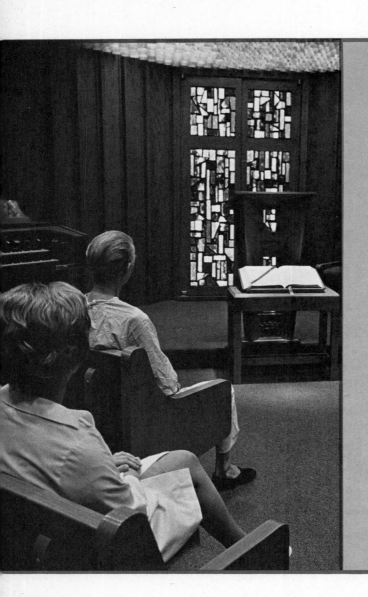

behavioral objectives

When mastery of content in this chapter is reached, the student will be able to

Define terms appearing in the glossary.

Explain why knowing one's own attitude toward impending death is important before caring for a terminally ill patient.

Discuss the stages of dying, as described by Dr. Elisabeth Kübler-Ross.

Describe various ways in which the nurse can help meet the emotional, spiritual, and physical needs of the terminally ill patient.

List signs of approaching death.

List signs of death.

Describe how the family of a terminally ill patient may be helped to face the loss of a loved one.

State various ways in which the nurse can help the family when a terminally ill patient is being cared for at home.

Describe the care of the body after death.

Explain the requirements for performing an autopsy and how the family can be helped to accept it.

Describe how governmental agencies use death certificates.

List typical agency policies concerning the handling of valuables of a patient who has died.

glossary

Autopsy The examination of organs and tissues of the human body after death.

Cryonics The freezing of the dead human body.

Euthanasia Painless or mercy killing.

Terminal Illness One from which recovery is beyond reasonable expectation.

Thanatology The study of death and its medical and psychological effects.

introduction

A **terminal illness** is one from which recovery is beyond reasonable expectation. The illness may be due to a disease condition or it may be the result of accident or injury. Errors of judgment concerning recovery sometimes are made. Some of you may recall from personal experiences patients whose illnesses were considered terminal, but who survived and lived for many years. Also, during the course of an illness medical progress may bring forth a means of saving a life. Many diabetics, for example, faced certain premature death until insulin was discovered. Hence, there is good reason to remain hopeful while caring for terminally ill patients. The patient and his family often find courage and support in knowing that everything possible is being done and that hope for recovery is not abandoned.

In the past health practitioners and agencies were so concerned with cures and health maintenance that death was often viewed as a personal failure on the part of health personnel. As a result, the terminally ill patient unfortunately was often avoided, except for essential physical care. Health personnel received little formal educational preparation for care of the dying person. There was generally a reluctance to discuss or acknowledge feelings about death with a patient or family members or even in professional conferences.

In recent years, there has been increased interest in the process of dying and death. The term **thanatology** refers to the study of death and its medical and psychological effects. Death and dying are commonly the focus of literature, conferences, and investigations, and are included in almost all programs designed to prepare health personnel. In some areas varied programs are also offered to family members during terminal illness of patients and following death. In some agencies, health team conferences for dealing constructively with health workers' feelings and for planning improved patient care are indications of changes which have occurred and which are influencing the care of terminally ill patients.

Everyone has the privilege and the right to meet death serenely and comfortably. The nurse can often do much to make this experience less fraught with sorrow, fear, and discomfort for all concerned. Both the patient and the family may turn to her for support and assistance.

Perhaps most of all, the nurse needs to be able to accept and support the individuality of the person, whether his beliefs or behavior coincide with her own. Provision of care may be easier when the nurse sees her purpose as that of assisting the patient to meet his physical and psychological needs, just as with any other patient. Her goal is to provide the support and assistance necessary to help the patient die with as much comfort and dignity as possible.

The nurse's attitude toward terminal illness

Impending death is accompanied by fear of the unknown and the natural instinct of all creatures to cling to life. It becomes particularly important for the nurse to understand her own feelings toward terminal illness, death, and its usual accompanying grief in order to help to meet the needs of the patients for whom she is caring.

Because in our culture, youth and productivity are highly valued in contrast to illness, aging, and dying, the nurse brings these influences with her when caring for terminally ill patients. The orientation of society and her educational background are strongly directed toward health and life. These experiences make dealing with death difficult. The nurse must also deal with her views and feelings regarding prolongation of life by artificial means and regarding **euthanasia,** that is, painless or mercy killing. Discussing one's feelings with others is one of the most effective ways of developing increased insight and of learning to handle personal emotions.

The nurse who neglects to deal with her feelings about life, dying, and death is in a questionable position to be able to meet the needs of patients who are facing death. The easy way to react is to ignore the feelings. Sadly enough, as a result, the dying person and his family are often emotionally abandoned and left to face a very lonely situation by themselves.

Responses to dying

While every person responds to the knowledge of impending death or to loss in a distinctive way, studies have shown that there is a common pattern. Dr. Elisabeth Kübler-Ross, a recognized authority on the subject, has described the psychological stages through which a dying person goes. The stages do not always follow one another; they may overlap. The duration of any stage can vary from being as brief as a few hours to being as lengthy as many months.

Dr. Kübler-Ross describes the stages as denial and isolation, anger, bargaining, depression, and acceptance. In the denial and isolation stage, the person usually reacts with feelings of loneliness and a type of response expressed by "No, not me. It must be a mistake." During the anger stage, his reaction is generally "Why me?" with expressions of hostility directed toward family members, friends, and health personnel. When he proceeds to the bargaining stage, he responds with a "Yes, me, but . . ." The bargain often is a promise to God in exchange for an extension of life. The depression stage is indicated by a "Yes, me" and general sadness. The final stage of acceptance is a positive feeling of "I'm ready."

To help the patient and his family, the nurse needs to try to identify the stage at which involved people are. Then she can better use her skills to provide appropriate support.

Helping the patient who has a terminal illness

Helping to Meet Emotional Needs. Hope is a desire with a feeling of anticipation. Without hope, despair exists. Hope, no matter how minimal, usually occurs in the patient, his family, and in the nurse. However, very often the patient's hope, the family's hope, and the nurse's hope are not the same. As the patient begins to face impending death, he may hope to be free of pain or nausea or to be able to walk down the hall one more time. His family may still be hoping for a miraculous cure. The nurse may be at some point in between. It is the patient's hope which should be identified and supported if realistic. The nurse will want to work toward fulfilling his hope and assisting the family to accept the patient's wishes.

Sharing fears and concerns with others generally makes dealing with them easier. There are few exceptions to the observation that most persons have some fear of dying. Communication between persons can have the effect of both decreasing anxiety and of increasing the ability to cope with it. Dying patients and family members often share their fears with the nurse. The nurse may also need to strengthen her resources through sharing her concerns with others.

As Chapter 3 pointed out, nonverbal communication often carries messages more readily than verbal communication. The nurse caring for a patient undergoing stresses will wish to tune in to the patient's nonverbal communication. Also, the patient will be aware of the nurse's nonverbal communication in many instances.

Philosophies of life and death differ. Most patients are afraid, while others may look forward to death as a relief from earthly suffering and sorrow. Some patients—often those with strong religious beliefs—have been observed to be ready to enter another life to which they look forward with joy. Others may treat death as an avenger and feel so depressed and desperate that they have suicidal tendencies. A strong influence on the patient's attitudes toward death may be his cultural background and conditioning.

The age of the patient often influences the manner in which terminal illness and death are accepted. Children usually approach death with little fear or sorrow. Teenagers and adults through middle age often consider death an injustice, for they yearn to continue the experience of life and are sad about leaving their loved ones. This earnestness to live almost always subsides as death approaches, but in some cases it may not. Older people more often face death as a friend. They may have little desire to live and often are lonesome and tired of life. This is especially true when loved ones have died before them. The nurse should be careful that she does not misjudge the patient, and if he is old, for example, expect him to have a peaceful attitude toward death. No two persons experience death in the same manner. As no two lives are lived the same, death too is an individualized experience.

A patient's reaction to death may change from day to day. A person may feel more discouraged one day and less so on another. The nurse must often develop great sensitivity in order to detect the patient's responses if she is to find clues for guiding her action.

Sometimes, a patient may mask his true feelings about death. Or, he may not really want to face the truth. He may claim to be unafraid and prepared for death when he really is fearful and trying to appear brave. Patience, careful observations, and listening in order to learn true feelings are a prerequisite if the nurse wishes to give sincere comfort and support to the dying patient.

The behavior of the patient facing death may not conform to what the nurse believes to be correct. But her actions must be guided by the patient's feelings and attitudes, not her own. Comfort, support, and encouragement are essential, but the manner in which they are offered depends on individual circumstances. In some instances, the nurse may find that it is best to say nothing and just listen. The patient may find comfort in having someone with whom he can talk out his feelings. The lonely patient may experience support and understanding by a simple handclasp.

The question usually arises concerning what to tell the terminally ill patient about his prognosis. It is the physician who usually is responsible for deciding what and how the patient shall be told. Usually he makes this decision after discussing the problem with the patient's family and after assessing the patient individually. The nurse, social worker, or clergyman may also be involved in making the decision and in discussing it with the patient.

In some situations, the physician may decide not to tell the patient his prognosis. He may feel that the experience of knowing may cause depression which may lead to suicide. At times this argument is no doubt valid. The knowledge of impending death may be too much for some to tolerate.

In other situations, the patient does have an interest and a desire to know. It is generally considered unkind and unjust to permit such a patient to die without his having known the seriousness of his condition. For example, by not knowing, he may have been denied the time to arrange important business affairs, papers, finances, and so on. Many people find comfort in the knowledge that, should they die, their "house is in order."

From many observations, it has been seen that most patients realize without being told that they are suffering from an incurable illness. The nonverbal communication of the patient's family and the health personnel often speak louder than their words. Patients often feel even more isolated, lonely, and rejected when the truth is withheld, especially when falsehoods are told them. After the prognosis has been discussed in an open and frank manner, health personnel must be prepared to offer the patient support. But usually the patient finds solace eventually in knowing and realizing that he will not be left to meet death alone.

The important thing for all involved persons is to know exactly what the patient and family have been told. Unless all persons are aware, they may be working at cross-purposes.

The adult patient has the ultimate right to refuse treatment. In dealing with the person with an incurable disease, health personnel sometimes find the patient's desire not to have further surgery or extensive treatments difficult to accept. At other times, the patient has uncertain feelings and needs the time and support necessary to explore them.

Many patients make decisions to donate various organs after death to organ banks for possible transplantation. The patient may ask the nurse questions about the technique and her views. He may be seeking information or he may wish to explore his feelings aloud. The nurse should assist him in these conversations rather than focus on her own beliefs. Legal documents permitting organ removal are available from most health agencies. Care should be taken to see that they are accurately completed if it is the patient's desire to donate organs.

Helping to Meet Spiritual Needs. Many terminally ill patients find great comfort in the support they receive from their religious faiths. It is important to help in obtaining the services of a clergyman as each situation indicates. In some instances, the nurse may offer to call a clergyman when the patient or family has not expressed a desire to see one. But this must be handled tactfully and in good judgment so that the patient is not frightened by the suggestion. However, it must be remembered that a religious faith is not an insurance policy guaranteeing security from the tragedy and loneliness of death. The chaplain's visit does not replace the kind words and the gentle touch of the nurse. Rather, he should be considered as one of the team assisting the patient to face terminal illness.

Helping to Meet Physical Needs. Unless death occurs suddenly, there are certain nursing problems concerning the patient's physical needs that the nurse usually can expect to encounter.

Nutrition

The patient who is terminally ill usually has little interest in food and fluids. His appetite fails, and often the physical effort to eat or drink is too great for him. Meeting the nutritional needs may in itself help to prolong life. It also often helps to make the patient more comfortable. Poor nutrition leads to exhaustion, infection, and other complications such as the development of decubitus ulcers. Therefore, maintaining the nutritional state of the patient plays an important part in sustaining energy and preventing additional discomfort. When the patient is unable to take fluids and food by mouth, the physician may order intravenous therapy or other means of maintaining nutrition and fluid intake.

When death is pending, the normal activities of the gastrointestinal tract decrease. Therefore, offering the patient large quantities of food may only predispose to distention and added discomfort.

If the swallowing reflex is present, offering sips of water at frequent intervals is helpful. As swallowing becomes difficult, aspiration may occur when fluids are given. The patient can suck on gauze soaked in water or on ice chips wrapped in gauze without difficulty since sucking is one of the last reflexes to disappear as death approaches.

Care of the mouth, nose, and eyes

If the patient is taking foods and fluids without difficulty, oral hygiene is similar to that offered other patients. However, as death approaches, the mouth usually needs additional care. Mucus that cannot be swallowed or expectorated accumulates in the mouth and throat and may need to be removed. The mouth can be wiped out with gauze. Or, suctioning may be necessary to remove mucus. Positioning the patient on his side very often helps in keeping the mouth and the throat free of accumulated mucus.

The mucous membranes should be kept free of dried secretions. Lubricating the mouth and the lips is helpful as well as comfortable for the patient.

The nostrils should be kept clean also and lubricated as necessary.

Sometimes, secretions from the eyes accumulate. The eyes may be wiped clean with tissues or cotton balls moistened in normal saline. If the eyes are dry, they tend to stay open. The instillation of a lubricant in the conjunctival sac may be indicated to prevent friction and possible ulceration of the cornea.

Care of the skin

As death approaches, the patient's temperature usually is elevated above normal. But, as circulation fails, the skin feels cold and the patient often perspires profusely. It is important to keep the bed linens and the bed clothing dry by bathing the patient and changing linens as necessary. Using light bed clothing and supporting it so that it does not rest on the patient's body usually give additional comfort. The patient often is restless and may be observed to pick at his bed clothing. This may be due to the fact that he feels too warm. Sponging him and keeping him dry often promote relaxation and quiet sleep.

Elimination

Some patients may be incontinent. Others may need to be observed for retention of urine and for constipation, both of which are uncomfortable. Cleansing enemas may be ordered. It should be remembered that if the patient is taking little nourishment, there may be only small amounts of fecal material in the intestine.

Catheterization at regular intervals, or an indwelling catheter may be necessary for some patients. If the patient is incontinent of urine and feces, care of the skin becomes particularly important to prevent odors and decubitus ulcers. Waterproof bedpads are easier to change than all of the bed linens. They make keeping the bed clean and dry less of a problem.

Positioning the patient

Good nursing care provides for proper positioning with frequent changes in position. The patient may not be able to express a desire to have his position changed. Or, he may feel that the effort is too great. Even though the patient appears to be unconscious, proper positioning is important. Poor positioning without adequate support is fatiguing as well as uncomfortable.

When dyspnea is present, the patient will be more comfortable when supported in the semisitting position. Noisy breathing frequently is relieved when the patient is placed on his side. This position helps to keep the tongue from obstructing the respiratory passageway. Proper positioning was discussed in Chapter 12. The same principles guide action in positioning the terminally ill patient.

Protecting the patient from harm

The terminally ill patient may be restless. In these instances, special precautions are necessary to protect him from harm. The use of bed siderails may be indicated. Restraining the patient usually is undesirable but may be necessary in some instances. The patient's relatives may offer to remain with him so that he does not injure himself. However, family members should not be left with the complete burden of the patient's safety. The nurse should check the patient frequently because the responsibility for his welfare still is hers. Well-meaning but unprepared, fatigued, and stressed family members sometimes use poor judgment in protecting the patient. Feeling the responsibility of care, or guilt if some unexpected occurrence results in injury, is an unfair price to expect family members to pay. If relatives or friends do stay with the patient, the nurse should see that they are relieved periodically. Remaining with a confused and restless terminally ill person can be both physically and emotionally taxing.

Care of the environment

It is economical of nursing time to place the hospitalized patient in a room that is convenient for giving nursing care and for observing him at frequent intervals. Very often, he is placed in a private room to avoid distressing other patients. However, this experience in itself may be upsetting to the patient.

Having familiar objects in view can help to make the patient feel more comfortable and secure. The family can be encouraged to make his room meaningful to him. Pictures, books, and other significant objects can be very important. Whether the patient is at home or in a health agency, it is desirable to have the environment reflect his preferences. Once the environment is pleasing to the patient, it can remain thus unless he chooses to make alterations. In this way, the patient is being given some degree of control over his environment when he has lost control of most other aspects of daily living. The home environment is generally not difficult to maintain according to the patient's wishes.

Normal lighting should be used in the patient's room. Terminally ill patients often complain of loneliness, fear, and poor vision, all of which are exaggerated by darkening the room. The room should be well ventilated, and the patient protected from drafts.

When conversing at the patient's bedside, it is preferable to speak in a normal tone of voice. Whispering can be annoying to the patient and may make him feel that secrets are being kept from him. It generally is believed that the sense of hearing is the last sense to leave the body, and many patients retain a sense of hearing almost to the moment of death. Therefore, care should be exercised concerning topics of conversation. Even when the patient appears to be unconscious, he may hear what is being said in his presence. It generally is comforting to the patient for others to say things which he may like to hear. Even when he cannot respond, it is kind and thoughtful to speak to him. It also remains important for the nurse to explain to the patient what she is going to do when giving nursing care or working in the unit so that the patient does not misunderstand her actions or become fearful.

Keeping the patient comfortable

Efforts to meet the physical needs of a terminally ill patient may still fall short of keeping him comfortable. In this case it becomes necessary to consider the use of medications to relieve pain and restlessness. In most instances, the physician will order a narcotic to help in relieving pain. Although such medications should be administered with the usual precautions, there appears to be little excuse for withholding their use until the patient suffers from discomfort. When pain is intense, relief is more difficult to obtain. Therefore, it is better to keep pain under control. The problem of drug addiction is present when it is expected that the patient may live with a terminal illness for a long period of time, but this problem decreases as death draws near.

It has been observed that complaints of pain sometimes are used to cover fear. However, pain is less likely to be overrated when the nurse has gained the patient's confidence. Persons working with the terminally ill have noted that patients experiencing good emotional support require less pain-relieving drug therapy.

Drugs may also be indicated for very anxious patients. It is often best to plan nursing care for these patients when drugs have reached peak action.

Some patients prefer and are able to control their own medication regimen. They can tolerate discomfort with greater ease when they know they can decide when more medication is needed. Other persons find tolerating pain more acceptable than the clouding of mental alertness and loss of awareness that come with use of the more potent drugs.

As circulation fails, the absorption of drugs given subcutaneously is impaired, and other routes of administering the drug may become necessary.

Signs of approaching death

In most instances, the process of dying occurs over a period of time. Most persons die gradually over a period of hours or even days and weeks. Human cells cease to live when there is lack of oxygen. The capacity of tissues varies as to the period of time they can live without oxygen. During the process of dying, there are signs that usually indicate rather clearly that death is imminent.

Motion and sensation are lost gradually. This usually begins in the extremities, particularly the feet and legs. The normal activities of the gastrointestinal tract begin to decrease, and reflexes gradually disappear.

Although the patient's temperature usually is elevated, he feels cold and clammy, beginning with his extremities and the tip of his nose. His skin is cyanosed, gray, or pale. The pulse becomes irregular, weak, and fast.

Respirations may be noisy and the "death rattle" may be heard. This is due to an accumulation of mucus in the respiratory tract which the patient is no longer able to raise and expectorate. Cheyne-Stokes respirations occur commonly.

As the blood pressure falls, circulation fails. Pain, if it has been present, usually subsides and there is mental cloudiness. The patient may or may not lose consciousness. The amount of mental alertness varies among patients, which is important to remember when giving care to the patient. It has been observed that some patients see visions just prior to death.

The jaw and facial muscles relax and the patient's expression which may have appeared anxious becomes peaceful. The eyes may remain partly open.

Even though these signs may be present, the nurse will realize that neither she nor any other member of the health team can predict the amount of time before death actually occurs. The family of a dying patient, because of fears and concerns, may ask the nurse how long she thinks the patient will live. The nurse's role at this time is to be supportive and to indicate that she is unable to give a realistic answer to the question. Keeping the families aware of changes that are occurring is generally helpful to assist them to prepare themselves for the patient's death.

Signs of death

In previous times, the person was considered dead when no pulse and respirations could be determined for a period of several minutes, even with auscultation. With extensive use of artificial means to maintain cardiac and respiratory activity, other means of determining death have had to be developed. The absence of all reflexes and of electrical currents normally set up in the brain for a period of 24 hours are generally considered as positive indications of death. Brain wave activity is determined with an electroencephalograph and recorded on an electroencephalogram. Certainty of death is present when the process of death becomes irreversible by whatever techniques of resuscitation that may be employed.

Helping the patient's family

Words of comfort are usually hard to find. The family is about to or has lost a loved one. Kindness and respect for their feelings expressed in dignified and tactful actions and words are important.

There are times when it may be best to say nothing and to be a listener if relatives wish to express their thoughts. Relatives often find comfort in feeling that they are assisting the patient, that everything possible is being done for him, and in knowing that he is being kept comfortable. Also, they need to be offered hope. They derive little comfort from efforts to cheer them and suggestions that they try to forget and think of something else. Sometimes, allowing a willing member of the family to assist with aspects of nursing care is comforting to the patient as well as to the relative. Nevertheless, as indicated earlier, the nurse needs to check the patient frequently to determine his condition as well as the relative's ability to cope with the situation. The nurse should help the relative to feel he can call for assistance at any time. The family needs to feel that when members leave, or are too tired to give care, a nurse will intervene. Some family members may not want to provide care but they may need help in knowing what to expect and what to say to the patient.

The considerate nurse will remember that as relatives become tired, they may also become critical of nursing care. The families may well be correct in their thinking, as research has shown that the dying patient's light is answered last. The nurse should spend time with the relative to determine the cause of critical comments.

There are instances when the nurse spends more time with the relatives than she does with the patient. This may occur especially when the patient becomes unconscious. It takes less nursing time to turn and position the patient than it does to be sufficiently supportive to the family waiting at the bedside.

Family members may need to be reminded to get rest and to eat. Occasionally, a family member will want to spend the night with the patient. When permitted, the nurse should provide as much comfort as possible for the relative.

Children too play an important role in the family of a dying person. When allowed to visit the hospitalized patient, they may help brighten his day. Children also usually benefit from seeing and knowing where the parent or grandparent is. Just as adults, children need honest information about what is happening.

Too many visitors may tire the patient and when explanations are offered, relatives usually understand this readily. When they wish to remain at the hospital, it is desirable to direct them to a place where it is quiet and they may relax.

The grief expressed at time of death depends on many factors. Often it is due to the fact that the loss is a great personal one and so, in a sense, one is feeling sorry for oneself. In other instances, the customs of a cultural group require that proper grief be shown for one who has died. Or, it may be feelings of guilt that cause the family to show great emotion. The nurse will want to recognize that there is no one approach to either the patient or his family. She will need to proceed carefully in the direction in which she feels she can serve both and keep her own feelings from interfering with her effectiveness.

Relatives of patients occasionally ask about a form of body preservation after death known as **cryonics.** The term refers to freezing of the dead human body. While freezing will slow tissue deterioration, there is no means at this time to prevent irreversible cell damage or to restore whole organs or bodies.

Home care of the terminally ill patient

In some cases, the terminally ill patient remains at home and the family assumes responsibility for his care. Various health agencies offer services for the care of the terminally ill at home. The nurse in the hospital may anticipate this need and assist the family in obtaining such services. Some hospitals permit nursing staff members to make home visits between hospitalizations to provide support and continuity of care.

When the terminally ill person is surrounded by his familiar home environment and has family members nearby, he usually feels more secure. He often can have his own routines maintained, have food that is familiar, and can maintain some degree of his family role. Family members have time to demonstrate their feelings of love without concern for agency regulations. Guilt feelings may be lessened by family members caring for the person. Children can participate more extensively in the last days and can be helped to understand death with less fear. Since the process of dying generally is a gradual one, family members can have the opportunity to work through some of the beginning phases of grieving that are often more difficult when the patient is in a health agency.

The nurse will want to remember that the care needed by some patients is too complex or demanding for family members. Some patients and family members find security in the facilities of a health agency. Families may have neither the physical nor emotional strength to deal with the terminally ill person in the home. The nurse must be careful that she does not unintentionally make the family feel guilty about not having the person at home.

Care of the body after death

After the physician has pronounced the patient dead, the nurse ordinarily is responsible for preparing the body for discharge from the health agency. The nurse will be guided by local procedure. Although these procedures vary with agencies and morticians, there are certain common elements.

To prevent discoloration from the pooling of blood, the body should be placed in normal anatomical position. Soiled dressings are replaced and any tubes removed. Inasmuch as the body is washed by the mortician, a complete bath is unnecessary. Hairpins should be removed to avoid scratching the face. Most morticians prefer that dentures not be replaced. It generally is considered better for the mortician to place the teeth in position in order to minimize possible tissue trauma. The nurse should see to it that dentures, properly identified, are given to the mortician when he calls for the body.

Double identification of the body is advised. One tag should be fastened securely to the shroud or garment in which the body is wrapped. The second one should be tied to the ankle. If it is tied to the wrist, the wrist should be padded first and the tag tied loosely around the padding to avoid damaging tissue from a tight band. *The importance of proper and complete identification of the body cannot be overstressed.* Mistakes which have occurred can cause embarrassment and added sorrow for all concerned.

The arms may be placed on the abdomen. Tying them in place can result in tissue damage. The legs may be tied together at the ankles. The body is then wrapped with a shroud or other garment provided by the agency. To facilitate moving the body from the bed, placing a full sheet around the body and tucking it securely in place prevents the extremities and head from falling out of place. Most morticians ask that the body be cooled as soon as possible. Morticians may take the body from the patient's room. Or, it may be removed to the hospital morgue refrigerator from where it will be taken to the mortuary.

When death occurs following certain communicable diseases, the body requires special handling to help in preventing the spread of the disease. The requirements are specified by local law and policy. The measures taken will depend on the causative organism, the mode of transmission, and other characteristics of the pathogen.

Autopsy

An **autopsy** is an examination of the organs and tissue of a human body following death. Consent for autopsy is a legal requirement. The person authorized to give approval varies. Generally the closest surviving family member or members have the authority to determine whether or not an autopsy is performed.

It is generally the physician's responsibility to obtain permission for an autopsy. Sometimes the patient may grant this permission before he dies. When permission is being sought from relatives of the patient, the nurse often can assist by helping to explain the reasons for an autopsy. This requires tact and good judgment. Many relatives will find comfort when they are told that an autopsy may help to further the development of medical science as well as to establish proof of the exact cause of death.

If death is caused by accident, suicide, homicide, or illegal therapeutic practice, the coroner must be notified according to law. The coroner may decide that an autopsy is advisable and can order that one be performed even though the family of the patient has refused consent. In many cases, a death occurring within 24 hours of admission to the hospital must be reported to the coroner.

Tissue and organ removal

Body organs and tissues are often used for transplants or for medical research and study. Permission must be secured for the removal of body parts. Prior to death, patients may grant such permission. However, in many states, after death the next of kin still must sign a permit and have it properly witnessed before tissue or organs can be removed from the body. The nurse will want to acquaint herself with local laws in relation to transplant permits, to help in avoiding the unpleasantness of possible legal action.

The death certificate

The laws of this country require that a death certificate be prepared for each person who has died. The laws specify the information that is needed. Death certificates are sent to local health departments. They compile statistics from the information that become important in identifying needs and problems in the fields of health and medicine.

The mortician assumes responsibility for handling and filing the death certificate with proper authorities. However, the physician's signature is required on the certificate, as well as that of the pathologist, the coroner, and others in special cases. The death certificate also carries the mortician's signature, and, in some states, his license number as well.

Care of valuables

Each agency has policies concerning the care of valuables when patients are admitted to the institution. Those which the patient has chosen to keep with him—usually rings, a wristwatch, money, and so on—require careful handling after death. Occasionally, the patient's family may take the valuables home when death becomes imminent. This should be noted on the form sheet which the agency specifies. If valuables are still with the patient at the time of death, they should be identified, accounted for, and sent to the appropriate department for safekeeping until the family claims them. If it is impossible to remove jewelry, such as a wedding ring, the fact that it remained on the body should be noted. As a further safeguard, the article should be secured with adhesive so that it becomes impossible for it to slip off and be lost. Loss of valuables is serious and can result in a legal suit. The nurse owes it to the patient's family as well as to the agency in which she works to use every precaution to prevent loss and misplacement of valuables.

Conclusion

Care of the patient who is dying requires delicate and demanding skill on the part of the nurse. She must be capable of giving supportive psychological and physical care. Often she is called upon to assist family members as well. To meet the patient's needs, she must come to grips with her own feelings about life and death. While care of the person who is dying is not easy, skillful nursing can contribute extensively to the comfort of both the patient and his family and can provide satisfaction for the nurse too.

References

Barnsteiner, Jane H., "Death and Dying: Anxieties, Needs and Responsibilities of the Nurse," *The Journal of Practical Nursing*, 24:28–30, June 1974.

Chura, Victoria, "Difficult Patients: Sarah Wanted to Die at Home—But Her Family Resisted," *Nursing '74*, 4:16–18, July 1974.

Fleming, Ruth P., "Good Physical Care, Priority for the Dying," *RN*, 37:46, 47, 48, 50, 53, April 1974.

Fletcher, Joseph, "Ethics and Euthanasia," *American Journal of Nursing*, 73:670–675, April 1973.

Gray, V. Ruth, "Grief," *Nursing '74*, 4:25–27, January 1974.

Griffin, Jerry J., "Family Decision: A Crucial Factor in Terminating Life," *American Journal of Nursing*, 75:794–796, May 1975.

Hampe, Sandra Oliver, "Needs of the Grieving Spouse in a Hospital Setting," *Nursing Research*, 24:113–120, March–April, 1975.

Hoevet, Sister Martha, "Dying Is Also Living," *Nursing Care*, 7:12–15, July 1974.

Ingles, Thelma, "St. Christopher's Hospice," *Nursing Outlook*, 22:759–763, December 1974.

Kübler-Ross, Elisabeth, *On Death And Dying*, The Macmillan Company, New York, New York, 1969, 260 p.

Lacasse, Christine Mitchell, "A Dying Adolescent," *American Journal of Nursing*, 75:433–434, March 1975.

Marino, Elizabeth Begg, "Difficult Patients: Vinnie Was Dying. But He Wasn't the Problem I Was," *Nursing '74*, 4:46–47, February 1974.

Murray, Ruth, "Illness as a Crisis: The Terminally Ill Child," *The Journal of Practical Nursing*, 23:22–25, March 1973.

Myers, Saul, "Effects of Death on the Living," *The Journal of Practical Nursing*, 25:31, 36, January 1975.

Northrup, Fran C., "The Dying Child," *American Journal of Nursing*, 74:1066–1068, June 1974.

Pienschke, Sr. Darlene, "Guardedness or Openness on the Cancer Unit," *Nursing Research*, 22:484–490, November–December 1973.

Rinear, Eileen E., "Helping The Survivors of Expected Death," *Nursing '75*, 5:60–65, March 1975.

Sobel, David E., "Death and Dying," *American Journal of Nursing*, 74:98–99, January 1974.

"The Dying Person's Bill of Rights," *American Journal of Nursing*, 75:99, January 1975.

Walker, Margaret, "The Last Hour Before Death," *American Journal of Nursing*, 73:1592–1593, September 1973.

Weber, Leonard J., "Ethics and Euthanasia: Another View," *American Journal of Nursing*, 73:1228–1231, July 1973.

Whitman, Helen H. and Lukes, Shelby J., "Behavior Modification for Terminally Ill Patients," *American Journal of Nursing*, 75:98–101, January 1975.

Wise, Doreen J., "Learning About Dying," *Nursing Outlook*, 22:42–44, January 1974.

Zopf, Dolores, "Speaking Out: The Dying Patient: Meeting His Needs Could be Easier Than You Think," *Nursing '75*, 5:16, March 1975.

index*